# LIFE SPAN MOTOR DEVELOPMENT

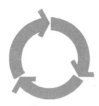

Kathleen M. Haywood, PhD
University of Missouri–St. Louis

**Human Kinetics Publishers**

**Library of Congress Cataloging-in-Publication Data**

Haywood, Kathleen.
    Life span motor development / Kathleen M. Haywood. -- 2nd ed.
        p.    cm.
    Includes bibliographical references and index.
    ISBN 0-87322-483-3
    1. Human growth.   2. Motor ability.   I. Title.
QP84.H34   1993
612.7'6--dc20                                                93-18656
                                                             CIP

ISBN: 0-87322-483-3

Acquisitions Editor: Richard D. Frey, PhD
Developmental Editor: Lori K. Garrett
Assistant Editors: Lisa Sotirelis, Julie Swadener, John Wentworth
Copyeditors: Barbara Walsh, Lisa Sotirelis
Proofreaders: Pam Johnson, Laurie McGee
Indexer: Barbara Cohen
Production Director: Ernie Noa
Typesetter: Sandra Meier
Text Design: Keith Blomberg
Text Layout: Denise Peters, Tara Welsch
Cover Design: Keith Blomberg
Cover Photo: F-Stock
Illustrations: Mary Yemma Long, Studio 2D
Printer: Edwards Brothers

Printed in the United States of America        10   9   8   7   6

**Human Kinetics**
Web site: http://www.humankinetics.com/

*United States:* Human Kinetics, P.O. Box 5076, Champaign, IL 61825-5076
1-800-747-4457
e-mail: humank@hkusa.com

*Canada:* Human Kinetics, 475 Devonshire Road, Unit 100, Windsor, ON N8Y 2L5
1-800-465-7301 (in Canada only)
e-mail: humank@hkcanada.com

*Europe:* Human Kinetics, P.O. Box IW14, Leeds LS16 6TR, United Kingdom
(44) 1132 781708
e-mail: humank@hkeurope.com

*Australia:* Human Kinetics, 57A Price Avenue, Lower Mitcham, South Australia 5062
(088) 277 1555
e-mail: humank@hkaustralia.com

*New Zealand:* Human Kinetics, P.O. Box 105-231, Auckland 1
(09) 523 3462
e-mail: humank@hknewz.com

To my family in return for their unwavering support

# Contents

# Preface

True to its name, the area of study termed *motor development* continues to develop! Just as with living organisms, the changes are exciting; they open up a new world of possibilities for researchers, instructors, and students alike. Because the process of change is ongoing, one could argue that any motor development text needs to be revised as soon as it is in print. But it does take a few years before the changes can be placed into perspective such that newcomers to motor development will benefit. The time has arrived when students can gain richer insights into motor development from new material and perspectives, and this second edition of *Life Span Motor Development* is the result.

Change in motor development has taken many forms. Foremost is the emergence of a new perspective—the dynamic systems, or ecological, perspective. This new theoretical approach, introduced in chapter 1, stimulates new questions about the developmental process, reveals limitations of other perspectives, and raises questions about assumptions with which we have become comfortable. I have taken the dynamic systems perspective in many places throughout this second edition, sometimes contrasting it with more traditional viewpoints.

New research instrumentation and statistical techniques have allowed data on motor development to be gathered and analyzed more quickly and accurately than ever before. Integrated video-computer systems now allow movement analysis at a speed and sophistication not previously possible. Though you will not be burdened with the details of this research, you will benefit in chapters 3 and 4 from the information obtained. A relatively new statistical technique, meta-analysis, has been used to examine gender differences in motor development, a topic discussed in chapter 5.

Continued research also changes our thinking about various aspects of development. For example, progressive resistance training has often been considered of little value to prepubescent children. However, you are likely to reach a different conclusion after reading chapter 7.

Research has been conducted on new topics in motor development and in correlated areas of study. For example, researchers have recently examined how children structure their knowledge about skills and sports. This material has been incorporated into chapter 8. And there is now sufficient material on the development of self-esteem for skill performance that an entirely new concept has been added to chapter 9.

Though revised, *Life Span Motor Development* is still intended for the newcomer to motor development. My goal has been to improve upon the first edition, providing a strong foundation in the basics along with the most current information. Several sections have been expanded, and the book's format redesigned into three parts. Part I consists of chapters 1 and 2, providing an overview of the study of motor development followed by a discussion of physical growth processes occurring in various body systems. Part II, comprised of chapters 3, 4, and 5, follows motor development from infancy through older adulthood. Part III, the final four chapters of the book, discusses how motor development is affected by perceptual and cognitive development, physiological responses to training, and psychosocial factors.

This second edition includes twice as many photos and more drawings, tables, and graphs. More learning tools have been incorporated. You will find key terms highlighted in the text and listed at the end of each chapter; these terms are defined, along with others, in the new glossary at the end of the book. Each chapter closes with a chapter summary, a list of key terms, discussion questions, and suggested readings. These elements will enhance your learning as you begin your exploration of the field of motor development.

The most enjoyable aspect of writing this book has been meeting and speaking with instructors and students who used the first edi-

tion. Associating actual names and faces with readers has been a tremendous help to me through the long revision process. I tend now to see *Life Span Motor Development* not merely as a text but, like motor development itself, as an ongoing process. I look forward to incorporating the research some of *you* will do and the suggestions many of *you* will make in the future.

# Preface to the First Edition

Change in motor behavior from infancy to older adulthood is a fascinating process to study. Just a few years ago, study in motor development was limited to children and adolescents. Today, however, motor development is an expanding area of study. Increasingly, motor development is recognized as a continuous developmental process that must include the study of motor behaviors over the entire life span. Certainly age-related changes in motor behavior and skill performance are not limited to persons under 20 years of age. It is important, then, that changes in motor development that occur throughout adulthood and older adulthood also are studied in a systematic way. *Life Span Motor Development* is intended to fill the need for a comprehensive motor development text that takes a life span view.

In 1982, several members of the Motor Development Academy of the American Alliance for Health, Physical Education, Recreation and Dance developed a list of minimum exit competencies appropriate for student coursework in motor development. These competencies include (a) the ability to formulate a developmental perspective, especially from a life span viewpoint; (b) knowledge of changing motor behavior across the life span; (c) knowledge of the factors affecting motor development, including physical growth and physiological change, perceptual change, cognitive change, sociocultural practices, and interventions; and (d) the ability to apply motor development knowledge. This text covers the suggested areas of knowledge; course instructors may wish to further enhance the application of motor development knowledge with supplemental activities in laboratory and clinical settings.

The text is written as an undergraduate introductory text, so little background knowledge in the movement sciences is required. Persons who are interested in motor behavior as it relates to physical education, developmental psychology, elementary education, early childhood education, special education, and gerontology should find this book instructive as well. It is assumed that most readers anticipate working with children, adolescents, and perhaps young adults. With the increasing proportion of adults in the population who are concerned with developing and maintaining an active lifestyle, the demand for individuals with knowledge of life span motor development will afford increased employment opportunities.

The breadth of information pertaining to motor development throughout the life span often seems overwhelming to beginning students. One way to handle the large volume of detailed information is to conceptualize how this information supports broader generalizations about motor development. A conceptual understanding of motor development is particularly useful for students whose application of this knowledge may occur in a wide array of professional settings. For this reason, *Life Span Motor Development* focuses on concepts in motor development throughout.

The book consists of nine chapters divided into two parts. Part I (chapters 1 to 5) concerns the developmental perspective on human behavior and includes changes in physical growth and aging and changes in motor performance. Part II (chapters 6 to 9) includes a consideration of the correlates of motor behaviors—that is, the factors that influence individual performance levels such as physiological, perceptual, and cognitive changes—and sociocultural influences. Featured within each chapter are several motor development concepts. After the concept is introduced and discussed, a brief summary is provided before moving on to the next concept.

The book's chapters and concepts are organized to provide a logical sequence of study beginning with parameters of physical growth and development, continuing with motor skill acquisition, and progressing to correlates of motor development. Other than in chapters 3, 4, and 5, which concern specific developmental periods, the discussion covers the entire life span. Concepts within the chapters are supported by discussions of relevant research and study and by specific examples of their application in natural settings. Instructors may wish to introduce additional materials for various chapters and concepts as appropriate; because each chapter is a complete unit, the chapters may be read in a different order than presented to meet the needs of individual instructors or students without jeopardizing the integrity of the book.

The concepts emphasized in *Life Span Motor Development* should help you make knowledgeable decisions concerning motor development. I hope that as you gain an understanding and appreciation of the process of developmental change in motor behavior, you will continue to seek new information in the study of motor development.

# Acknowledgments

As with any work this size, many people provided valuable assistance. Several professionals read first edition chapters for accuracy: John Strupel, MD and Elizabeth Sweeney, BSN read chapter 2; Bruce Clark, PhD read chapter 7; and Susan Greendorfer, PhD offered valuable suggestions on chapter 9. Mary Ann Roberton, PhD furnished materials from which many of the chapter 4 illustrations were drawn.

The photographs in chapter 2 were taken by Brian Speicher. Michael, Douglas, and Jennifer Imergoot; and Matthew and Christina Haywood posed for the pictures. Laura Haywood posed for the pictures in chapter 3. Ann Wagner typed many of the manuscript tables and figure captions for the first edition. Cynthia Haywood assisted in checking the reference list. The support of Elizabeth Sweeney, Lynn Imergoot, Stephanie Ross, Cathy Lewis, and members of the Motor Development Research Consortium with the first edition is gratefully acknowledged.

Many colleagues made contributions to the second edition. Special thanks to Jane Clark for help with incorporating the dynamic systems perspective. Maureen Weiss was kind enough to provide much of the material for the new concept in chapter 9. Thanks, too, to Kathleen Williams and Ann VanSant for collaborating on some of the new research added to chapter 5. Continued thanks to Mary Ann Roberton for her helpful suggestions.

William Long, OD, PhD provided a new photograph for the second edition of chapter 9 and did much of the photo development work on the new photographs. Anna Tramelli posed for the new photos in chapter 3 and Cathy Lewis for all the "grasp and grip" photos. John Haubenstricker, Ann VanSant, and Jill Whitall provided film tracings for new figures in chapter 4. Thanks once again to all my motor development colleagues whose many helpful comments along the way have made this a better text.

# Part I
# Foundations of
# Motor Development

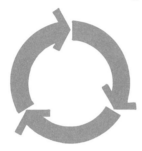

Part I sets the stage for our discussion of motor development. We begin, in chapter 1, with a definition of motor development and why it applies beyond childhood to the entire life span. We also review some of the field's basic terms. With the history of motor development as a guide, you'll learn that as knowledge about motor development has changed over time, so too have people's perspectives and that interpretations of motor behavior over the years have often been colored by the prevailing viewpoint. We end this chapter by reviewing several critical issues debated throughout the history of motor development.

In chapter 2 we explore physical growth and aging. Growth and age-related changes in skill performance are so entwined that it makes little sense to study motor development without a thorough knowledge of growth and the aging process. You will learn about overall body growth as well as growth and aging in each of the relevant body systems so that we can link the advancement in the various systems with the appearance of new motor skills. We also examine factors that specifically affect physical growth and aging.

## Chapter 1

# The Developmental Perspective

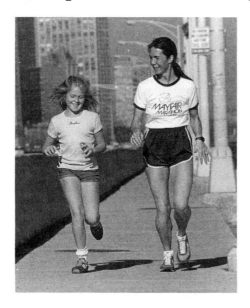

## CHAPTER CONCEPTS

**1.1**
Motor performance undergoes many age-related changes during an individual's life span.

**1.2**
To understand motor development, you must understand the terminology used in the field.

**1.3**
We can view motor development from many different theoretical perspectives.

**1.4**
Some aspects of development are topics of discussion and debate.

Learning and performing motor skills is a lifelong challenge. The process begins early in life with the attainment of postural control and grasping skills. It continues with the acquisition of locomotor skills and manipulative skills, such as throwing. During childhood, basic skills are refined and combined into movement sequences to produce complex skills. Adolescents continue to acquire movement sequences and improve their abilities to match motor skills to the goal of a task and the environment in which it is performed. Throughout infancy, childhood, and adolescence, the physical body is growing and maturing. Perception of the surrounding world becomes keener, and mental capacity increases as mental skills improve. Social skills, too, are acquired as new relationships are formed. With all these changes, the performance of motor skills must be accommodated and modified.

Motor skills are usually perfected during late adolescence and young adulthood. Elite athletes exemplify the ultimate in motor skill development. Such skilled performers have maximized their motor performance based on their physical size and condition and their cognitive and social experiences. Developmental changes are most dramatic early in life, but they do not cease with adulthood—physiological changes continue to occur, and environmental experiences refine individuals' perceptions, mental skills, and social relationships. Perhaps adults attempt to perform skills in new ways, but both new and well-learned skills must continue to accommodate these ongoing, though subtle, changes. This is particularly true as individuals age beyond young adulthood, and the pace of physical, mental, and social changes increases.

## THE LIFE SPAN PERSPECTIVE

Movement patterns change continually over the life span. This ongoing change poses important questions for educators. For example, what influences the potential for skilled performance? Is it determined by genetics, or can parents and educators provide experiences to promote skill development? Does skilled performance necessarily decline after young adulthood? By studying the developmental process with its many facets and intricacies, we can begin to unravel the answers to questions such as these.

> **CONCEPT 1.1**
> Motor performance undergoes many age-related changes during an individual's life span.

### Traditional Focus on Children

It is traditional to think of *motor development* solely as the process of skill acquisition in children—that is, the progression from unskilled performance in very young children to intermediate skill mastery during childhood, to relatively skilled performance during late adolescence. Working from this perspective, a motor developmentalist studies motor behavior by testing children of different ages and monitoring the course of their skill acquisition. The presumption that motor development concerns only children and adolescents has developed because the majority of study in motor development has concentrated on the early years of the life span. But researchers now recognize that the study of development in general and motor development in particular should encompass the entire life span. By studying the processes underlying behavioral change throughout the life span, motor developmentalists seek not only to describe such changes but also to explain them.

---

In this text, the field of motor development concerns the study of processes underlying behavioral change throughout the life span.

---

## Increasing Interest in Older Adults

A growing segment of the human population consists of older adults. Increasingly, older adults seek to improve the quality of their lives through healthful and enjoyable physical activities, so we can no longer view older adulthood as a period of sedentary living and illness. We recognize that development does not stop at puberty with the cessation of physical growth, or at age 21, or at any other landmark of young adulthood. Changes in motor behavior, both substantive and qualitative, occur during older adulthood, too. Motor patterns vary with age from birth to death (VanSant, 1989). Because the earliest developmental research focused on children's motor behavior, many aspects of motor behavior in older adults are largely unexplored, and specific scientific knowledge of changes in motor skill is sparse. Gaining more complex knowledge and a better understanding

of motor behavior in older adults is an important challenge for motor developmentalists.

## Significance of the Life Span Perspective

Students—even those who anticipate working only with children or adolescents—can gain a fuller appreciation of motor development by viewing it from a *life span perspective*. Consider, for example, that children and older adults often display similar motor behavior. Both groups are relatively slower than young adults in their reaction time to a visual stimulus (see Figure 1.1). But are the causes of this difference in behavior the same for children and older adults? No. Children and older adults cognitively process information about the visual stimulus in different ways. We will discuss differential causes of behavior in more detail throughout the text.

---

Behavior is the product of many influences.

---

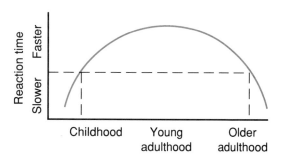

**Figure 1.1** Behavior might be identical at two points of the life span but the underlying processes contributing to that behavior might be different. Reaction time has been observed to improve during childhood and adolescence, reach its fastest in young adulthood, and slow in older adulthood. This is represented in the theoretical model above. At two ages, the average reaction time could be the same, yet developmentalists believe different processes bring about the relatively slower reaction times in childhood and older adulthood.

Our understanding of behavior is based on the integration of many influences—psychological, sociological, biological, physiological, cognitive, mechanical, and so on. Similarly, our greatest understanding of motor development is based on the integration of many behavior changes within a phase of development. We cannot possibly study all behavioral influences at once. Even though the discussions in this text may focus for a time on a particular aspect of behavioral change, the goal of developmentalists is to explain behavioral change throughout life from a global viewpoint. We encounter a broader range of causes and effects from this viewpoint, which in turn provides the basis for a more complete understanding of the factors involved in behavioral changes. More importantly, perhaps, a life span perspective enables students of motor development to better understand motor behavior and to consider how educators and health professionals might be able to influence individuals' optimal motor development throughout life.

## REVIEW 1.1

In discussing motor development in this text, we emphasize a life span perspective that relates to the processes underlying changes in motor behavior throughout life. The study of motor development involves both the description and the explanation of changes in motor behavior. Ultimately, motor developmentalists integrate knowledge of various biological, psychological, sociological, cognitive, and mechanical factors that influence behavior at particular levels of development. This method is quite different from studying changes as a function of time, such as when we study a particular motor behavior in several age groups to identify the differences among those groups or to establish norms or averages for particular ages. Developmentalists go beyond this descriptive level to study the processes underlying change that account for age-group differences.

Because changes in motor behavior occur from infancy through older adulthood, we must consider a broad range of influences on behavioral change. Consequently, we view motor skill development with a knowledge of preceding processes as well as potential effects.

## TERMINOLOGY IN MOTOR DEVELOPMENT

Understanding the terms used in the study of the developmental process will facilitate your learning. Every field of study develops its own terminology. Sometimes these terms hinder students' ability to read and comprehend pertinent literature, especially students new to the field. It can be frustrating to discover that a word you use in everyday conversation has a specific, different meaning when used in a scientific context. Yet precise communication among those interested in the topic often requires these specific meanings. Let's examine some common motor development terms.

> **CONCEPT 1.2**
> To understand motor development, you must understand the terminology used in the field.

## Growth and Development

Two basic concepts discussed in this text focus on the terms *growth* and *development*.

### Growth

Although *growth* and *development* are sometimes used interchangeably, *growth* means a quantitative increase in size. With physical growth, the increase in size or body mass results from an increase in complete biological units—that is, already-formed body parts (Timiras, 1972). This means that growth in height, for example, does not occur by adding a new section to each leg; rather, the legs, as biological units or body parts, grow longer. When each unit or part increases its size as a whole, the body increases its size, keeping its form.

Sometimes *growth* also is used to refer to an increase in the magnitude of intellectual ability or in social aptitudes (Rogers, 1982). In this text, however, we use the term to refer to physical growth, not social or cognitive growth. The physical growth period (change in absolute size) for humans is typically between conception and ages 19 to 22.

## Development

As a complement to *growth*, *development* implies a continuous process of change leading to a state of organized and specialized functional capacity—that is, a state wherein an individual can fully carry out an intended role (Timiras, 1972). Development may occur in the form of quantitative change, qualitative change, or both. Motor development, then, is the sequential, continuous age-related process whereby an individual progresses from simple movements to highly organized, complex motor skills, and finally to the adjustment of skills that accompanies aging. This process is not limited to the physical growth period; development continues throughout a person's life.

## Motor Development

The term *motor*, when used with other terms such as *development* and *learning*, refers to movement. Hence, *motor learning* deals with aspects of learning involving body movement and is not necessarily age-related. In discussions of both the development and learning of

movement, the term *motor behavior* is often used. Newcomers to the study of motor development often find it difficult to distinguish between motor development and motor learning. Roberton (1988, p. 130) suggests we apply three questions to make this distinction:

1. What is behavior like now, and why?
2. What was behavior like before, and why?
3. How is behavior going to change in the future, and why?

Specialists in both motor learning and motor development ask the first question, but only the developmentalist goes on to ask the second and third questions. The motor learning specialist studies motor behavior in the short term, as a function of practice of a certain skill or the instructional strategies used by teachers. The developmentalist is interested in present behavior only as a point on a continuum of change.

## Maturation

Another term often used along with *growth* is *maturation* or, more specifically, physiological or physical maturation. Physical maturation is a qualitative advancement in biological makeup and may refer to cell, organ, or system advancement in biochemical composition rather than to size alone (Teeple, 1978). Typically, maturation connotes progress toward physical maturity, which is the state of optimal functional integration of an individual's body systems and the ability to reproduce.

## Aging

Physiological changes occur throughout life, although these changes take place much more slowly after the physical growth period. The term *aging* used broadly, applies to the process of growing older regardless of chronological age. More specifically, *physical aging* refers to continuing molecular, cellular, and organismic differentiation. Aging changes reflect an earlier state of development and foreshadow future changes; hence, physical aging is inseparable from the developmental processes (Timiras, 1972).

## Age Periods

Developmentalists describe specific *age periods* by delineating characteristics of growth and development that set these age periods apart. Researchers define the age periods somewhat differently because rarely are sharp, clear divisions discernible between the periods. Aside from events such as birth and menarche (the first menstrual cycle in girls), the age periods blend from one to another, reflecting the continuous nature of growth, development, and maturation. In a few cases, common terms apply to more than one chronological age period, as you will see by examining the time frames listed in Table 1.1. Note also that some age periods, such as childhood, are subdivided.

## Stages

Students of development frequently encounter the phrase *stage of development*. Developmentalists have yet to adopt a standard definition and usage for the term *stage*; hence, they have used it in different ways. Most developmentalists agree that *stages* should describe qualitative differences in overall behavior, yet some use the term to describe change in individual behaviors—for example, in grasping. Still others favor the term to describe change in two or more variables developing in parallel. In this sense, a stage unites a set of behaviors (Wohlwill, 1973).

Because of the inconsistent use of this phrase, many developmentalists question the value of the *stage* label. Although the term is used often and loosely in developmental litera-

**Table 1.1　Chronological Ages for Various Developmental Periods**

| Developmental period | Approximate chronological age |
|---|---|
| Prenatal | |
| 　Embryo | 2 weeks to 8 weeks |
| 　Fetus | 8 weeks to birth |
| Neonate | Birth to 4 weeks |
| Infancy | Birth to 1 year |
| Childhood | |
| 　Early childhood | |
| 　　(preschool) | 1 to 6 years |
| 　Late childhood | |
| 　　(preadolescence) | 6 to 10 years |
| Adolescence | |
| 　Girls | 8 or 10 to 18 years |
| 　Boys | 10 or 12 to 20 years |
| Adulthood | |
| 　Young adulthood | 18 to 40 years |
| 　Middle adulthood | 40 to 60 years |
| 　Older adulthood | 60 years and over |

ture, we would benefit from defining the concept more precisely and moving toward a more accurate usage. Piaget outlined the most detailed set of criteria for defining the developmental process as stages (Miller, 1983; Salkind, 1981; Wohlwill, 1973). As a result, the term *stage* is most often used in the context described by Piaget, as outlined here:

• The major characteristic of a stage is qualitative change—that is, a stage contains new behavior previously unobserved rather than more of an earlier behavior. For example, at some point a child who could not previously jump off the ground with both feet at once can do so. In contrast, a quantitative change would be a child jumping 5 cm farther than before.

• Subsequent stages grow out of and incorporate previous stages, a characteristic that is termed *hierarchical integration*. Again in the case of jumping, a child progresses from a one-foot takeoff to a two-foot takeoff. One stage builds upon another.

• Behaviors within a stage emerge gradually and mix with the behaviors of the previous stage through a *consolidation* process. For example, when a child throws overhead, he or she progresses from taking a step with the foot on the same side as the throwing arm to taking a step with the opposite foot. Typically, at some time in development a child will step with one foot one time but with the other foot the next, and so on.

• Eventually, the individual reworks the previous stage behaviors so that regression to the previous stage is impossible.

• Stages are intransitive; that is, they lead to one another and cannot be reordered. If the stages are assigned numbers, for example, individuals advance from Stage 1 to 2 to 3, and so on. Individuals never move from 1 to 3, then back to 2.

• All individuals must progress through stages in the same universal order, and stages cannot be skipped.

• Movement to a new stage is stimulated by an imbalance between the individual's mental structures and the environment. This equilibration process is manifested in periods of relative stability at the end of each stage followed by periods of instability during the transition between stages. Children exhibit consistent behavior at the end of a stage, but in moving to the next stage they might exhibit variable behavior.

• The individual maintains what Piaget termed *structural wholeness* as the patterns of behavior or operations within each stage interconnect to form an organized whole. Various modes of behavior all exhibit the behavior characteristic of the stage.

• It is possible for individuals to acquire a given pattern of behavior or level of thought but not immediately apply the new behavior to all the possible tasks or situations they encounter. This time lag in the application of new behaviors within a stage is referred to as *horizontal decalage* (day-ca-'laj).

Sequential changes in behavior that conform to these characteristics, then, can be called stages. Behaviors that make qualitative transitions over time but do not meet the criteria for stages can be labeled *sequences*, *patterns*, *steps*, or *phases*. On occasion, *step* is used to describe a change within a stage. It is more appropriate to use these terms unless the behavioral transitions meet the stage criteria. Students of motor development, however, should expect to find these terms and the term *stage* sometimes used interchangeably in the literature.

## Research Methodology Terms

Through research, developmentalists improve our knowledge and understanding of developmental processes. To appreciate developmental research, we must understand the three designs researchers use in planning developmental studies.

### Longitudinal Research

The best design for studying human development is *longitudinal research*, in which measures on individuals are repeated periodically over the course of their development. Hence, change is observed directly rather than implied. Unfortunately, the advantages of longitudinal research also create problems. Such research usually takes years, making it difficult for researchers to keep in contact with subjects and increasing costs. Also, many years pass before the study results are available. Results may become distorted because of a practice effect, which occurs when the individuals being studied become overly familiar with the assessment device. In addition, a measurement tool appropriate for assessing young children may be inappropriate for older ones. Think how difficult it is to measure throwing accuracy from age 2 to age 10. An appropriate test for a 2-year-old would be far too easy for a 10-year-old!

## Cross-Sectional Research

To avoid these drawbacks to longitudinal research, many researchers adopt the *cross-sectional research* method. A cross-sectional study enables an experimenter to test individuals of different ages at the same time and then infer developmental change if performance trends appear across the different age groups.

Although it shortcuts many of the problems associated with longitudinal research, the cross-sectional technique also has weaknesses; developmental change must be inferred from group averages, which sacrifices attention to individuals (Wohlwill, 1973). The individuals in a cross-sectional study also come from different *cohorts*, that is, different groups who share a common characteristic, such as age. Researchers using the cross-sectional approach must remember that significant changes in nutrition, health care, education, toys, and social attitudes occur over the years. If factors such as these might affect the behavior studied, a change in behavior across age groups cannot be attributed solely to development. The change could result from an intervening variable. For example, suppose a researcher is interested in the age at which children can use two legs together to pedal their cycles. The researcher might reach one conclusion studying a cohort of children who used only traditional tricycles (with seats high off the ground), and a different conclusion studying a cohort that grew up riding Big Wheel tricycles (with seats low to the ground). For these reasons, when we interpret the traditional research methods in development—longitudinal and cross-sectional studies—we must consider the effects of such practices as repetitious testing and mixing different cohorts.

## Sequential Research

*Sequential research* is a third methodology; it has been suggested as a way to overcome longitudinal and cross-sectional problems. Sequential research combines longitudinal and cross-sectional designs. One type of sequential design includes three factors (Schaie, 1965):

1. Cohort
2. Time of measurement
3. Age

A model of this design is presented in Figure 1.2. This example shows four cohorts, one born in each year—1960, 1965, 1970, and 1975. Each cohort is tested at three times: 1980, 1985, and 1990. Each row, then, is a short longitudinal study. For example, the group born in 1975 is tested at age 5, at age 10, and finally at age 15. Each column is a cross-sectional study. In 1980 four age groups are tested, as they are in 1985 and 1990.

The advantage of this design is the time lag component, shown as the diagonal arrows in Figure 1.2. Three cohorts are tested at the same age but in different years. This component allows researchers to compare individuals from different cohorts at the same chronological age to identify any existing cohort differences. For example, suppose Big Wheel tricycles had been introduced halfway through a sequential study of cycling skill in children. If the three cohorts did not display identical behavior at the same age, a researcher would suspect that some factor other than skill influenced the study's outcome. The cohort that had learned early to pedal the new type of tricycle would perform better than the other cohorts.

Nevertheless, this model has disadvantages as well. A major drawback is the difficulty researchers have in analyzing the statistical results of such a study. For a more thorough discussion of this analysis problem and others concerning sequential designs, see articles by Kausler (1982) and Wohlwill (1973). Despite the disadvantages of the sequential design, studies using it make valuable contributions to our understanding of development.

Each research strategy has strengths as well as weaknesses (see Table 1.2). The particular strategy a researcher selects depends in part on the behavior to be studied and the factors expected to influence that behavior. Ideally, researchers should confirm results by two or more research strategies.

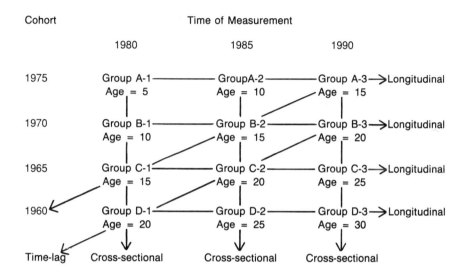

**Figure 1.2**   A model of sequential research design. Note that each row is a short longitudinal study and that each column is a cross-sectional study. The time lag component, shown by the two diagonal lines, allows comparison of different cohorts at the same chronological age, thus identifying any cohort differences.

**Table 1.2   Developmental Research Designs**

| Research design | Advantages | Disadvantages |
|---|---|---|
| Longitudinal | • Development is observed directly<br>• Researcher can note individual variation | • Results are not available for a long time<br>• Subject attrition limits results<br>• Process is expensive<br>• Practice effects are possible<br>• Measurement tool might not remain appropriate over age span tested |
| Cross-sectional | • Results are available immediately<br>• Repeated testing is not necessary | • Change must be inferred<br>• Cohort effects might influence results<br>• Individual variation is masked |
| Sequential | • Development is observed directly but the time required is short<br>• Time lag component identifies cohort effects | • Statistical analyses are problematic |

Development is a complex, continuous process. Using precise terminology helps us to distinguish the many aspects of development and the subtle differences and changes in growth and development. We need this precise interpretation of common vocabulary to comprehend specific facts and research studies about growth as well as various theoretical viewpoints that guide the study of development. In this book as well as in related readings, you will encounter terms not discussed here. You will find them in the glossary at the end of this text.

## THEORETICAL PERSPECTIVES

Consider the many factors contributing to development—biological, perceptual, and social, to name a few—that one must synthesize to form a total conceptualization of development. Is it any wonder that most developmentalists choose to study one aspect of development at a time? In doing so, developmentalists usually adopt a frame of reference or theoretical perspective. Though no single frame of reference can encompass all of the details of development, adopting a perspective is advantageous because it permits researchers to identify and structure a finite set of hypotheses or questions that they can begin to test. A disadvantage of adopting one perspective is that our knowledge of some aspects of development comes almost solely from one perspective. Sometimes, research conducted from two different perspectives yields conflicting results. Although this can be frustrating to readers new to motor development, developmentalists often advance our knowledge of developmental processes when they conduct further research in an attempt to resolve conflicting results. Knowing the major perspectives or frames of reference in development

helps us understand explanations of behavior. This knowledge is especially useful when two or more explanations conflict.

## Biological Versus Psychological Perspectives

Development is generally viewed from either a *biological* or a *psychological perspective*. In the former, the body's parts and systems are studied, sometimes at a cellular level, sometimes at an organismic level. In the psychological perspective, an individual is studied as a thinking, emotional being (Rogers, 1982) whose behavior is observed as a reflection of the developmental process.

Both perspectives are important in the study of motor development. A full understanding of motor development requires knowledge of physical growth, including growth of the body's systems, and of age-related changes to the physiological demands of vigorous activity. Therefore, we must adopt a biological viewpoint to study many aspects of motor development.

At the same time, it is important to understand behavior resulting from an individual's decisions and feelings. Such behavior plays an important role in an individual's choice to be active, the success of skill performance, and the extent of participation. So, we must adopt the psychological (and psychosocial) perspective to study still other aspects of motor development. Ultimately, we must view individuals from both perspectives, biological and psychological. For example, a 12-year-old boy who is reluctant to participate in physical activities might feel inadequate because he is smaller than other boys his age. His physical size affects his social relationships and, in turn, his motivation to participate in physical activities. His teachers and parents must understand his situation from both viewpoints if they are to help him find a way to take part in and enjoy healthful physical activities.

---

*The biological and psychological perspectives of development are complementary, and consideration of both views contributes to a greater understanding of the total person.*

---

## Developmental Theories

The psychological frame of reference on development, known as developmental psychology, includes several important theoretical perspectives that have implications for motor development (see Figure 1.3). Additionally, several theoretical perspectives have emerged from the study of motor behavior. We could study each perspective in great detail; however, this discussion focuses on the implications for motor development.

### The Maturation Perspective

The *maturation perspective* emerged during the 1930s, led by Arnold Gesell (Gesell, 1928,

1954; Salkind, 1981). His important developmental viewpoint was influenced by recapitulation theory—the notion that ontogeny, the individual's development, recapitulates or reflects phylogeny, the species' development. Gesell believed that the biological and evolutionary history of a species (e.g., humans) determined its orderly and invariable sequence of development and that the rate of the developmental sequence was individually determined. He explained maturation as a process controlled by internal (genetic) rather than external (environmental) factors. Environmental factors, he thought, affected developmental rate but only temporarily, because hereditary factors were in ultimate control of development.

Using identical twins as subjects, Gesell and his co-workers introduced the *co-twin control strategy* to developmental research. In this strategy, one twin receives specific training (the experimental treatment), while the other (called the control) receives no special training (the control treatment) and is allowed to develop as natural circumstances and opportunities dictate. After a specific period, the twins are measured and compared on certain previously determined developmental criteria. In an alternate version of this research technique, the experimental treatment is applied to the control twin at an older age, after which the twins are again compared. The co-twin control research strategy provided significant contributions to

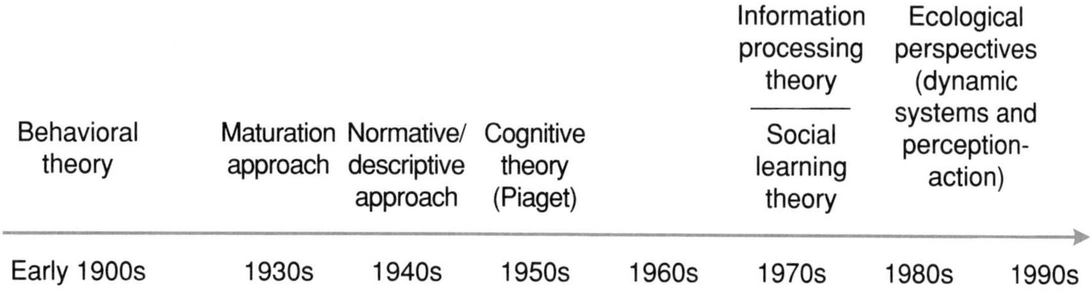

| Behavioral theory | Maturation approach | Normative/ descriptive approach | Cognitive theory (Piaget) | | Information processing theory ——— Social learning theory | Ecological perspectives (dynamic systems and perception-action) | |
|---|---|---|---|---|---|---|---|
| Early 1900s | 1930s | 1940s | 1950s | 1960s | 1970s | 1980s | 1990s |

**Figure 1.3** Various theories and perspectives have emerged in the history of developmental psychology and motor development. Although a perspective may dominate only for a time, its influence can be felt even as other perspectives emerge.

the study of development. It had particular impact on the study of basic motor skills that emerge during infancy and childhood, because developmentalists began identifying the sequence of skill development, noting variations in the rate of skill onset.

Although maturationists described the course of motor development, many of them were interested in the processes underlying development as well. Myrtle McGraw, for example, associated changes in motor behavior with development of the nervous system. She considered maturation of the central nervous system to be the trigger for the emergence of new skills. McGraw also was interested in learning, but those who followed in the study of development generally overlooked this aspect of her work (Clark & Whitall, 1989a).

It is important that we appreciate the maturation approach because it has continued to influence thinking about motor development. Often the influence takes the form not of what the maturationists actually proposed, but of interpretations of their perspective. The focus on

maturation as the primary developmental process led many researchers to assume that basic motor skills automatically emerge. Neither special training nor mild deprivation of experience were believed to alter the emergence of new skills except by small variations in age at onset. Hence, even today many researchers feel it is unnecessary to facilitate development of basic skills. In addition, the maturationists' emphasis on the nervous system as the one system triggering behavioral advancement evolved to almost single-minded emphasis on that system, nearly to the exclusion of other systems. Only recently have developmentalists associated the advancements in other systems with the onset of new behaviors. Finally, the descriptive methodology that characterized the work of the maturationists resulted in other scientists' associating developmentalists with only that methodology.

By the mid-1940s developmental psychologists turned to an interaction approach in which they credited the environment with a larger role in development. As their interest in motor

## Are Skills Learned Automatically?

The basic assumptions of the maturation perspective continue to influence thoughts about skill development. The maturationists focused their attention on infancy and were struck by the universality of motor development. They observed that all human infants develop postural skills, like sitting and standing, and the movement patterns specific to humans, especially two-legged walking. Moreover, these skills develop in the same order in all infants despite variations in an individual infant's experience and surroundings. Based on these findings, many researchers assumed that all motor skills develop automatically and that instruction and structured practice of motor skills are unnecessary.

The notion of automatic skill development, or the maturation of skills, pervades thinking today about the importance of physical education in the basic school curriculum. If one believes motor skills develop automatically, physical education becomes an extra that can be eliminated to save money. If one believes that instruction and structured practice (experience) are necessary for children to fully develop skills, and that it is important for children to have these skills, physical education becomes an integral part of the curriculum. Keep this issue in mind as you learn more about motor development. Perhaps you will change the way you view school physical education programs!

development waned, physical educators took up the study of motor development. The maturation perspective continued to influence the approach of these physical educators, and their study of motor development entered a descriptive period.

## The Descriptive Perspective

From the mid-1940s to 1970, the *descriptive perspective*, which emphasizes the qualitative description of movement and the identification of age group norms, dominated the study of motor development (Clark & Whitall, 1989a). During this time motor developmentalists from the physical education discipline focused their attention on school-age children.

### Normative Description

Anna Espenschade, Ruth Glassow, and G. Lawrence Rarick led a *normative description* movement during this era. In the 1950s, standardized tests and norms became a concern in education. Consistent with this concern, motor developmentalists began to describe children's average performance in terms of quantitative scores on motor performance tests. For example, they described the average running speed, jumping distance, and throwing distance of children at specific ages. Although these motor developmentalists were influenced by the maturation perspective, they focused on the products of development rather than on the underlying developmental processes contributing to quantitative scores. We will discuss some of this work in more detail in chapter 5.

### Biomechanical Description

Ruth Glassow led another descriptive movement during this era. Glassow made careful *biomechanical descriptions* of the movement patterns children used in performing fundamental skills such as jumping. Lolas Halverson and others continued these biomechanical descriptions with longitudinal observations of chil-

dren. As a result, the developmentalists were able to identify the course of sequential improvement through which children moved in attaining biomechanically efficient movement patterns. We will review some of these sequences in chapter 4.

The knowledge obtained from the normative/descriptive perspective was valuable in that it provided educators with information on age-related changes in motor development. Because description prevailed during both the maturation and descriptive eras, motor development as a field of study came to be labeled as descriptive. Interest in the processes underlying age-related changes, which had been so meticulously recorded in this period of history, seemed to disappear.

## The Behavioral Perspective

Another major developmental perspective consists of behavioral, or environmental, theories. Several articulations of the *behavioral perspective* exist, most of which tend to view the individual as reactive—that is, subject to influence by external stimulation. Hence, stimulus-response associations are the basic behavioral units. Ivan Pavlov, John Watson, Edward Thorndike, B.F. Skinner, and Sidney Bijou with Don Baer are among the psychologists who outlined early behavioral theories. More recently, the work of Albert Bandura reflects a movement by behaviorists away from the notion of a strictly passive, reactive individual. The example presented here is Bandura's social learning theory (Bandura, 1977), on which most of the research on imitation and motor performance has been based (Weiss, 1983).

Bandura views reinforcement of a response to a stimulus as a powerful means to shape behavior, but he also attributes much of learned behavior to the imitation of successful (rewarded) models. In other words, vicarious reinforcement is as valuable as direct reinforcement. Behaviorists, in contrast to maturationists (such as Gesell), emphasize environmental influences in development. Bandura moderates this behavioral tenet by stressing the concept of reciprocity between the individual and the environment. For example, a learner does not simply observe a model and then imitate behavior. Instead, the learner first internalizes the model's behavior and then attempts to match this internal representation through progressive approximations of the model's behavior. Reinforcement (reward) is used to refine the approximations until they match the internalized behavior (Salkind, 1981). Researchers often explain the process whereby children begin to participate and imitate others in sport from the social learning viewpoint, which we will discuss in more depth in chapter 9.

## The Cognitive Perspective

Another perspective emerging from developmental psychology is the *cognitive*, or organismic, *perspective*, whose chief proponent was Jean Piaget (Piaget, 1952). Piaget theorized that an individual can act upon the environment and the environment can act upon the individual so that an interaction occurs between the two. This position contrasts sharply with most behavioral theories (though not Bandura's social learning theory), because it states that the individual is not passive but actively attends to certain aspects of the environment, screens out other aspects, and reformulates incoming information (Endler, Boulter, & Osser, 1976). For Piaget, the developmental process encompasses biological growth, children's experiences, social transferral of information and attitudes from adults (especially parents) to children, and the inherent tendency for persons to seek equilibrium with the environment and within themselves (Salkind, 1981).

One of Piaget's significant contributions to developmental study is the notion of stages—that is, times when children's thinking and behavior reflect a certain type of underlying structure (Miller, 1983). Although other develop-

mentalists before Piaget had used the concept of stages, Piaget envisioned stages based on qualitative, structural changes that (a) have a fixed order and (b) cannot be skipped. Piaget's primary interest was the development of intelligence and the source of knowledge. However, because performing motor skills requires information to be processed, Piaget's theory has implications for motor development.

## The Information Processing Perspective

In the *information processing perspective*, researchers attempt to explain behavior on the basis of *perceptual-cognitive processes* that are based on a computer model of the brain (Clark & Whitall, 1989a). This approach emerged around 1970 and became the dominant perspective among experimental psychologists, developmental psychologists, and motor learning scientists specializing in physical education. Behaviorism influenced the information processing theory through its emphasis on stimulus-response associations and feedback and knowledge of results (Pick, 1989). Although some motor developmentalists continued with the product-oriented work of the normative/descriptive era, others adopted the information processing perspective. Researchers studied many aspects of performance, such as attention, memory, and effects of feedback, across age levels. Motor learning researchers and experimental psychologists tended to study a perceptual-cognitive mechanism in young adults first. Then, developmentalists studied children and older adults, comparing them to the young adults. In this way, they could identify the processes that control movement and change with development (Clark & Whitall, 1989a). Today, the information processing perspective is still a viable approach to the study of motor development. We will use the information processing perspective in chapter 8 to review the perceptual-cognitive and memory aspects of motor performance.

Within the framework of information processing, some developmentalists also continued to study perceptual-motor development in children. This work began in the 1960s with proposals that linked learning disabilities to children's delayed perceptual-motor development. Early research focused on this link; by the 1970s, researchers had turned their attention to the development of sensory and perceptual abilities, adopting information processing paradigms (Clark & Whitall, 1989a). Therefore, much of what we know about perceptual-motor development resulted from the work of researchers who adopted the information processing perspective. We will review perceptual-motor development in chapter 6.

## The Ecological Perspective

A new perspective on development emerged during the 1980s and is attracting increased attention in the 1990s. This approach is broadly termed the *ecological perspective* because it stresses the interrelationship between the individual and the environment. There are two branches of the ecological perspective—one concerned with perception and the other with motor control and coordination. The two branches are linked by several fundamental assumptions that differ notably from the maturation and information processing perspectives. In contrast to the maturation theory, both branches consider motor development to be the development of multiple systems rather than only one (the central nervous system—CNS). In information processing theory, an "executive" function is thought to decide all action, based on calculations of perceptual information and resulting in hundreds of commands to control the individual muscles. The ecological perspective maintains that a central executive would be overwhelmed by this task. Rather, perception of the environment is direct, and muscles self-assemble into groups, reducing the number of decisions required of

the higher brain centers (Konczak, 1990). Let us look more closely at each branch of the ecological perspective.

### The Dynamic Systems Perspective

One branch of the ecological perspective is *dynamic systems theory*. Peter Kugler, Scott Kelso, and Michael Turvey (1980, 1982) gave shape to this perspective on movement control and coordination (Clark & Whitall, 1989a). Following the writings of the Soviet physiologist Nikolai Bernstein, they suggested that the very organization of physical and chemical systems constrains or restricts behavior to certain limits. In that an infinite number of possibilities is therefore restricted to a manageable set, groupings of the muscles could execute coordinated movement without the extensive and detailed neural commands from the central nervous system that would be necessary if the behavioral possibilities were limitless.

The collection of muscles that assembles for a particular situation and task is termed a *coordinative structure*. This possibility for spontaneous self-organization, or self-assembly, of body systems is the first of the fundamental tenets of dynamic systems theory. Note, though, that a resulting movement emerges from

1. self-organization of body systems,
2. the nature of the performer's environment, and
3. the demands of the task.

All three of these components give rise to a particular movement behavior. For example, a person might be able to move a particular limb in one body position or posture but not another—you can kick both legs while lying on your back but not when you're standing. Hence, we see the close interrelationship among the individual, the environment, and the task in this perspective.

A second fundamental assumption of the dynamic systems theory is that individuals are composed of many complex, cooperative systems (Thelen, Ulrich, & Jensen, 1989). Even the simplest movement requires the cooperation of many systems: the muscle system to move the skeletal system; the postural system to balance or maintain position; the sensory and perceptual systems to provide information about the environment; the cardiovascular system to supply oxygen to the muscles; and so on.

The body's systems do not develop together. Some might mature quickly, others more slowly. Consider the hypothetical example graphed in Figure 1.4. The development of four hypothetical systems is pictured in each of the small graphs numbered 1 to 4. As time passes, the development of System 1 plateaus. System 2 plateaus, advances in a large step, then plateaus again. System 3 advances gradually, whereas System 4 alternately advances and plateaus. The exhibited behavior, represented in the large graph, is the product of all the individual systems. An individual might begin to perform some new skill, such as walking, only when the slowest of the necessary systems for that skill reaches a certain point.

Any such system or set of systems is known as a *rate controller* for that skill because that system's development controls the individual's rate of development at that time. Suppose that System 4 in Figure 1.4 is the muscular system. Perhaps an infant's muscular strength must reach a certain plateau before the legs are strong enough to support the infant's weight on one leg to walk. Hence, muscular strength would be a rate controller for walking.

These tenets of dynamic systems theory differ significantly from those of the maturation theory. Maturationists tended to focus on the central nervous system as the only system relevant to development and the only rate controller. Dynamic systems theory focuses on many systems and acknowledges that different systems might be rate controllers for different skills.

The last fundamental assumption of dynamic systems theory that we will consider here is the discontinuous nature of development. Qualitative changes in skill performance can be discontinuous even with an accompanying, continuous increase or decrease in a factor such as

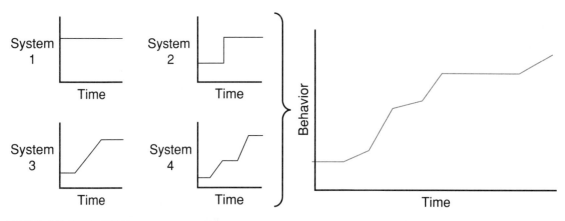

**Figure 1.4**    The dynamic systems perspective views development as parallel developing systems, each with its own course of development. A system that develops later might act as a rate controller, limiting the rate at which the individual develops. Here, four developing systems are depicted as contributing to behavior within an environmental context and for some particular task. The horizontal axis is time, and the vertical axis is some quantity of a system or behavior.
(Adapted by permission from Thelen, Ulrich, & Jensen, 1989.)

speed. An example often cited is a horse that shifts from a walk to a trot (opposite front and back legs moving forward together) to a gallop (the two front legs moving together but opposite the two back legs, which move together) as it goes faster. Hence, a continuing steady increase in speed at some point causes the horse to change its leg movement pattern from linking opposite-side front and back limbs to linking the front limbs together and the back limbs together. Likewise, in human motor development we might see new movement patterns emerge as children gradually become capable of exerting more force and increasing their speed and momentum in executing skills.

---

The three fundamental principles of dynamic systems theory are as follows:

1. Body systems are capable of spontaneous self-organization, or self-assembly.
2. Individuals are composed of many complex, cooperative systems.
3. Development has a discontinuous nature; thus new movement patterns replace old ones.

---

Many of the developmental perspectives do not address aging. Dynamic systems theory accounts for changes in older adults as well as advancement in youths. Figure 1.5 presents a hypothetical example of aging in the body's systems. System 1 declines steadily but then improves with a treatment or rehabilitation program. (For example, an individual could regain lost flexibility through a flexibility exercise program.) System 2 experiences a sharp decline, perhaps due to disease, whereas System 3 declines gradually, perhaps from disuse. System 4 alternately declines and plateaus. Behavior is the product of all the individual systems.

The concept of a system acting as a rate controller for a movement behavior applies in this example as well. When one or more of an individual's systems declines to a critical point, a change in behavior might occur. This system is a rate controller; it is the first to decline to some critical point, and it triggers the reorganization of a movement to a less efficient pattern. For example, if an individual's shoulder joint deteriorates due to arthritis and loses flexibility, at some point that individual might have to use a different overhead throwing motion or even

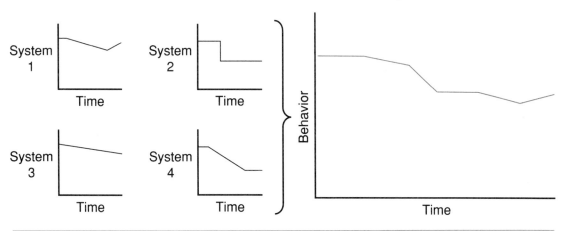

**Figure 1.5** The dynamic systems perspective can account for declines and improvements in behavior with aging. Contributing systems might decline or be rehabilitated, as depicted here. Early decline, onset of disease, or a sudden injury in one system might trigger a decline in some behavior. This system then acts as a rate controller. Rehabilitation of a system might trigger an improvement in some behavior.

throw underhand. The dynamic systems approach is very appropriate because changes do not necessarily occur in all systems over the entire span of older adulthood. Disease or injury might strike one system, or systems might be differentially affected by lifestyle. An active older adult who maintains a regular and balanced exercise program might experience less decline in many of the systems than a sedentary peer.

### The Perception-Action Perspective

The second branch of the ecological perspective is the *perception-action perspective*. J.J. Gibson proposed this model in his writings during the 1960s and 1970s (1966, 1979) but those who study movement have only recently adopted this perspective. Gibson proposed that a close interrelationship exists between the perceptual system and the motor system, emphasizing that they evolved together in animals and humans. In this perspective, we cannot study perception independent of movement if our findings are to be ecologically valid—that is, applicable to real-world movement behavior. Likewise, the development of perception and the development of movement must be studied together. And we cannot study the individual while ignoring the surrounding environment.

Gibson used the term *affordance* to describe the functions environmental objects provide to an individual of a certain size and shape within a particular setting. For example, a horizontal surface affords a human a place to sit, but a vertical surface does not. A squirrel can rest on a vertical tree trunk, so a vertical surface affords a squirrel a resting place. A baseball bat affords an adult, but not an infant, the opportunity to swing. Hence, the relationship between individual and environment is so intertwined that one's characteristics define objects' meanings. This implies that people assess environmental properties in relation to themselves, not an objective standard (Konczak, 1990). For example, an individual perceiving whether he or she can

walk up a flight of stairs with alternate footsteps considers not just the height of each stair alone, but the height of each stair in relation to the climber's body size. Obviously, a comfortable step height for an adult is not the same as that for a toddler. The use of intrinsic (relative to body size) rather than extrinsic dimensions is termed *body scaling*.

The implications of these ideas for development are that affordances might change as individuals change; therefore, new movement patterns emerge. Growth in size or enhanced movement capabilities might allow actions not previously afforded. Eventually a toddler grows to a size that makes climbing stairs with alternate footsteps easy. Additionally, scaling environmental objects to one's body size permits actions that are otherwise impossible.

Body scaling also applies to other age periods. For example, steps that are an appropriate height for most adults might be too high for an older adult with arthritis to climb comfortably with alternate footsteps. A wall-mounted telephone might be at a comfortable height for most adults, but it may be a frustrating inch too high for someone in a wheelchair. At any age, achievement of a movement goal relates to the individual, who is a certain shape and size, and to environmental objects, which afford certain movements to that individual.

Gibson also rejected the notion of a CNS executive that performs almost limitless calculations on stimulus information to determine the speed and direction of both the person and the moving objects. The information processing perspective holds that such calculations are used to anticipate future positions so that we can reach up to catch a thrown ball, for example. Instead, according to Gibson, individuals perceive their environment directly by constantly moving their eyes, heads, and bodies. This activity creates an optic flow field that provides both space and time information. For example, the image of a baseball approaching a batter not only indicates the ball's location, but the image expands on the eye's retina. The

## Body Scaling in Youth Sport Programs

Physical educators in elementary schools and youth sport coordinators often adapt equipment and games to take body scaling into account. For example, they have children use basketballs that are smaller and lighter than standard basketballs. Because children have small hands, a basketball scaled to their hand size rather than to an adult's affords them a better opportunity to handle the smaller ball the way an adult handles a larger ball. The lighter weight affords children a better opportunity to learn a one-handed shot. Using a heavy ball, a child would need to heave it up to the basket with two hands. Equipment size and weight and distances (basket heights, base paths, soccer field dimensions, etc.) can be increased as children grow in size and strength.

Parents and youth sport coaches sometimes debate the value of scaling down equipment and distances. They fear that young athletes will have difficulty adapting to "official" sizes and dimensions later. However, when we apply Gibson's notion of affordances and body scaling to this issue, we can see that scaling equipment size and playing distances to young participants results in playing environments that are consistent across age groups.

batter uses this rate of image expansion to time his swing—that is, the rate of expansion gives the batter's central nervous system direct information about when the ball will be in range. Likewise, the expansion rate of an oncoming car's image on a driver's retina yields the "time to collision." From Gibson's perspective, an individual can perceive this so-called time to collision directly and does not need to perform a complicated calculation of speeds and distances to predict where and when collisions and interceptions will occur.

Researchers often cite the interception movements of animals as support for Gibson's notion of direct perception. For example, a dog can jump to catch a ball or frisbee. And certain insects strike to catch their prey only when the prey comes within striking distance. Insects and animals that lack humans' mental capacity obviously can intercept objects. Hence, there must exist means of perceiving movement and taking appropriate action that do not require complex calculations of speed and distance.

The influence of the ecological perspectives is just taking hold in motor development research. Developmentalists are beginning new types of research studies (Clark & Whitall,

1989a). Although the areas investigated thus far are limited in number, the ecological perspectives encourage professionals to view developing individuals in a very different way than before. As a result, these perspectives will both excite and challenge students in the field. In many sections of this text, we will contrast the maturation and dynamic systems approaches on a particular issue and highlight the differences between these perspectives.

## REVIEW 1.3

The theoretical approaches reviewed here often have very different basic assumptions as well as common views (see Table 1.3). Maturation theorists emphasize biological development. Behaviorists stress the importance of the environment. Cognitivists assume an incorporated biological and psychological influence on development. Maturation and information processing theorists emphasize the nervous system. Ecological theorists stress all the body systems and the inseparable nature of the individual and the environment. Behaviorists and information processing theorists view an individual as reactive, whereas cognitivists and

**Table 1.3  Theoretical Perspectives in Motor Development**

| Perspective | Author | Basic principles |
|---|---|---|
| Maturation | Gesell (1928, 1954) | "Ontogeny recapitulates phylogeny"<br>Development is ultimately controlled by heredity<br>Central nervous system is the major rate-controlling system |
| Descriptive—normative branch | Espenschade, Glassow, Rarick (1950s) | Motor development can be described through age group norms |
| Descriptive—biomechanical branch | Glassow, Halverson (1960s) | Motor development can be described through sequential improvements in movement patterns |
| Behaviorism—social learning branch | Bandura (1977) | Behavior is shaped by both direct and vicarious reinforcement |
| Cognitivism | Piaget (1952) | Development involves individuals acting upon the environment<br>Development occurs in stages |
| Information processing | Connolly (1970) | Information is manipulated in humans through a series of operations leading to a (movement) response |
| Ecological psychology—dynamic systems branch | Kugler, Kelso, Turvey (1980, 1982) | Body systems can spontaneously self-organize<br>Individuals are composed of cooperative systems<br>Development is discontinuous |
| Ecological psychology—perception-action branch | Gibson (1966, 1979) | Environment affords certain movements to individuals<br>Movement is perceived directly by the central nervous system |

Based on Clark and Whitall (1989a).

ecologists see the individual as active. Behaviorists believe, too, that development is a process of quantitative change wherein learning episodes accumulate with time; thus to them the description of stages is counterproductive (Miller, 1983). Maturationists, on the other hand, emphasize development as qualitative change by describing the sequence in which new skills emerge. Cognitivists focus on qualitative changes that take place as an individual moves from stage to stage; further, cognitivists acknowledge that quantitative changes occur in the developmental process as behavior patterns and cognitive skills become stronger, more consistent, and more efficient (Miller, 1983).

Diametrically opposed perspectives cannot be merged, but students of motor development are free to view behavior from different perspectives. It is important to remember that these theoretical viewpoints often focus only on specific aspects of development; that is, developmentalists with a particular perspective tend to study certain behaviors or age spans. The maturationists focused on infancy, whereas the descriptive developmentalists focused on late childhood and adolescence. Information processing theorists searched for age differences, whereas ecologists studied transitions from one skill to another (crawling to walking, for example). As students of motor development, you must be able to interpret knowledge of development in light of the perspective of those generating that knowledge. You must identify biases in interpreting data that result from a certain perspective and realize the benefits and limitations of adopting a single perspective. Professionals may need to combine aspects of several viewpoints to understand and explain global motor behavior. In keeping with this line of reasoning, basic concepts of motor development discussed in this text reflect a variety of theoretical perspectives.

## CONTEMPORARY ISSUES

It would be ideal if the scientific information educators and health care professionals use were complete, accurate, and proven. Unfortunately, this is seldom the case, especially in the area of development. Although some of the cornerstone research in motor development was conducted in the 1930s, many questions central to development remain unanswered.

These gaps in developmental knowledge exist for many reasons. First, scientific research on a particular question simply may not have been conducted, as with study of the mechanics of older adults' motor skill performance. Another reason is that the technology for conducting a given type of research may not exist, or the existing technology may limit the amount and depth of research possible. For example, initial attempts to analyze motor skill performance via high-speed filming were limited. Before digital and computer film analysis systems were available, researchers meticulously analyzed and measured film by hand, a time-consuming process. Developmentalists also often examine an issue using basic assumptions from conflicting theoretical viewpoints. Some developmentalists believe heredity is the major influence in development and conduct their research from this perspective, whereas others believe the environment is the major influence.

As with any area of study, it is important for students of motor development to recognize the limitations of the information currently available. They must be aware of the unsettled issues and be alert to research findings that they must interpret with caution. Toward that end, the following discussion examines a few of the major unresolved issues that have implications for the study of motor development.

---

> **CONCEPT 1.4**
> Some aspects of development are topics of discussion and debate.

---

## Nature Versus Nurture

One of the longest standing issues in motor development is that of nature versus nurture, sometimes called heredity versus environment or nativism versus empiricism. One of humankind's fundamental questions has concerned the source of new behaviors (Thelen, 1989). How does a person come to execute a new skill, such as walking, when that person was not capable of it earlier? Traditional explanations centered on either hereditary or environmental factors as the major source of new behavior. Nativists claimed that new behaviors are stored in the genes and appear with maturation. Empiricists held that absorption of information from the environment brings about new behaviors. This issue has far-reaching implications for motor development. For example, if environmental factors are the chief determinants of motor behavior, parents who want to raise a successful athlete might structure their infant's environment in a certain way. On the other hand, if genetic factors predominate and great athletes are born, not made, a parent or educator could do little to enhance the talents of a child beyond his or her innate ability.

Today, few theorists and teachers adopt the extreme position of one or the other, because neither position has been proven exclusively. Thus, greater attention must shift toward the mechanisms that mediate development (Endler et al., 1976); that is, how do nature and nurture interact to produce developmental change?

---

*The contemporary approach recognizes that heredity and environment are intertwined and that motor behavior is influenced by the interaction of heredity and environment.*

---

## Sensitive Periods

A critical or sensitive period is a time span during which an individual is most susceptible to the influence of an event or mitigating factor. This period may not be the only time when an event is influential, but it is the time when the individual is most likely to be affected by it. To illustrate the concept, suppose that a truly *critical period* exists between 4 and 8 months of age for an infant to acquire reaching and grasping skills. If the supposition is correct, an infant who does not have an opportunity to learn these skills during this span may never be as proficient as if he or she had acquired them during the critical time. If the period between 4 and 8 months is only a *sensitive period*, the infant might later acquire reaching and grasping skills, but not to the level possible if the infant had had experience in reaching and grasping during that span.

Developmentalists disagree about whether critical periods truly exist. Although considerable evidence is available for the existence of critical periods in animals, the hypothesis re-

mains difficult to test in humans for both ethical and moral reasons. For humans, then, the term *critical* is probably a misnomer, and *sensitive* is the preferred term. Behaviorists strongly disagree that an individual is susceptible to influence during a biologically based time span, because they argue in favor of developmental control by environmental factors. This controversy is especially relevant to the acquisition of basic motor skills. Consequently, we will discuss this topic further in chapter 3.

## Discontinuity Versus Continuity

Accounting for both the sudden appearance of new behaviors and the continuous advancement of developmental processes is a puzzle for developmentalists (Thelen & Ulrich, 1991). The emergence of discrete, new skills is a discontinuous process: A child begins to sit unsupported, to stand alone, to walk, to speak a first word. Hence, it is possible to view development in terms of stages centered around these new behaviors. Most theoretical accounts of development include the notion of developmental stages.

At the same time, individuals and their body systems are continuously changing, perhaps not at the same rate at all times, but changing nevertheless. To add to the dilemma, consider that the emergence of new skills often is tied to the context or situation. A child does not learn to ride a bicycle unless he or she has a bicycle to ride. If one child learns to ride at a younger age than another, the first child is not necessarily more developmentally advanced than the second child. Perhaps the first child had the opportunity to ride at a younger age.

Some developmentalists use "stages" as a convenient system of categorizing development rather than as a characteristic of development. Others focus on the stagelike quality of development. Accounting for both continuity and discontinuity in development remains a challenge for developmentalists.

## Viewing Behavior Through Tinted Glasses

Developmentalist Jane Clark suggested that adopting theoretical perspectives is like putting on a pair of tinted glasses. Suppose you are looking at a piece of multicolored fabric. If you look through a pair of blue-tinted glasses, the fabric looks a certain way to you. If you take off the blue glasses and replace them with yellow-tinted ones, the fabric looks different.

So too with theoretical perspectives! If you adopt a particular perspective, you might explain a given behavior one way. If you adopt a different perspective, you might explain that same behavior another way. Remember that developmentalists' explanations of behavior are colored by their theoretical perspectives. Take this into account when reading scientific literature, and try to identify which "color" you are looking through when you explain the developmental behavior you observe.

## Universality Versus Variability

Another paradox in development centers around the universality of development as opposed to individual differences (Thelen & Ulrich, 1991). Individuals in a species show great similarity in their development, following an almost stereotypical course. Stages, of course, describe the emergence of universal behaviors. Those who anticipate working with individuals in a particular age range often are interested in the behaviors typical of those in that range.

Yet individual differences in development exist. Any individual we might observe is more likely to be above or below average, or to achieve a milestone earlier or later than average, than to be exactly average. And children can arrive at the same point in development by very different pathways (Siegler & Jenkins, 1989). Every individual has different experiences, even twins. Those who work with any group of individuals supposedly at the same stage of development usually are amazed by the variability within the group.

Developmentalists, educators, parents, and health professionals must be able to consider an individual's behavior in the context of both universal behaviors and individual differences. It also is important to recognize when others use a perspective that focuses on the universality of behavior and when they are focusing on variability in behavior.

### REVIEW 1.4

It would be wonderful if all the controversial issues in development were settled, but in fact many still are being debated. It is valuable to identify the differing perspectives and viewpoints that relate to growth and development. Doing so allows us to better understand the different positions developmentalists have taken on these unresolved issues. We can better untangle the controversies surrounding growth and development and sort through the various pieces of information to form a clearer picture of the developing individual as a whole. In addition, we are less susceptible to the influence of a particular bias.

### SUMMARY

Readers new to a field of study often expect that field to be complete. They expect researchers to have asked all the important questions and found all the important answers. This is rarely the case, however. Many areas of study, including motor development, are still evolving. Research is ongoing, and important issues remain unresolved.

Motor development is a product of its history. Various theoretical perspectives have dominated thinking in motor development for a time, only to be replaced eventually by another perspective. Students of motor development must realize that new perspectives often advance our knowledge by introducing fresh ideas and new explanations of behavior. Explanations of behavior are always derived from a particular perspective. Professionals must be aware of this and interpret explanations accordingly.

To read motor development literature, we must grasp the terminology used in the field and appreciate the fundamental developmental perspective. Remember that developmentalists, no matter what their theoretical perspectives, view behavior as a point on a continuum of change. They relate observed behavior to the behavior that preceded it and to the behavior that will likely follow it.

The human body and its component systems are always changing. Naturally, then, physical growth and aging impact motor development. In the next chapter, we will take a biological approach to the basic concepts of physical growth and aging.

## Key Terms

affordance
aging
cohort
consolidation
coordinative structure
critical period
cross-sectional research
development
dynamic systems theory
growth
information processing perspective
longitudinal research
maturation
motor behavior
motor development
motor learning
perception-action perspective
rate controller
sensitive period
sequential research
stage

## Discussion Questions

1. Choose two theoretical perspectives. Compare and contrast them, indicating areas of similarity or agreement (if any) and areas of disagreement. Remember that not all theoretical perspectives address the same aspects of motor development.

2. What is the fundamental developmental perspective that separates motor development from other subdisciplines of the movement sciences?

3. Suppose that an educator is interested in comparing a new teaching method to a traditional one. The educator pretests two classes of students; teaches one class using the traditional method and the other using the new method, both for 6 weeks; and then tests the classes again. Would this be a developmental research study? Why or why not?

4. Why might a person planning a career teaching children study older adults?

5. Which theoretical perspective(s) is (are) likely to emphasize the universality of behavior and deemphasize individual differences?

## Suggested Readings

Clark, J.E., & Whitall, J. (1989). What is motor development? The lessons of history. *Quest*, **41**, 183-202.

Endler, N.S., Boulter, L.R., & Osser, H. (1976). *Contemporary issues in developmental psychology* (2nd ed.). New York: Holt, Rinehart and Winston.

Kausler, D.H. (1982). *Experimental psychology and human aging*. New York: John Wiley & Sons.

Miller, P.H. (1983). *Theories of developmental psychology*. San Francisco: W.H. Freeman.

Rogers, D. (1982). *Life-span human development*. Monterey, CA: Brooks/Cole.

Salkind, N.J. (1981). *Theories of human development*. New York: D. Van Nostrand.

Thelen, E., & Ulrich, B.D. (1991). Hidden skills. *Monographs of the Society for Research in Child Development*, **56** (1, Serial no. 223).

Wohlwill, J.F. (1973). *The study of behavioral development*. New York: Academic Press.

## Chapter 2

# Physical Growth, Maturation, and Aging

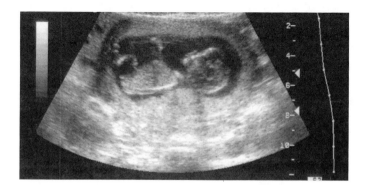

## CHAPTER CONCEPTS

**2.1**
We can assess physical growth and maturation in many ways.

**2.2**
Both genetic and environmental factors influence normal embryonic and fetal growth.

**2.3**
Abnormal prenatal development can result from either genetic or environmental factors.

**2.4**
Postnatal growth proceeds in precise and orderly patterns that differ among the body systems.

**2.5**
Environmental factors become more important as postnatal growth and maturation proceed.

Should parents be concerned if their 12-month-old infant is not walking yet? Is a 6-year-old physically ready for youth league soccer? The answers to these questions relate partly to each child's physical maturity and partly to each child's exposure to and experience in a particular setting. To determine children's potential to perform particular motor skills at a given age, we must consider their physical growth and maturation. This includes the extent of growth and maturation of the body systems. Infants' bone and muscle strength, for example, must develop to some minimal level before their legs can support their weight. Their nervous systems must develop sufficiently to allow them to walk voluntarily.

Attempting to teach children skills before they are physically ready is often frustrating and can sometimes be harmful if they have not yet developed the skeletal and muscular strength necessary for the skills. Growth and maturation of the body and its systems tend to advance as children get older, but not necessarily at a steady rate. Some systems advance before others do, so developmentalists need a complete understanding of the course of development in each system. We will consider the influence of experience more fully in later chapters.

Children are not all the same. We cannot measure one 6-year-old to determine the growth status of all 6-year-olds. Children typically grow either faster or slower than "average for age" growth. Before we can assess an individual's potential for skill performance, we must know the course of normal growth and the normal variations of growth for persons of a given age. We can then determine if a particular 6-year-old is about the same height and weight as other 6-year-olds, or bigger or smaller. Parents and recreation leaders can consider this and other information when deciding if a child is ready for youth league soccer.

## ASSESSING GROWTH AND MATURATION

Assessing children's physical growth and maturation requires a knowledge of normal growth patterns and an understanding of growth measures. Normal growth includes not only the average extent of growth at a given age but also the normal variations of growth. These standards identify the range within which children's measurements should fall at a given age if their bodies are growing properly.

An examiner must also understand the advantages and disadvantages of the many ways to measure growth. Some measures are useful for children of one age but not another, some are influenced more by genetic inheritance than by the child's environment, and others are influenced more by the environment than by heredity. Being aware of the strengths and weaknesses of each measure allows the examiner to use the information gained from the measure appropriately.

The following discussion deals with the normal patterns of growth obtained with growth measures. This knowledge is helpful to those who teach skills because it allows their instruction and expectations of students to be individualized based on the progress of each child's physical growth. Additionally, educators can identify children growing abnormally and refer them to medical personnel for further evaluation.

You might think that once an individual becomes an adult, there is little reason to measure height, weight, and so on. But the body is not static in adulthood. There may be many changes, especially in body weight and composition, such as the amount of fat weight. Many of the measures we discuss are also useful with adults.

---

**CONCEPT 2.1**

We can assess physical growth and maturation in many ways.

---

## Growth Measures: Anthropometry

The branch of science involving human growth and body measurement is termed *anthropometry.* Anthropometric measures include

- height,
- weight,
- segment length,
- body breadth, and
- circumferences.

Although most of us would consider these measures fairly routine, such measures must be pre-

cise if they are to provide us with reliable information about human growth (Boyd, 1929). Examiners should rigidly follow standard procedures for taking growth measures; these are available in the *Anthropometric Standardization Reference Manual* (Lohman, Roche, & Martorell, 1988). Following are several common growth and maturation measures, including the accepted assessment procedure.

### Height

One of the most useful and common measures of growth is that of body height, or stature. Children up to 3 years old are measured lying down. Thereafter, the individual being measured stands erect on a stadiometer. This instrument consists of a vertical rule and a horizontal headboard that contacts the highest point (vertex) of the person's head. In a clinical setting, a right triangle placed flat against the rule can be used as a headboard (see Figure 2.1). The person stands erect with arms at the sides, and barefoot with heels together and touching the vertical board. The shoulder blades and

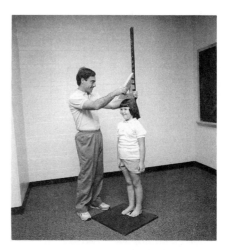

**Figure 2.1** The measurement of standing height with inexpensive equipment. When the triangle is held against the measurement scale a level reading is assured.

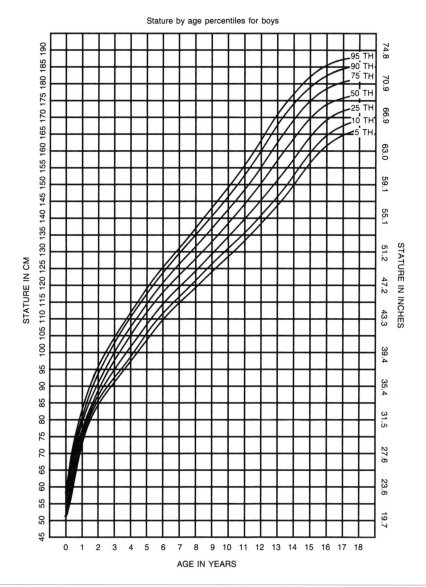

Stature by age percentiles for boys

**Figure 2.2a** Stature (standing height) by age percentiles for boys. Note the sigmoid or "s" shape of the curves.
(Reprinted by permission from Hamill, 1977.)

buttocks also touch the vertical board. Just before taking the measurement, the examiner asks the person to take a deep breath.

Anthropometrists have measured large groups of children and adolescents at various ages to determine average heights for different ages. These averages and the range of height are often plotted against age, as in Figures 2.2a and 2.2b. The range of scores is expressed in percentiles that show relative position. For example, in a group of a hundred 8-year-olds, a child whose height measured at the 50th per-

Stature by age percentiles for girls

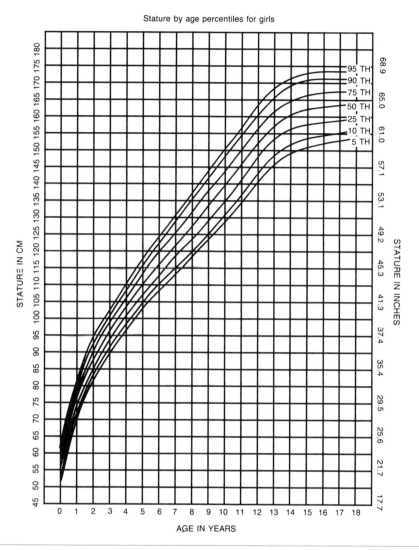

**Figure 2.2b**  Stature (standing height) by age percentiles for girls.
(Reprinted by permission from Hamill, 1977.)

centile would be taller than 49 of the children and shorter than 50 of the children in the group.

We can measure an individual's height and compare it to the charted values for chronological age. We must use caution, however, in interpreting deviations from the average. For example, if the height of an 8-year-old boy falls at the 25th percentile, we may wonder if he is a late maturer, if he is growing abnormally, or if he will be a relatively short adult as dictated by his genetic inheritance. There is no way to answer this question from the height measure alone, though, so we must take care not to jump to incorrect conclusions. Despite the limitations outlined, measures of stature are easy to take

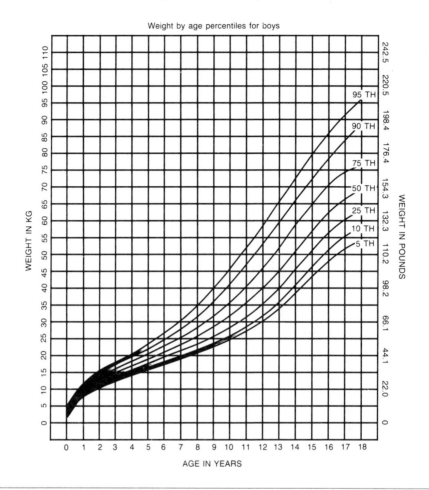

**Figure 2.3a**  Weight by age percentiles for boys.
(Reprinted by permission from Hamill, 1977.)

and helpful in assessing growth and screening for disease or malnutrition (Gordon, Chumlea, & Roche, 1988).

It is important to recognize that some height charts are based on individuals of a particular race and socioeconomic background. The most accurate comparisons are those made to data taken on a group similar to that of the measured individual.

### Weight

Weight is a common anthropometric measure. Measuring weight requires an accurate scale, preferably a platform model with a beam and movable weights (Gordon, Chumlea, & Roche, 1988). The person to be weighed wears minimal (or no) clothing and stands in the center of the scale platform. Height and weight fluctuate slightly throughout the day, so if the individual is to be measured repeatedly and the results compared to previous measurements, the ex-

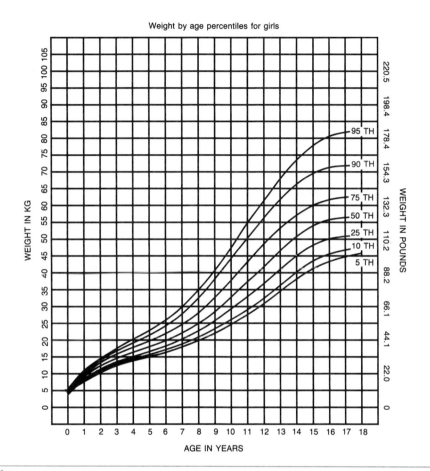

**Figure 2.3b** Weight by age percentiles for girls.
(Reprinted by permission from Hamill, 1977.)

aminer should measure both height and weight at the same time of day for consistency.

As with stature, average weights for different ages are often plotted graphically, as in Figures 2.3a and 2.3b. Here, too, we must exercise caution in interpreting deviations from the average, because weight values give no information about body composition (leanness or fatness). Think about a 16-year-old boy whose weight is at the 85th percentile. This teenager might be overweight, might be heavily muscled, or might have reached his adult size before most of this peers. Again, we cannot tell from the weight measure alone.

## Body Composition

To obtain more information about growth related to weight, examiners make estimates of leanness or fatness—*body composition*. They divide body weight into fat weight (adipose tissue) and fat-free or lean body weight. Lean body weight includes

- bone,
- muscle,
- organs, and
- tissues other than fat.

Directly measuring the amount of body fat in a living individual is difficult, but we can predict it by several methods.

## Underwater Weighing

We can estimate body denseness by contrasting body weight measured normally with body weight measured under water. Muscle is denser than fat, so a heavily muscled person with little fat will weigh more under water than a person of identical weight who has more fat. To obtain an accurate underwater measurement, you must make sure the individual is completely submerged and then expels the air in the lungs. Because this method is especially difficult for young children, it is rarely used with them.

## Potassium 40

Another body composition measure assesses the amount of potassium 40 that a person's body naturally emits, because that amount is proportional to the lean body mass. This is a simple method—the person being measured lies in a whole-body counter that scans the body and records the potassium 40 radiation levels. However, these counters are expensive and not widely available.

## Skinfold Thickness

Skinfold thickness measures are the most practical way to estimate body composition in educational and recreational settings. The examiner measures skinfold thickness by placing a caliper over a fold of skin and the underlying fat tissue, lifted between the examiner's thumb and forefinger at clearly specified body sites (see Figure 2.4). The examiner then enters the measures into mathematical equations that estimate body density and fat weight. These equations are, ideally, specific to age group, race, fitness level, and gender, especially after puberty. For example, children have a higher water content and lower bone mineral content than adults. Using adult equations overesti-

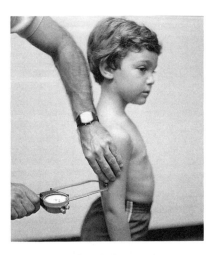

**Figure 2.4**   A skinfold measurement taken over the triceps muscle in the back of the upper arm.

mates percent body fat in children (Boileau, Lohman, Slaughter, Horswill, & Stillman, 1988). Equations are available for older children and adolescents (Boileau et al., 1984; Slaughter et al., 1988), but equations for children under 7 years are still needed (Lohman, 1989).

## Circumference

Circumference measurements reflect cross-sectional size; we can use them alone or along with skinfold measurements to assess growth, fat patterns, or nutritional status. An examiner should use a nonstretchable tape measure for circumference measurements. It is important to measure at a standard site, making certain the tape measure is horizontal to the body segment, and to hold the tape snugly, but not so tight as to indent the skin.

Common circumference measurements include the following:

- Head
- Neck
- Waist
- Hip

- Thigh
- Calf
- Arm

Due to variations in inspiration and in breast development, chest measures are often inaccurate; thus, chest girth is less desirable as a growth measure than other circumference measures.

Head circumference is an important dimension in the growth of infants and young children. This measurement is taken just above the bony ridge over the eyes (see Figure 2.5). Normal head-circumference measures fall within a fairly narrow range for any given age, so marked deviations might imply neurologic abnormalities. For example, an abnormally rapid increase in head measurements taken at periodic intervals might indicate that a child has hydrocephalus ("water on the brain"), an accumulation of excess cerebrospinal fluid. This liquid surrounds and protects the brain and spinal cord, but too much fluid puts pressure on the brain and can eventually lead to brain damage. In some cases, small head circumference for age has been associated with mental retardation, but notable exceptions occur, and

therefore we should exercise caution in interpreting small head-circumference measures. However, head circumference does serve as a valuable screening measure that may indicate the need for medical examination (Brandt, 1978).

## Breadth

Breadth measures are useful in assessing growth, particularly in body build, or physique. An examiner takes them with a breadth caliper or blade anthropometer at palpable bone locations, such as the acromion processes (shoulders) or the iliac crests (hips) (see Figure 2.6). It might be difficult to locate these bony sites in obese individuals. While sliding the blades of the caliper into place, the examiner applies pressure to assure that soft tissues make minimal contributions to the measure (Wilmore et al., 1988). The most common measures are biacromial breadth (shoulder width) and biiliac or bicristal breadth (hip width). Biacromial width divided by the bicristal width (biacromial/bicristal ratio) provides a useful ratio we can use to observe proportional changes in physique.

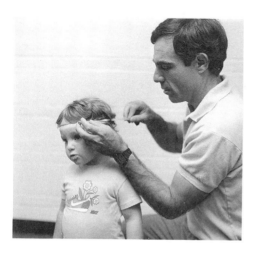

**Figure 2.5**  Measurement of head circumference with a spring-loaded steel tape measure.

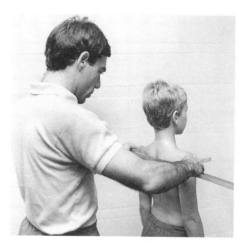

**Figure 2.6**  A breadth measurement taken at the shoulders, the biacromial breadth.

sique. This ratio dramatically illustrates gender differences in growth at puberty. Men tend to have a greater ratio than women, reflecting their relatively wider shoulders and narrower hips. The pelvis grows proportionately wider in women to accommodate childbirth, yielding a smaller shoulder-to-hip width ratio. Other measures include wrist breadth, knee breadth, and bitrochanteric (greater trochanter of the thighbone) breadth.

## Segment Length

Besides breadth measures, we can also assess the length of various body segments, such as sitting height. We can then determine the contribution of certain body segments to overall size. Researchers also use segment lengths to study differential rates of growth in various body segments and variation in individual physique. Segment lengths are measured either between two bony landmarks or between a flat surface and a bony landmark. For example, calf length can be measured between the top of the tibia (shankbone) and distal tip of the medial malleolus (inner anklebone). It can also be measured between the top of the lateral side of the tibia and the floor when a person is standing erect (see Figure 2.7). An examiner typically uses an *anthropometer* to measure segment lengths. Techniques for locating bony landmarks should be followed carefully (Martin, Carter, Hendy, & Malina, 1988).

Observing an individual's *sitting height* can help us describe body proportions during growth. The procedure for measuring sitting height is identical to that for stature except the individual is seated with the feet hanging freely. We can estimate leg length by subtracting the sitting height from standing height (termed functional leg length), or we can measure it directly from the lateral malleolus (outer anklebone) to the greater trochanter of the femur (thighbone). We can then calculate a ratio of sitting height to stature. This ratio is large in

infancy and decreases throughout childhood as the legs grow more rapidly to catch up with the trunk and head, which are proportionately longer early in life. We will discuss further the differential growth of body segments in a later section.

## Maturation Measures

Maturation is progress toward maturity by qualitative rather than quantitative advancement. It is ideal to assess maturation directly because maturation and chronological age are not related to one another exactly. A person's chronological age is the number of years and days elapsed since birth. Yet two children who are the same age can have dramatically different levels of physical maturity. One could be an early maturer—a child whose rate of maturation is faster than average, resulting in physical maturity more advanced than that of most children of the same chronological age. The other could be a late maturer. It is difficult to infer maturity from size alone.

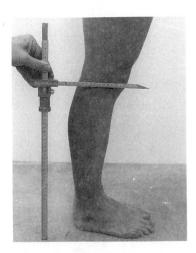

**Figure 2.7** Segment lengths, such as a direct calf length measurement, are typically measured with an anthropometer.
(Reprinted by permission from Lohman, Roche, & Martorell, 1988.)

An individual child can appear to be small and slight of build but may actually be relatively mature for his or her chronological age.

Suppose you measure a child's height, weight, biacromial breadth, and so on and compare these values to those on standard growth charts for the child's age. If most of the body dimensions fall within the upper percentiles, you might conclude that the child is an early maturer. In concluding this, though, you may overlook other factors, such as the child's genetic inheritance or excess fat weight. For example, a child whose genetic potential is to be tall might appear to be an early maturer because of his or her size, but the child actually may be maturing at an average rate, because maturation is a qualitative rather than a quantitative advancement. Obviously, it is best to assess maturation directly, because maturation and chronological age do not correspond exactly. In the following review of the direct measures of maturation, you will learn the advantages as well as the shortcomings of these assessments.

## Skeletal Age

The most useful method of assessing maturation is to determine *skeletal age* by taking radiographs (x-rays), usually of the bones of the wrist but occasionally of the long bones or teeth. Wrist and hand radiographs have been standardized to identify skeletal maturation at 6-month and 1-year intervals (Greulich & Pyle, 1959). To determine a child's skeletal age, for example, you must compare his or her radiograph to the standard radiographs of bone development. Figure 2.8a and Figure 2.8b show

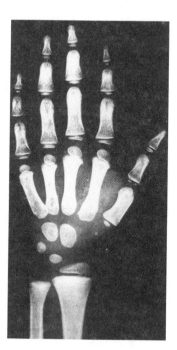

**Figure 2.8a**  An x-ray of the hand, skeletal age 48 months for boys and 37 months for girls. (Reprinted by permission from Pyle, 1971.)

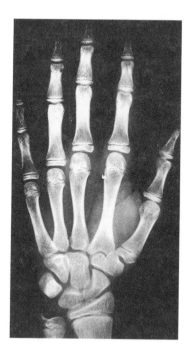

**Figure 2.8b**  An x-ray of the hand, skeletal age 156 months for boys and 128 months for girls. (Reprinted by permission from Pyle, 1971.)

wrist and hand radiographs that reveal the differences in bone development between a younger child and an older one. Areas that appear as black or grayish spaces in the wrist are actually cartilaginous bone not yet calcified.

As each cartilaginous wristbone begins to ossify, it becomes denser and appears as a visible opaque area in the x-ray. The number of ossification centers and the size of the ossified area in each wristbone increase as a child matures. Greater calcification in the *epiphyses* (ends) of long bones in the hand and forearm also indicate advanced development in a physically more mature child. If we analyzed a wrist and hand x-ray of a girl and decided it was closer in appearance to the x-ray in Figure 2.8b than to any other in the set of standards, we would assign the girl a skeletal age of 128 months (10 years, 8 months). If her actual chronological age was 9 years, we would consider her an early maturer; on the other hand, if she was 11-1/2 years old, her skeletal age would indicate she is a late maturer.

The difficulties in assessing skeletal age, aside from technical problems and the accuracy of the person rating the x-ray, include the expense of this method and the doubtful advisability of repeated, unnecessary x-ray exposure. Consequently, wrist and hand x-rays are rarely available to researchers and educators in large numbers. Hand and wrist radiographs of adults are also useful, to measure not the degree of physical maturity but rather the extent of *osteoporosis* (bone loss). We can analyze bone density using the radiograph measurement of the width of the bone cortex, the compact bone surrounding the marrow cavity (Brewer, Meyer, Keele, Upton, & Hagan, 1983; Oyster, Morton, & Linnell, 1984). Hence, hand and wrist radiographs are informative at various times in an individual's life.

### Dental Eruption

Another direct measure assesses maturation by dental eruption (appearance of teeth), but this method is restricted to two age spans: between approximately 6 months and 3 years, when deciduous (baby) teeth first appear, and between approximately 6 and 13 years, when permanent teeth appear. The appearance of both baby and permanent teeth follows a typical order. For early maturers, teeth appear at a younger age than for late maturers.

### Secondary Sex Characteristics

Another simple, straightforward method of maturity assessment rates the appearance of *secondary sex characteristics*: pubic hair and genital development in boys, and pubic hair and breast development in girls. We can assign a rating from 1 to 5 for each measure by comparing an individual's development to standard photographs (Tanner, 1962; Weiner & Lourie, 1981). Axillary and facial hair development also may be rated. As with dental eruption, such ratings are useful only within a specific age period, in this case adolescence.

Direct measures are preferable for assessing maturation, but because they are not always available or applicable for use over wide age spans, we must sometimes infer maturation from an individual's size for chronological age. We should base such an inference on as many anthropometric measures as feasible and be sure to keep the limitations of this method in mind.

## Plotting Growth

Anthropometric measures are often charted in relation to age, as illustrated earlier in Figures 2.2a, 2.2b, 2.3a, and 2.3b.

### The Distance Curve

The curve derived from this process is termed a *distance curve* because the absolute amount, or total accumulation of growth, is represented over regular time intervals, such as months or years. You might think of parents who mark their child's height on a wall chart every birthday. The distance from the floor to the mark increases as the child grows.

Several features of a distance curve are important. One is the rate, or speed, of growth. Where the curve is steep, growth is rapid; where it is relatively flat, growth is slow. Figure 2.9a is a distance curve for height. Note that the curve is particularly steep between 12 and 13 years, but it flattens out between 14 and 16 years. Another feature of the distance curve is the location of inflection points—that is, places where a transition exists from faster to slower growth, or vice versa. An inflection point in the distance curve of Figure 2.9a is at approximately 12.3 years.

## The Velocity Curve

We can highlight the rate of growth and the inflection points of a distance curve by plotting a *velocity curve*. We obtain the velocity curve by plotting the rate of incremental change in growth, rather than accumulated growth, over time. For example, if a person grows 2 cm between ages 11 and 12, a point is plotted at 2 cm on the vertical, or "height gained," axis and at the midpoint of the growth interval, 11.5 years of age, on the horizontal axis. If the child grows 3 cm between ages 12 and 13, another point is plotted at 3 cm on the vertical axis and at 12.5 years on the horizontal axis. We continue the process and connect the points by a smooth curve, the velocity curve. Figure 2.9b is the velocity curve that corresponds to the distance curve in Figure 2.9a. Note that rapid growth is indicated by the portion of the velocity curve high on the graph, and slower growth by the portion of the curve low on the graph. The inflection point of the distance curve is a peak in the velocity curve and is called the *peak velocity*.

## The Acceleration Curve

We can obtain an *acceleration curve* that illustrates the rate of growth change by repeating

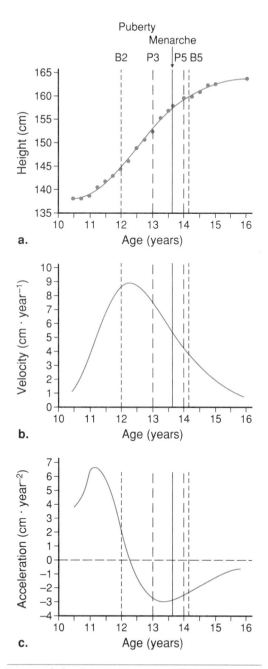

**Figure 2.9** (a) Height attained, (b) height velocity, and (c) height acceleration curves for a girl at adolescence. Note menarche came after peak height velocity. B2 marks beginning of breast development, B5, adult form. P3 marks intermediate stage of pubic hair development, P5, adult form. (Reprinted by permission from Maclaren, 1967.)

# A Longitudinal Study of Belgian Boys

A longitudinal study of adolescent boys living in Belgium (Beunen et al., 1988) is a good example of the type of information that growth measurements can provide. In this study researchers measured approximately 300 boys annually between the ages of 12 and 19 years. The measurements included 16 growth measures and nine motor performance tests. Velocity curves also were plotted from the longitudinal measurements.

These measurements allowed investigators to describe the extent and rate of growth relative to the boys' chronological ages and to examine changes in motor performance relative to age at peak height and peak weight velocity. Among the investigators' findings were the following:

1. The fastest rate of growth occurred between the ages of 14 and 15.
2. Skinfold measurements had a unique pattern of change relative to other growth measurements. Trunk skinfolds increased whereas limb skinfolds decreased during adolescence.
3. Peak velocity in strength motor performance measurements occurred at an age closer to peak weight velocity than to peak height velocity. (This topic also is discussed in chapter 7.)

4. The motor performance tests involving speed of movement revealed that the boys reached their maximum velocities before they experienced their peak height and weight increases.

By measuring both growth and motor performance, the investigators were able to address two often quoted but unproven notions about physical growth. First, no period of adolescent awkwardness or clumsiness occurred. Scores on the motor performance tests increased at every age, even during a spurt in height. Second, the investigators found no evidence that the boys "outgrew" their strength—that is, grew in height without increasing in strength. Strength measures showed improvement throughout the study.

Another important finding of this study pertains to maturation and skill proficiency. Those boys who experienced their adolescent growth spurt at a young age scored better on the motor performance items until the later maturing boys caught up to them in size and strength. Therefore, educators working with children and adolescents should keep in mind that individual differences in maturation rate often influence motor test performance.

the process of plotting change, this time from the velocity curve rather than the distance curve. The acceleration curve, shown in Figure 2.9c, emphasizes the age periods when the rate of change in growth is constant, speeding up, or slowing down.

## REVIEW 2.1

We study physical growth through careful and repeated measurement of body dimensions.

Researchers can easily obtain such growth measures, and standard growth curves can be derived from studies of large numbers of children. We can then measure an individual child and compare the results to the standard range for a given chronological age. Maturation level, the level of qualitative advancement of body tissues, can be inferred from dimensional growth measures with caution. Direct measures of maturation are more desirable but are often impractical.

Growth assessment is a valuable tool for educators. Much of a child's progress in skill development is related to physical size and maturity. Although size and maturity tend to increase with chronological age, they do so at a unique rate for each child. Educators can then more realistically estimate capabilities according to each child's level of physical maturity. This enables them to set realistic expectations and plan physical activities accordingly.

## NORMAL PRENATAL DEVELOPMENT

The growth process begins the instant an ovum (egg) and spermatozoan fuse in fertilization. Early development is astonishingly precise, carried out under the control of genes. Genes, then, determine both the normal aspects of development and inherited abnormal development. At the same time, the growing embryo, and later the fetus, is very sensitive to environmental factors. These include the environment in which the fetus is growing—the amniotic sac in the uterus—and the nutrients delivered to the fetus via the mother's circulation and the placenta. Some environmental factors, such as abnormal external pressure applied to the mother's abdomen or the presence of certain viruses and drugs in the mother's bloodstream, are detrimental to the fetus. Other factors, such as delivery of all the proper nutrients, enhance the fetus's growth.

Environmental factors can positively or negatively affect growth and maturation.

Ideally, growth and development proceed normally in an environment that maximizes genetic potential. It is possible, however, for the fetus to develop anomalies or be exposed to detrimental environmental influences. This can affect the potential to function normally in life and participate fully in a wide range of physical activities; factors that affect prenatal growth might later affect skill potential. Thus, to completely understand the active individual, we must first completely understand the normal developmental process. Beyond this, knowing the environmental conditions that can affect growth and development and knowing how they do so is also valuable. Moving, active individuals are products of their genetic inheritance and the environmental factors present throughout their development. With such knowledge, we can reduce risks to growing individuals and prescribe appropriate activities for those whose potential for physical performance may be limited by genetic or environmental factors. These two aspects of prenatal growth—the normal process of development and the environmental factors influencing it—are discussed next.

> **CONCEPT 2.2**
> Both genetic and environmental factors influence normal embryonic and fetal growth.

## Embryonic Development

Development begins with the fusion of two sex cells, an ovum from the female and a spermatozoan from the male. But how is the genetic inheritance of the new individual determined?

### Formation of Sex Cells

The genetic information that determines hair and eye color, height potential, skeletal structure, and many other characteristics is contained in genes in the form of DNA (deoxyribonucleic acid) molecules. The genes are located on chromosomes, filament-like bodies within the cell's nucleus. Human beings have 23 pairs of chromosomes in all of their cells, except for the sex cells, when they are formed. The sex cells are specialized cells formed by a type of cell-reduction division termed *meiosis*. In meiosis, each sex cell divides into two "daughter" sex cells, and only one chromosome from each of the 23 pairs migrates to each daughter cell. Which one of the pair a daughter cell receives is a matter of chance; thus, there is a great deal of variability possible in the offspring of any set of parents. When an ovum and spermatozoan unite in fertilization, each donates the "chance" set of 23 chromosomes, reestablishing the total of 46 chromosomes (23 pairs). When we understand that each human chromosome has 30,000 or more pairs of genes, it is no wonder that each human being is unique!

## Cell Growth and Differentiation

The genes also direct the continuous development of the embryo in a precise and predictable pattern. The fertilized egg, or zygote, divides into two cells, then four, then eight, and so on, all by mitotic cell division (*mitosis*). In mitotic division, the dividing cell passes the complete set of 46 chromosomes to each of its daughter cells. After about 4 days, the cell mass is transformed into a sphere termed a blastocyst (see Figures 2.10 and 2.11). By this time, the blastocyst contains about 60 cells, 5 of which form the inner cell mass. It implants itself in the uterus when it is about 5 to 6 days old.

The inner cell mass forms three layers of tissues through continued cell division and through the migration (movement) of cells to a new location. These three tissues—the ectoderm, the endoderm, and the mesoderm—give rise to all the various tissues and organs of the body. The ectoderm layer eventually becomes skin, tooth enamel, the nervous system, parts of different glands, and parts of the sensory receptors. The endoderm is the origin of the epithelial linings (avascular cellular layers) of many structures such as the auditory tube, larynx, urinary bladder, urethra, and prostate. The remaining body tissues and organs originate from the mesoderm. These include muscles, the blood, all connective tissues, the teeth, the

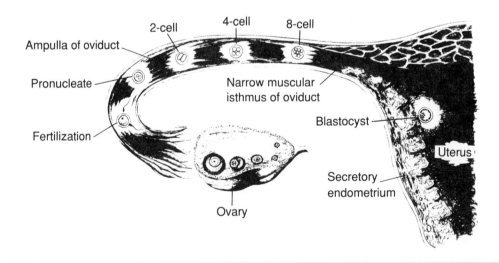

**Figure 2.10** Movement of a human embryo through the oviduct and its implantation in the uterus. (Reprinted by permission from Edwards, 1981.)

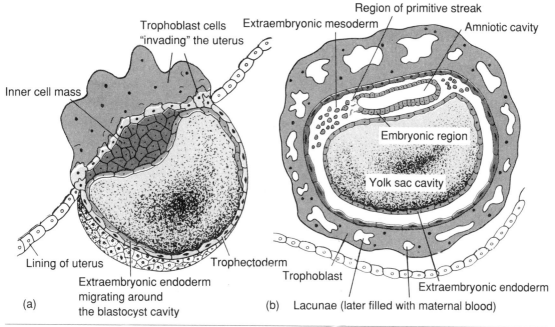

Trophoblast cells "invading" the uterus

Region of primitive streak

Extraembryonic mesoderm

Amniotic cavity

Inner cell mass

Embryonic region

Yolk sac cavity

Lining of uterus

Trophectoderm

Extraembryonic endoderm migrating around the blastocyst cavity

Trophoblast

Extraembryonic endoderm

(a)

(b)    Lacunae (later filled with maternal blood)

**Figure 2.11**    Diagrams of human embryos: (a) 9 days after fertilization, (b) 12 days after fertilization. The embryo by this time is embedded in the uterus. (Reprinted by permission from Edwards, 1981.)

adrenal cortex, and the skeleton (Timiras, 1972). The process whereby cells become specialized and form specific tissues and organs is called *differentiation*.

In general, the cells differentiate into the various body organs and form the human shape during the first 8 weeks after conception.

Formation of the tissues and organs proceeds in a predictable time line, summarized in Table 2.1. The limbs are roughly formed and the heartbeat begins at 4 weeks. The eyes, ears, nose, mouth, fingers, and toes are formed at approximately 8 weeks. During this time, the organism is an embryo, and this period (weeks 2 through 8) is termed the embryonic stage.

## Fetal Development

The period following the embryonic stage, the fetal stage, is characterized by further growth and cell differentiation of the fetus, leading to functional capacity. This continued growth of the organs and tissues occurs in two ways: by *hyperplasia*, an increase in the absolute number of cells, such as in blood, bone, or liver tissue; and by *hypertrophy*, an increase in the relative size of each individual cell, such as in the brain or lungs. If you examine the landmarks of growth carefully, you also see that growth tends to proceed in two directions. One direction is *cephalocaudal* (head to tail), meaning that the head and facial structures grow fastest, then the upper body, followed by the relatively slow-growing lower body. At the same time, growth is *proximodistal* (near to far) in direction, meaning the trunk tends to advance, then the

**Table 2.1  Landmarks in Embryonic and Fetal Growth**

| Age (wks) | Length | Weight | Appearance | Internal development |
|---|---|---|---|---|
| 3 | 3 mm | | Head, tail folds formed | Optic vesicles, head recognizable |
| 4 | 4 mm | 0.4 g | Limb rudiments formed | Heartbeat begins, organs recognizable |
| 8 | 3.5 cm | 2 g | Eyes, ears, nose, mouth, digits formed | Sensory organs developing, some bone ossification beginning |
| 12 | 11.5 cm | 19 g | Sex externally recognizable, head very large for body | Brain configuration nearly complete, blood forming in bone marrow |
| 16 | 19 cm | 100 g | Motor activity; scalp hair present; trunk size gaining on head size | Heart muscle developed; sense organs formed |
| 20 | 22 cm | 300 g | Legs have grown appreciably | Myelination of spinal cord begins |
| 24 | 32 cm | 600 g | Respiratory-like movements begin | Cerebral cortex layers formed |
| 28 | 36 cm | 1,100 g | Increasing fat tissue development | Retina layered and light-receptive; cerebral convolutions appearing |
| 32 | 41 cm | 1,800 g | Weight increasing more than length | Taste sense operative |
| 36 | 46 cm | 2,200 g | Body more rounded | Ossification begins in distal femur |
| 40 | 52 cm | 3,200 g | Skin smooth and pink, at least moderate head hair | Proximal tibia begins ossification; myelination of brain begins; pulmonary branching 2/3 complete |

Adapted by permission from Timiras, 1972.

nearest parts of the limbs, and finally the distal parts of the limbs.

Although cells differentiate during growth to perform a specialized function, some cells have an amazing quality termed *plasticity*, the capability to take on a new function. If some of the cells in a system are injured, for example, the remaining cells might be stimulated to perform the role the damaged cells ordinarily carry out. The cells of the central nervous system have a high degree of plasticity, and their structure, chemistry, and function can be modified pre- and postnatally (Timiras, 1972).

## Environmental Factors and Prenatal Growth

Many characteristics of the fetal environment have the potential to affect growth, either posi-

tively or negatively. The nourishment system is the environmental factor that has the most impact on fetal development; thus it is helpful to know how the fetus is nourished.

### Fetal Nourishment

The structure involved in fetal nourishment is the placenta, a network of blood capillaries that is formed early in development from a part of the embryo's outer membrane and some maternal tissue. The placenta actually consists of two parallel "plates" separated by a maternal blood-filled space (see Figure 2.12). Villi (vascular fingerlike projections) extend into the space, thereby increasing the surface area for fetal-maternal exchanges. Fetal blood flows through the umbilical cord to capillaries within the villi. Maternal blood is brought to the placenta by an artery and fills the space around

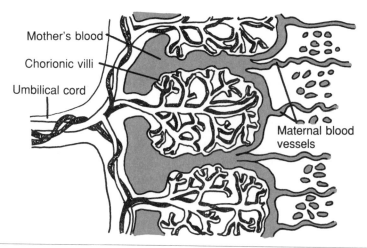

**Figure 2.12** A diagram of the placenta showing the two circulations (mother and fetus), which are intimate but never mingle.
(Reprinted by permission from Rhodes, 1969.)

the villi. Respiratory and nutritive exchanges take place via diffusion between fetal blood in the capillaries and maternal blood in the space without the direct mixing of the two blood supplies. One of the most important exchanges is that of oxygen to the fetus and carbon dioxide to the mother for elimination by her respiratory system. Nutrients transferred to the fetus via the placenta include the following:

- Proteins
- Amino acids
- Polypeptides
- Carbohydrates
- Water
- Inorganic ions (sodium, potassium, iron, etc.)
- Vitamins

Excretory by-products of fetal metabolism are removed from the fetus by this process as well.

## Maternal Health Status

Among the demands pregnancy places on a woman are

- increased energy requirements,
- increased nutrient requirements,
- greater oxygen consumption, and
- increased cardiorespiratory function (Malina & Bouchard, 1991).

The growing fetus needs energy, nutrients, and oxygen. If these are in short supply, mother and fetus compete for limited resources, possibly compromising the needs of the fetus.

Women at lower socioeconomic levels typically give birth to lighter infants than do women from higher socioeconomic levels. This is significant because low-birth-weight infants are at greater risk of disease, infection, and death in the weeks after birth than are normal-weight infants. Though birth weight is certainly related to both maternal and fetal nutrition, it is likely that overall maternal health status also plays a role in assuring normal prenatal development. A woman living in better conditions and receiving early prenatal health care is more likely than a woman living in poorer conditions to meet the oxygen, energy, and nutrient needs of the fetus. She is also more likely to be at lower risk for illnesses and infections that might compromise the needs of the fetus.

**REVIEW 2.2**

Fertilization begins a process of growth and development that is affected by both genetics and the environment. Early in embryonic life the pattern and timing of organ and tissue formation are remarkably precise and predictable. Functional capacity is achieved during the fetal stage. Cells of the organs and tissues grow by hyperplasia and hypertrophy. The upper and central parts of the body grow faster than the lower body and limbs. This gives the fetus its characteristic form, a large head and shoulders but small hips and limbs. Although the genes direct this orderly and precise course of development, environmental factors can affect growth and development. The chief mode of environmental influence is the nourishment that the placenta delivers. Respiratory, nutritive, and excretory exchanges take place here through diffusion between the maternal and fetal bloodstreams. A fetus that receives appropriate levels of oxygen and nutrients has the best chance of reaching its full genetic potential. Unfortunately, harmful substances also can reach the fetus through the nourishment system. Next we will consider those factors that might cause abnormal development during the prenatal period.

## ABNORMAL PRENATAL DEVELOPMENT

Normal prenatal growth occurs in a predictable pattern and on a predictable time line, under genetic control. But the growth of some individuals does not proceed normally. Abnormal growth may arise from either genetic or environmental factors. Genetic abnormalities are inherited and can be immediately apparent or can remain undetected until well into postnatal growth. A host of environmental factors also can negatively affect the fetus. A few examples include drugs and chemicals in the mother's bloodstream, viruses in the mother's bloodstream, and excessive pressure applied to the

mother's abdomen. Anomalies or defects present at birth are termed *congenital* whether their causes are genetic or environmental. Let's consider some examples of congenital defects in more detail.

---

**CONCEPT 2.3**
Abnormal prenatal development can result from either genetic or environmental factors.

---

## Genetic Causes of Abnormal Prenatal Development

An individual may inherit genetic abnormalities as dominant or recessive (including sex-linked) disorders. Dominant disorders result when one parent passes on a defective gene. Recessive disorders occur in children who inherit a defective gene from each parent.

### Dominant Disorders

*Dominant disorders* are so named because carriers have one normal copy of the involved gene and one abnormal copy. The defective gene dominates or overrides the normal gene. Children of an affected parent have a 50% chance of inheriting the defective gene. Examples of dominant disorders include hereditary multiple exostosis (formation of a tumor on a bony surface) and sickle-cell anemia.

### Recessive Disorders

A *recessive disorder* occurs when a child receives a defective gene from each parent. The parents carry the defective gene along with a normal gene and are unaffected because the defective gene is recessive and thus is masked by the normal gene. Children who inherit a normal gene from each parent or a normal gene from one parent but a defective gene from the other parent are unaffected, although the latter continue to be carriers. Approximately one in four children inherit a defective gene from each parent and are consequently affected. An example of a recessive disorder is phenylketonuria (PKU), a condition in which phenylketonuric acid may accumulate, damaging the nervous system and resulting in mental retardation. Another recessive disorder is Down syndrome (trisomy 21), in which three chromosomes rather than two are present in one chromosome "pair," giving the individual a total of 47. Characteristics of Down syndrome include mental retardation, cardiac abnormalities, and short stature. Cystic fibrosis also is a recessive disorder.

## Sex-Linked Recessive Disorders

*Sex-linked disorders* involve a defective gene on the X chromosome. Women have two X chromosomes, and men have one X and one Y chromosome. Children receiving an X chromosome from each parent are female, whereas those receiving an X chromosome from their mother and a Y chromosome from their father are male. Approximately one in four children inherits a defective gene on the X chromosome. Hence, these disorders are termed *sex-linked* or *X-linked*. Girls with the defective gene are unaffected carriers because this recessive gene is dominated by their other, normal gene. Boys are affected because they do not have another dominant, normal X chromosome but instead have a Y chromosome. Examples of sex-linked disorders are color blindness and some forms of muscular dystrophy.

## Mutations

Genetic abnormalities also can result from a new *mutation*, the alteration or deletion of a gene during formation of the egg or sperm cell. Researchers suspect irradiation and certain hazardous environmental chemicals of causing genetic mutations, and the potential for genetic damage to sex cells increases with advancing maternal and paternal age (Nyhan, 1990). Mutations also can occur spontaneously, without cause. A spontaneous mutation is most likely the cause of a genetic disorder in a child born to a family without a history of that disorder.

## Variability of Genetic Disorders

Both new mutations and inherited disorders can result in single or multiple malformations of an organ, limb, or body region; deformations of a body part; or disruptions in development resulting from the breakdown of normal tissue. Many of these abnormalities are obvious at birth, but some do not appear until later. An infant with Tay-Sachs disease appears normal through the first several months after birth but by 1 or 2 years of age is blind and without cerebral function. From these examples you can see that genetic abnormalities vary considerably in both appearance and severity.

# Environmental Causes of Abnormal Prenatal Development

Our earlier discussion of fetal nourishment revealed how dependent the fetus is upon the mother for the oxygen and nutrients it needs. Unfortunately, fetal nourishment can also deliver harmful substances to the fetus. In addition, a variety of factors can potentially affect the fetus's physical environment and thereby its growth and development.

---

It is important to understand how environmental factors affect a fetus. Congenital disorders arising from environmental factors can affect the potential for postnatal growth and development. Moreover, when medical professionals are aware of negative influences, they can manage these influences to minimize the risk to the fetus.

---

## Teratogens

In addition to oxygen and nutrients necessary for fetal life and growth, other substances can diffuse across the placenta. Among these are viruses, drugs, and chemicals. Sometimes, either too much or too little of the necessary vitamins, nutrients, and hormones are delivered to the fetus through the placenta. Some of these substances act as malformation-producing agents, or *teratogens*. You can find a partial list of the known teratogens and their possible effects on growth and development in Table 2.2. The specific effect a teratogen has on the fetus depends on the stage of fetal development when the substance is introduced as well as the amount of the substance.

**Table 2.2  A Partial List of Teratogens and Their Possible Effects**

| Teratogen | Possible effect on fetus |
| --- | --- |
| Nutritional deficiencies Vitamin A, vitamin E, riboflavin, fatty acids, glucose | General influence on all aspects of growth and development, including low birth weight; possible effect on placental function; possible malformations |
| Hypervitaminosis Excess vitamin D | Cardiac defects, mental retardation, sensory abnormalities |
| Drugs Cocaine/Alkaloid (crack) cocaine | Retarded growth, increased irritability, muscular rigidity, increased risk of sudden infant death |
| Retinoic acid (to treat acne) | Facial abnormalities, ear deformations, central nervous system damage, cardiovascular anomalies |
| Morphine/heroine addiction | Addiction in infant |

| Teratogen | Possible effect on fetus |
| --- | --- |
| Barbiturates | Depression of central nervous system |
| Antibiotics | Sensory disorders, deafness |
| Tetracycline | Impaired growth |
| Antithyroid medications | Thyroid gland enlargement, mental retardation |
| Alcohol | Fetal alcohol syndrome; in extreme alcoholism, low birth weight, suppressed growth, mental retardation, physical deformities |
| Thalidomide | Various malformations (limbs, heart, viscera) |
| LSD | Chromosomal damage |
| Nicotine/heavy smoking | Growth retardation, low birth weight, spontaneous abortion, premature birth |
| Infections Human immunodeficiency virus (HIV) | Heights, weights, and head circumferences below third percentile, head and facial abnormalities |
| Rubella | Cardiac defects, impaired growth, mental retardation, cataracts, deafness |
| Cytomegalic inclusion disease | Mental retardation, microcephaly |
| Excess hormones Androgens | Masculinization of female fetus |
| ACTN | Cleft palate |
| Hormonal deficiencies Alloxan diabetes | Suppressed growth |

Data from Timiras, 1972.

Any tissues undergoing rapid development when a teratogen is introduced are especially susceptible to malformation. The fetus is particularly vulnerable in the early stages of development (the first 16 weeks) when organs and limbs are forming. Some teratogens have specific actions on certain tissues or cells, affecting one kind of tissue at a certain stage of development and another tissue at another time. In other words, there are critical periods, periods of particular vulnerability to change, for the growth and development of tissues and organs. For example, the rubella virus is harmful if the embryo is exposed to it during the first 4 weeks of pregnancy. The earlier the infection, the more serious the resulting abnormalities. Very early exposure can result in miscarriage. Other possible abnormalities are listed in Table 2.2. Some, like deafness, occur more frequently than others.

Some malformation-producing or growth-retarding conditions arise because a nutrient is delivered to the embryo or fetus through the placenta in an insufficient amount. Other abnormal conditions arise if too much of a substance is present. Vitamins are an excellent example. Note in Table 2.2 the effects of a deficiency of vitamin A and an excess of vitamin D.

Still other congenital defects result from the mere presence of a harmful substance in the maternal blood. Whether the fetus is exposed depends on the size of the substance. For example, small virus particles, such as rubella, present in maternal blood can cross the placenta and harm the fetus. Human immunodeficiency virus (HIV), the causative agent in acquired immunodeficiency syndrome (AIDS), also can infect a fetus, resulting in an infant who is HIV positive. Fetal exposure to HIV can also cause growth retardation, short stature, and facial abnormalities (Nyhan, 1990). Drugs with molecular weights under 1,000 cross the placenta easily whereas those with molecular weights over 1,000 do not.

The drug thalidomide was tested extensively on adult animals and humans. It caused no toxic effects and was subsequently sold without prescription as a sleeping pill, tranquilizer, and sedative. After statistics revealed that many women who used thalidomide gave birth to infants with limb deformities, the medical community realized that this drug diffused across the placenta and acted as a teratogen, especially if the mother ingested it, even in small doses, between the 27th and 33rd days after conception. If the drug was taken early in this period, ear defects were most likely; if taken midway through, arm defects; and if taken late in this period, leg defects. After the thalidomide experience, medical personnel recognized more and more that they could not extrapolate adult data safely to the fetus (Timaras, 1972). Teratogens often have little or no effect on the mother. For this reason, they have been difficult to identify and, therefore, difficult to guard against.

Although government agencies can regulate prescription drugs, some harmful drugs are available illegally. Crack cocaine is a particular concern. Many fetuses are exposed to this drug through its presence in their mothers' blood streams. Fetal exposure results in infants who are born addicted and at higher risk of sudden infant death. Years later, these children have difficulty learning in school, in part because of attentional deficits.

In contrast to illegal drugs, some harmful substances are sold legally and are widely used in society. As seen in Table 2.2, alcohol and nicotine can affect a fetus. Today, product labels often contain warnings about use during pregnancy, but abstaining is difficult for women who are habitual consumers.

A mother can maximize fetal growth and development by avoiding substances that might be teratogenic and maintaining a diet that supplies adequate but not excessive nutrients. Otherwise, the fetus might develop a specific malformation or be generally retarded in growth and small for age at birth. It is important to recognize that these conditions, including low birth weight, can affect postnatal growth and development.

## Other Prenatal Environmental Factors

Malformation, retarded growth, or life-threatening conditions can also result from external factors affecting the fetus's environment. Examples include

1. external or internal pressure on the infant, including pressure from another fetus in utero;
2. extreme internal environmental temperature, as when the mother suffers from high fever or hypothermia;
3. exposure to x-rays or gamma rays;
4. changes in atmospheric pressure, especially those leading to *hypoxia* (oxygen deficiency) in the fetus; and
5. environmental pollutants.

The precise effects of these factors also depend upon the fetus's stage of development. Like teratogens, external factors have the potential to affect both present and future growth and development.

---

### REVIEW 2.3

Prenatal abnormalities can arise from two sources—genetic inheritance and environmental factors. Some abnormal conditions are a product of both genetic inheritance and the environment; that is, a tendency for a disease might be inherited, and subsequently the disease will appear only under certain environmental conditions (Timiras, 1972). A healthy environment maximizes the fetus's chance of reaching its full genetic potential. Individuals involved in taking care of the fetus can attempt to control environmental factors known to influence fetal growth and development. A proper diet is important, as is avoiding illness, smoking, alcohol, and harmful drugs.

We should view physical growth and development, then, as a continuous process that begins at conception. Individuals are, in part, products of the factors that affected their prenatal growth and development. Either the fetus has grown in an environment that maximizes its chances of survival and of reaching full growth, or it may already have been harmed or placed at risk during birth and the days thereafter. Next on the growth continuum, birth and postnatal growth and development are examined.

# NORMAL POSTNATAL DEVELOPMENT

Is an 11-year-old capable of long-distance runs? How about a 60-year-old? Of course, no one answer applies to all 11-year-olds or all 60-year-olds. Educators often need to evaluate an individual's status and potential to help him or her set reasonable personal goals. As discussed in concept 2.1, this evaluation includes assessing physical maturity. It is important that educators be aware of the average pattern of postnatal growth and the typical pattern of aging in adults. They must be able to compare an individual with the average and adjust expectations for performance accordingly. Educators must also know the growth rates and maturation patterns of various body tissues and systems.

- Does one system advance more slowly than the others and delay the onset of a behavior?
- Does muscle growth keep pace with whole-body growth?
- Do the muscles and skeletal framework maintain their young-adult levels of strength with aging?
- Does the musculoskeletal system weaken and cause a decline in performance?

To plan appropriate activities, educators must recognize when the different body systems are changing.

> **CONCEPT 2.4**
>
> Postnatal growth proceeds in precise and orderly patterns that differ among the body systems.

## Overall Growth

Body growth after birth is a continuation of prenatal growth. The growth pattern is predictable and consistent but not linear, no matter which measure of overall growth we choose to study. For example, look back at the growth curves for height and weight in Figures 2.2 and 2.3. They are characterized by rapid growth after birth, followed by gradual but steady growth, rapid growth during early adolescence, and then a leveling off. Thus, the curves are roughly *s-shaped*. We call this pattern of overall body growth a *sigmoid curve*, after the Greek letter for *s*. Although a normal growth curve is always sigmoid, the timing of a particular individual's spurts and steady growth periods is likely to vary from the average. For example, one girl might begin her adolescent growth spurt at 8 years, whereas another might begin hers at 10. Note that the range of variation, the gap between the 5th and 95th percentiles, widens with age, especially for weight (Malina & Bouchard, 1991).

---

Individual variability is increasingly obvious with advancing age.

---

## Gender

Gender is a major factor in the timing as well as the extent of growth. Gender differences are minimal in early childhood, with boys being very slightly taller and heavier. Throughout childhood, though, girls tend to mature at a faster rate than boys so that at any given age, girls as a group are biologically more mature than boys. Important gender differences in growth and development are especially pronounced at adolescence. Girls begin their adolescent growth spurt when they are about 9 years old (often termed the *age at takeoff*), whereas boys begin theirs at about 11. Note that these ages are group averages. About two thirds of all adolescents will initiate their growth spurts during the year before or the year after these averages.

### Height

On the average, girls reach their peak height velocity at 11.5 to 12.0 years (see Figure 2.13).

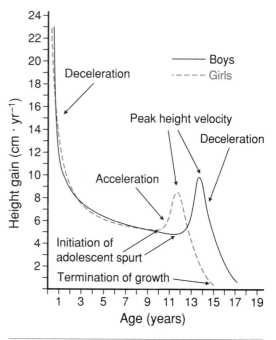

**Figure 2.13**  Velocity curves for height of British boys and girls in the 1960s. Note the age at takeoff of the growth spurt in height and the peak height velocity. These ages and the peak height velocities are slightly different for this sample than for the population averages discussed in the text, but the shape of the velocity curves is the same. (Reprinted by permission from Tanner, Whitehouse, & Takaishi, 1966.)

Their growth in height then tapers off at approximately age 14, with notable increases in height ending around age 16. Boys reach their peak height velocity at 13.5 to 14.0 years; this velocity is somewhat faster than that of girls—approximately 9 cm/yr for boys compared to 8 cm/yr for girls (Beunen & Malina, 1988). Boys' growth tapers off at 17 years, with notable increases ending by age 18. Note that males have about 2 more years of growth than females, amounting to 10 to 13 cm of height. This longer growth period accounts for much of the average absolute height difference between adult men and women.

Both men and women grow slightly in height into their 20s. Trunk length may even increase very slightly into the mid-40s. Aside from these small increases, height is stable through adulthood. It is common for an individual's stature to decrease slightly in older adulthood. Some of this decrease is due to the compression and flattening of the body's connective tissues, especially the cartilage pads between the vertebrae in the spinal column. The result is a compression of the spinal column and a decrease in trunk length. The bones also lose density as a result of progressive modifications in the protein matrix of the skeleton (Timiras, 1972). This breakdown is more severe in persons with osteoporosis and can result in the collapse of one or more vertebrae. If this occurs, the loss of stature is pronounced (see Figure 2.14).

### Weight

Peak weight velocity follows peak height velocity in adolescents by 2.5 to 5.0 months in boys and 3.5 to 10.5 months in girls. Sometimes, the growth of various segment lengths and breadths reach peak velocity before the individual reaches peak height velocity and sometimes after, but all reach their peak before or at peak weight velocity (Beunen et al., 1988).

Adults typically start gaining weight in their early 20s. This is related to changes in lifestyle. Young adults who begin careers and families

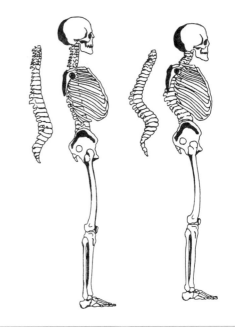

**Figure 2.14** Loss of height in those with osteoporosis can be pronounced. Compression fractures of the vertebrae lead to kyphosis (dowager's hump) and pressure on the viscera, causing in turn abdominal distension.
(Reprinted by permission from Aloia, 1989.)

commonly take less time to exercise and prepare healthy meals. In contrast, adults who exercise regularly and eat wisely often maintain their weight or even gain muscle and lose fat. Older adults sometimes lose weight, probably the result of inactivity and a consequent loss of muscle tissue. Loss of appetite accompanying lifestyle changes also can be factor. Again, active older adults are not as likely to lose muscle weight.

### Secondary Sex Characteristics

During the adolescent growth spurt, secondary sex characteristics appear. In girls, the breasts enlarge; pubic hair appears; and menarche, the first menstrual cycle, occurs. Regardless of the exact chronological age when a girl begins her growth spurt, menarche typically follows the peak height velocity by 11 to 12 months (see Figure 2.9). The average age of menarche therefore is 12.5 to 13.0 years. In boys, the testes and scrotum grow in size, and pubic hair appears. Boys have no landmark comparable to girls' menarche for puberty; the production of viable sperm is a gradual process.

## Environmental Factors and Postnatal Growth

Genetics control the timing and rate of an individual's growth, but environmental factors also can have a great impact, especially those influencing body metabolism. During the periods when the most rapid growth occurs—just after birth and in early adolescence—growth is particularly sensitive to alteration by environmental factors. The phenomenon of *catch-up growth* illustrates the susceptibility of body growth to environmental influence. A child might experience catch-up growth after suffering a period of severe malnutrition or a bout with a severe disorder such as chronic renal failure. During such a period, body growth is retarded. After the diet is improved or the child recovers from the disorder (i.e., a positive environment for growth is restored), growth rate increases until the child approaches or catches up to what otherwise would have been the extent of growth during that period (Prader, Tanner, & von Harnack, 1963) (see Figure 2.15). Whether the child recovers some or all of the growth depends on the timing, duration, and severity of the negative environmental condition.

Another example of environmental influence is the suggestion that a girl must attain a critical body weight before menarche can occur (Frisch, 1972). Though this proposal is unproven, if a relationship between age at menarche and critical body weight exists, environmental factors such as nutrition might influence menarche. Girls who are anorexic and consequently underweight, or young female athletes,

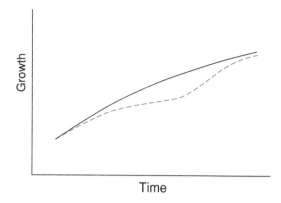

**Figure 2.15** A hypothetical illustration of catch-up growth. The solid line represents the course of normal growth, the dotted line actual growth. A negative environmental influence can cause a retardation of growth compared to the "normal" course growth would have taken. If the negative factor is removed, catch-up growth might occur to restore eventual growth to its normal or near-normal level.

such as gymnasts or dancers, who train strenuously and eat little, might experience delayed menarche.

## Regular Growth Assessment

A regular program of assessing children's growth and comparing the results with average values can help detect abnormal growth. Medical or environmental factors influencing abnormal growth can then be identified and corrected. Of course, such growth measures reflect the individual's genetic potential for height and body build (which often correspond to the parents' height and build) as well as the individual's personal growth timing. Children and teens who measure above the 90th or below the 10th percentile for their age, especially those whose parents are not exceptionally tall or short, respectively, should be referred to medical personnel for examination (Lowrey, 1973). Children also tend to maintain their relative position in comparison to height percentiles after they are 2 or 3 years old; that is, a 3-year-old child in the 75th percentile for height is most likely to measure around the 75th percentile throughout childhood. A large fluctuation in relative position could indicate that some environmental factor is influencing growth (Martorell, Malina, Castillo, Mendoza, & Pawson, 1988), and medical examination is warranted.

Teachers are in a particularly good position to regularly assess children's height and weight. Besides detecting possible growth problems, they can use height and weight data to teach children basic concepts about hereditary and environmental influences. Children who learn about the growth process can feel less anxiety about body size, especially regarding differences in maturation rates. For example, a late-maturing 13-year-old boy could be 20 cm (approximately 8 in.) shorter than his friends who are early maturers, and he may not yet possess any of the secondary sex characteristics such as a deepened voice. Without knowing what normal growth encompasses, the late maturer may feel inadequate or inferior.

Teachers can make children aware of the changes their bodies will likely undergo and help them set reasonable goals for their physical activities as they approach adulthood.

## Relative Growth

Although the body as a whole consistently follows the sigmoid growth pattern, specific body parts, tissues, and organs have differential rates of growth. In other words, each part of the growing individual has its own precise and orderly growth rate. These differential growth rates can result in notable changes in the body's appearance as a whole. Observe how the proportions illustrated in Figure 2.16 change dramatically throughout life. The head is one fourth of the total height at birth but only one eighth of adult height. The legs are about three eighths of the height at birth but almost half of adult height. Body proportions at birth reflect the cephalocaudal (head to tail) and proximodistal (near to far) directions of prenatal growth.

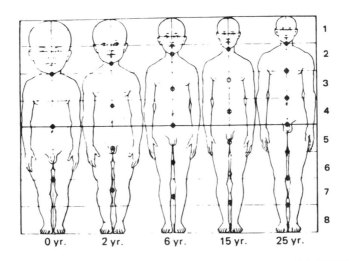

0 yr.     2 yr.     6 yr.     15 yr.     25 yr.

**Figure 2.16** Postnatal body proportion changes. (Reprinted by permission from Timiras, 1972.)

Therefore, the newborn has a form quite different from that of an adult.

When individuals are very young, body form might have implications for skill performance. For example, even if 5-month-old infants were neurologically ready to coordinate and control the walking pattern, it is unlikely that they could balance their top-heavy bodies on such thin, short legs and small feet. Note in Figure 2.16 that a 6-year-old still does not have adult form, although the differences are less dramatic. Form differences may possibly account for some of the differences between the skill performances of adults and children. Varying limb lengths and weights can affect balance, momentum, and potential speed in ballistic skills such as throwing. No researchers, however, have quantified a performance difference attributable to the proportional differences in form in children (Haywood & Patryla, 1978).

For an individual to achieve adult proportions, some body parts must grow faster than others during postnatal growth. For example, the legs grow faster than the trunk in infancy and childhood, and they undergo a growth spurt early in adolescence. Growth in height results mostly from an increase in trunk length during late adolescence and early adulthood. Boys and girls have similar proportions in childhood, but by the time they are adults, relative growth of some body areas brings about noticeable differences between the sexes. In girls, biacromial and biiliac breadth increase at about the same rate, so their biacromial/biiliac ratio is fairly stable during growth. Boys undergo a substantial increase in biacromial breadth during their growth spurt, so their ratio changes as they move into adolescence.

Specific tissues and organs also grow differentially. Although their prenatal growth tends to follow the increase in body weight, the postnatal growth of some tissues and systems follows unique patterns, as we see in Figure 2.17. Compare the growth of the systems graphed in Figure 2.17 with the s-shaped curve for body weight, including splanchnic (internal organ) weight. The brain, for example, achieves over 80% of its adult weight by the time the individual reaches age 4, but the weight of the suprarenal glands is minimal until it increases rapidly during the individual's teenage years. The thymus, a gland of the lymphatic system located within the thorax, grows rapidly in childhood, then decreases in relative size during late adolescence. It then involutes and is gradually replaced by adipose tissue in adults. Because various tissues of the body grow differentially after birth, we can best examine postnatal growth by considering the body systems individually.

---

*In planning vigorous activities for children, it is important to know if some systems, such as the skeletal or circulatory system, keep pace with whole-body growth.*

---

In understanding how and when children acquire certain skills and movement patterns, it is helpful to know if one system's advancement triggers changes in movement patterns. A discussion of the normal pattern of growth in individual systems—skeletal, muscular, adipose, endocrine, and nervous—is in order before we can deal with the environmental influences that can alter this growth.

## The Skeletal System

Early in embryonic life the skeletal system exists as a ''cartilage model'' of the bones. At the fetal age of 2 months, *primary ossification centers* appear in the midportions of the long bones such as the humerus (upper arm) and femur (thigh) and begin to form bone cells (see Figure 2.18). The bone shafts ossify outward in both directions from these primary centers until the entire shafts are ossified at birth. Thereafter, postnatal bone growth in length

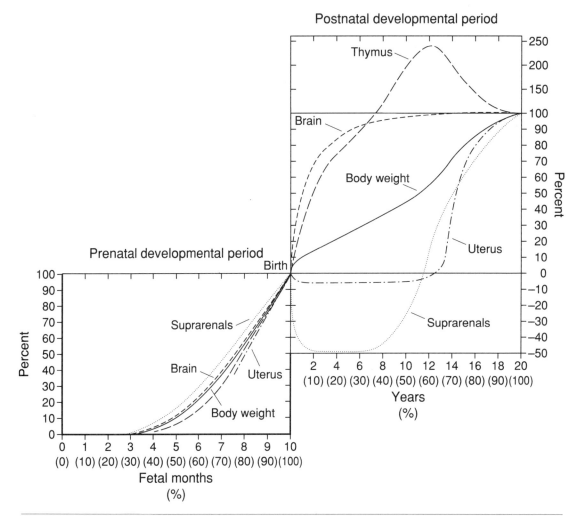

**Figure 2.17** Growth in weight of the body and selected tissues during prenatal and postnatal growth. The ordinate indicates size attained in percentage of final weight (100%). (Reprinted by permission from Timiras, 1972.)

occurs at a *secondary ossification center* at each end of the shaft, termed the *epiphyseal plate*, growth plate, or pressure epiphysis (see Figure 2.19).

The epiphyseal plate has many cellular layers, as seen in Figure 2.20. The outermost layer is the zone of resting cells, which serves as a reservoir for future cartilage cells and is nourished by a blood supply from the epiphysis

(end of the bone). In the next layer, the proliferative zone, cartilage cells increase in size, forming an extracellular cartilage matrix. In the adjoining layer, or hypertrophic zone, cartilage cells arrange themselves in vertical columns. In the calcified cartilage zone, cartilage cells erode, and bone is deposited by osteoblasts (cells engaged in making new bone) on the walls of cavities in the cartilage. Bone is thus laid

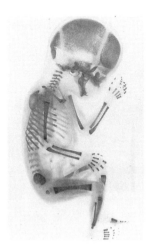

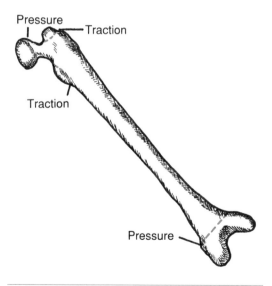

Pressure

Traction

Traction

Pressure

**Figure 2.19** The pressure epiphyses are located at the ends of long bones, such as the femur (thigh bone) pictured here. Epiphyses also occur at muscle tendon attachment sites, called traction epiphyses.

down at the epiphyseal plates. This process depends on nourishment through the blood supply, shown as the capillary invasion zone in Figure 2.20. Small round bones, like those in the wrist, ossify from the center outward.

At birth, about 400 ossification centers exist. Another 400 appear after birth. The various centers appear at earlier chronological ages in girls than in boys. Growth at the ossification centers ceases at different times in various bones. At the epiphyseal plates, the cartilage zone eventually disappears, and the shaft, or *diaphysis*, of the bone fuses with the epiphysis; this, too, usually occurs at a younger age in girls than in boys. For example, epiphyseal union at the head of the humerus occurs in girls at 15.5 years but in boys at 18.1 years, on the average (Hansman, 1962). Once the epiphyseal plates of a long bone fuse, the length of the bone is fixed. Almost all epiphyseal plates are closed by age 18 or 19.

Though the long bones are growing in length, they also increase in girth, a process called *appositional growth*. This is achieved by the addition of new tissue layers under the periosteum, a very thin outer covering of the bone, much like a tree adds to its girth under its bark. The shaft of a long bone is narrower than the ends. Therefore, the bone must be reshaped as it grows in length through a resorption process in the metaphyseal region between the diaphysis (shaft) and epiphysis (see Figure 2.20).

As discussed earlier, we can use this process of bone growth to assess skeletal age. The appearance of various ossification centers and later of epiphyseal union can indicate how an individual's skeletal development compares to the average rate of development. Skeletal age can easily be a year or more ahead of or behind chronological age, meaning that within a group of children who are the same chronological age, skeletal maturation could vary by 3 years or more. This certainly emphasizes the need to assess children's physical maturity individually.

Because linear growth is almost completely the result of skeletal growth, measures of stature reflect the linear growth of bone. In the absence of a direct measure of maturation such as a radiograph, height can imply maturation within the limits discussed in concept 2.1.

### Skeletal Injuries

Injuries to the growing skeleton rarely have a lifelong impact. In a young body, for example, broken bones typically heal quickly and efficiently. The potential exists, though, for severe injury to the epiphyseal plate. Such an injury can cut off the blood supply in the capillary invasion zone and result in the early cessation of growth at the site. A significant difference in the eventual length of the right and left limbs is possible if the injury occurs early in the growth period. Fortunately, epiphyseal injuries are not common, and those that do occur rarely involve the blood supply. Some injuries can be surgically repaired. Still, even the rare occurrence of epiphyseal injuries should give educators reason to question the wisdom of program-

ming certain activities, such as contact sports, for young children.

In addition to the epiphyseal plates, epiphyses exist at the sites where muscle tendons attach to the bones (see Figure 2.19). These *traction epiphyses* are also subject to irritation and injury. For example, in throwing, an individual can injure or irritate the traction epiphysis at the attachment site of the flexor-pronator muscles of the forearm (the medial epicondyle of the humerus) (see Figure 2.21). In a study of 162 male baseball players, 9 to 14 years old, all 80 of those who pitched had some irritation of this epiphysis (Adams, 1965). Of those who played baseball but did not pitch and those who did not play, few showed inflammation. Findings such as this have led many youth baseball programs to establish guidelines for the frequency and amount of overhand pitching.

Another familiar example of epiphyseal irritation is the tenderness of the tibial tuberosity (below the knee) at the patellar tendon attachment, known as Osgood-Schlatter disease. Treatment for this condition might include refraining from vigorous, especially weight-bearing, activities.

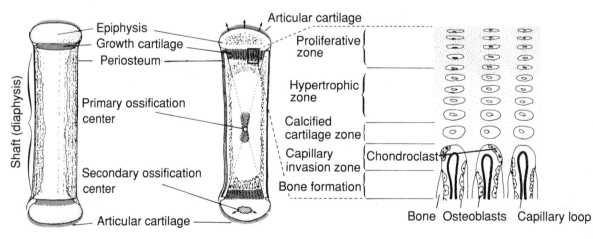

**Figure 2.20**  Development of a long bone in childhood. The epiphyseal growth plate, between the epiphysis and shaft, is enlarged on the right to show the zones wherein new cells ossify. (Reprinted by permission from Pritchard, 1979.)

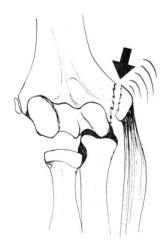

**Figure 2.21**   A drawing of an elbow joint. An injury to growth plate of the medial epiphysis (a traction epiphysis) has occurred from a violent contraction of the flexor-pronator muscle group in the act of throwing.
(Reprinted by permission from Rarick, 1973.)

Just like adults, children and adolescents can suffer overuse injuries such as stress fractures. The potential for such injuries rises with the use of repetitive training activities. As organized youth sport and exercise programs have increasingly used repetitive training, the incidence of overuse injuries has increased (Micheli, 1989).

## The Skeletal System in Older Adults

The skeletal structure changes little in young adulthood, although at any age poor posture can lead to skeletal misalignment. Researchers who have studied aging believe that some bone loss naturally occurs in the aging process (Smith, Sempos, & Purvis, 1981). They have also found evidence of change in bone composition. Children have essentially equal amounts of inorganic and organic components in their bone tissue, but older adults have seven times more inorganic material (Astrand & Rodahl, 1986; Exton-Smith, 1985). Beyond this, many older adults suffer from a major bone mineral disorder, osteoporosis, that is characterized by a loss of bone mass and, consequently, bone strength. The bone becomes abnormally porous through the enlargement of the canals or the formation of spaces in the bone. This condition increases the risk of fractures, especially at the hip, and adds to the difficulty of fracture repair (Timiras, 1972).

Prolonged deficiency of calcium in the diet is a major factor in osteoporosis, although many factors, either alone or in combination, can contribute to its occurrence. Deficient osteoblastic activity might be involved. In postmenopausal women, decreased levels of estrogen are implicated because estrogen hormones stimulate osteoblastic activity. This might account for the higher incidence of osteoporosis in older adult women than in men.

Treatments for osteoporosis include dietary supplements of calcium, vitamin D, and fluoride. Estrogen supplements are sometimes prescribed for postmenopausal women, but estrogen therapy is associated with increased risk of endometrial cancer. Concurrent use of progestogens can reduce this risk. Evidence also indicates that physically active women, both pre- and postmenopausal, have significantly less osteoporosis and bone loss than sedentary women have (Brewer et al., 1983; Oyster et al., 1984). When a person engages in physical activity, the mechanical forces applied to the bones help to maintain bone thickness and density. Even moderate physical activity prevents bone loss in adults and increases bone mineral content in older adults (Krolner, Tondevold, Toft, Berthelen, & Nielsen, 1982; Smith, Reddan, & Smith, 1981).

## The Muscular System

Muscle fibers (cells) grow during prenatal life by hyperplasia, an increase in the number of muscle cells, and by hypertrophy, an increase in muscle cell size. At birth, muscle mass accounts for 23% to 25% of body weight. Hyperplasia continues for a short time after birth, but thereafter muscle growth occurs predominantly by hypertrophy (Malina, 1978). An increase in the number of fiber nuclei accompanies muscle growth. Increases in muscle fiber diameter come with age and increased body size but are related also to the intensity of activity to which the muscle is subjected during growth. Naturally, muscles must increase in length as the skeleton grows, and this occurs by the addition of sarcomeres (contractile units; see Figure 2.22) at the muscle-tendon junction as well as by the lengthening of the sarcomeres (Malina & Bouchard, 1991).

Gender differences in muscle mass and number of fiber nuclei are minimal during childhood, with muscle mass constituting a slightly greater proportion of body weight in boys. During and after adolescence, however, gender differences are marked. Muscle mass increases rapidly in boys up to about age 17 and ultimately accounts for 54% of men's body weight. In sharp contrast, girls add muscle mass only until age 13, on the average, and muscle mass is only 45% of women's body weight (Malina, 1978). Men also have more fiber nuclei than women. The large gender differences in muscle mass involve upper body musculature more than leg musculature. For example, the rate of growth in arm musculature is nearly twice as high for males as for females, but the difference in calf muscle growth is relatively small. These gender differences in the addition of muscle mass are related to hormonal influences, which we will discuss later in this chapter.

## Muscle Fiber Type

Adult muscle consists of three main types of fibers: Type I (slow-twitch) fibers that are suited to endurance activities, and Types IIa and IIb (fast-twitch) fibers that are suited to short-duration, intense activity (see Figure 2.23). In

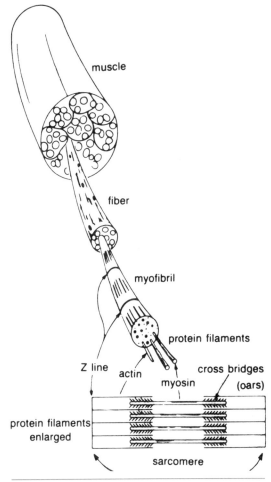

**Figure 2.22**  Muscle architecture. Note the basic unit, the sarcomere.
(Reprinted by permission from Sharkey, 1984.)

this context, a twitch is a brief period of contraction followed by relaxation of the muscle fiber. At birth, 15% to 20% of the muscle fibers have yet to differentiate into Type I, Type IIa, or Type IIb fibers (Baldwin, 1984; Colling-Saltin, 1980). This has led to speculation that an infant's early activities might influence the ultimate proportion of the three types of fibers, but this issue remains unresolved.

The proportion of Type I fibers is fixed by age 1. The percentage of Type IIa fibers com-

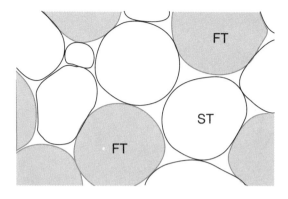

**Figure 2.23** A cross section of muscle showing that fast-twitch (FT) and slow-twitch (ST) fibers are intermingled.
(Reprinted by permission from Sharkey, 1984.)

pared to Type IIb fibers is greater in adults than in children, implying that this proportion is not fixed during childhood, but it is difficult for researchers to measure the number of Type IIb fibers accurately. Proportions also vary greatly among individuals (Malina & Bouchard, 1991), so the shift in proportion could reflect the makeup of groups tested by researchers. Questions about the alteration of fiber type proportions must await further research on the biochemical factors involved in muscle development (Baldwin, 1984).

## Motor Units

All of the muscle fibers that are innervated by a single motor neuron comprise a *motor unit*. We can also categorize motor units as either fast-twitch or slow-twitch by their speed of contraction and relaxation. Many human muscles are composed of both fast- and slow-twitch motor units. At birth, these mixed-composition muscles are composed predominantly of fast-twitch units. During the first 2 years of postnatal life, some units become slow-twitch (Malina & Bouchard, 1991). This transition also leads to speculation that the ultimate proportions can

be influenced during early development, but far more research is needed before we can consider this suggestion seriously.

## The Muscular System in Older Adults

In the average young adult, the percentage of body weight that is muscle decreases. This reflects not a loss of muscle but an increase in fat weight. Changes in diet and physical activity level are probably responsible for this shift. In old age, both the number and the diameter (size) of muscle fibers appear to gradually decrease. Type II fibers undergo a greater loss of size than Type I fibers. By very old age, an individual can lose as much as 50% of the muscle mass possessed in young adulthood. Although these trends describe the average growth and decline of muscle, remember that muscle mass is influenced by a variety of factors, including genetic inheritance, insulin level, growth hormone level, sex hormone level, nutrition, and activity or training level.

## Cardiac Muscle

The heart is muscle tissue, too. Like skeletal muscle, it grows by hyperplasia and hypertrophy, with an accompanying increase in fiber nuclei. The right ventricle (lower chamber) is larger than the left ventricle at birth, but the left ventricle catches up after birth by growing more rapidly than the right so that the heart soon reaches adult proportions (see Figure 2.24). The heart generally follows the sigmoid pattern of whole-body growth, including a growth spurt in adolescence, such that the ratio of heart volume to body weight remains approximately the same throughout growth.

Early in the 20th century some researchers thought that the large blood vessels around the heart developed more slowly than the heart itself. This implied that children who engaged in vigorous activity might be at risk. Later, it was shown that this myth had resulted from a

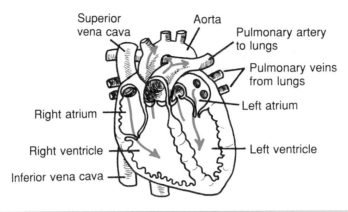

**Figure 2.24**   The human heart.
(Reprinted by permission from Sharkey, 1984.)

misinterpretation of measurements taken in the late 1800s; in fact, blood vessel growth is proportional to that of the heart (Karpovich, 1937, 1991). Yet, even recently, at least one author cited the original mistaken data as a reason to limit children's vigorous activity.

In old age, the heart's ability to adapt to an increased work load declines. This might relate in part to degeneration of the heart muscle, a decrease in elasticity, and changes in the fibers of the heart valves (Shephard, 1981). The major blood vessels also lose elasticity.

---

It has been difficult for researchers to distinguish the changes that are an inevitable result of age from those that reflect the average older adult's lack of fitness or poor diet.

---

## The Adipose System

A common misconception about adipose (fat) tissue is that its presence in any amount is undesirable. In reality, adipose tissue plays a vital role in energy storage, insulation, and protection, and the amount of adipose tissue necessarily increases in early life. Adipose tissue first appears in the fetus at 3.5 months and increases rapidly during the last 2 prenatal months. Even so, adipose tissue accounts for only 0.5 kg (1.1 lb) of body weight at birth. After a rapid increase of fat during the first 6 postnatal months, fat mass increases gradually until age 8 in both boys and girls. In boys, adipose tissue continues to gradually increase through adolescence, but girls experience a more dramatic increase. As a result, adult women have more fat weight than adult men, with averages of 14 kg and 10 kg, respectively. Fat weight during growth increases by both hyperplasia and hypertrophy, but cell size does not increase significantly until puberty.

Individual fatness varies widely during infancy and early childhood. A fat baby will not necessarily become a fat child. After 7 to 8 years of age, though, it is more likely that individuals maintain their relative fatness. An overweight 8-year-old has a high risk of becoming an overweight adult.

### Fat Distribution

The distribution of fat in the body changes during growth. During childhood, internal fat (fat around the viscera) increases faster than subcutaneous fat, which actually decreases until age 6 or 7. Both boys and girls then have an increase in subcutaneous fat until they are 12 or 13. This increase in subcutaneous fat continues in girls, but boys typically lose subcutaneous fat in midadolescence. Adolescent boys also tend to add more subcutaneous fat to their trunks than to their limbs, whereas girls have increased subcutaneous fat at both sites. Note in Figure 2.25 that skinfold measures for boys' extremities (solid line) actually decrease, except during the growth spurt. Trunk skinfolds tend to hold steady but also increase during the growth spurt. Girls' skinfold measures (dashed line) increase steadily for both trunk and limbs, especially after age 7. Girls usually add more subcutaneous fat to their legs than to their arms.

## Research Questions

Researchers are currently examining many aspects of adipose tissue development, including maternal weight gain during pregnancy, early infant feeding, and genetic factors. Of particular interest are the two periods when the number of adipose cells increases: during the first 6 postnatal months, and around puberty. Increases in cell number are significant because once they are formed, adipose cells persist, even with malnutrition; that is, the cells may be "empty" of fat, but they still exist. Therefore these two periods may be critical in the control of obesity.

## Adipose Tissue in Older Adults

Both sexes tend to gain fat weight during the adult years, reflecting changes in nutrition and activity level. The average person gains approximately 12 kg (Brozek, 1952). Total body weight begins to decline after age 50, but this may reflect loss of bone and muscle rather than fat.

It is difficult to identify the typical pattern of adipose tissue gain or loss in older adults. Because obese individuals have a higher mortality rate, either lighter individuals survive to

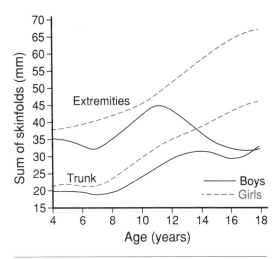

**Figure 2.25**   The changes in fat distribution during growth are illustrated by plotting the sum of five trunk skinfold measurements and five extremity skinfold measurements.
(Reprinted by permission from Malina & Bouchard, 1988.)

be included in studies of older adults whereas obese individuals do not, or thinner adults are more eager to participate in research studies. It appears that an increase in fat weight with aging is not inevitable; for example, lumberjacks in Norway, persons from undernourished parts of the world, and Masters-class athletes do not demonstrate such gains (Shephard, 1978b; Skrobak-Kaczynski & Andersen, 1975). Typically, though, most older adults add some fat weight as they age, with active older adults adding less than their sedentary peers.

## The Endocrine System

Hormones have an important role in regulating growth and maturation. Regulation of growth, though, is a complex and delicate interaction of hormones, genes, nutrients, and environmental factors. This discussion highlights only the major features of endocrine growth regulation.

Although many hormones are involved in the regulation of growth and maturation, three major types of hormones are discussed here:

1. Pituitary growth hormone (GH)
2. The thyroid hormones (thyroxine, tri-iodothyronine, thyrocalcitonin)
3. Two gonadal hormones (androgen, estrogen) (Timiras, 1972)

Either an excess or a deficiency of these hormones may disturb the normal process of growth and development. Although different in their chemical structure, all three promote growth in the same way: They stimulate protein anabolism (constructive metabolism), resulting in the retention of substances needed to build tissues. Each hormone plays a unique role in growth at a unique time.

## Growth Hormone

Growth hormone (GH) influences growth during childhood and adolescence by stimulating protein anabolism so that new tissue can be built. Under the control of the central nervous system, GH is secreted by the anterior pituitary gland (see Figure 2.26) via a substance called the GH-releasing factor. GH enhances the mobilization of stored fat while conserving carbohydrates. The body needs this hormone for normal growth after birth. A deficiency or absence of GH results in growth abnormalities and in some cases the cessation of linear growth. The anterior pituitary gland secretes five other hormones called the tropic hormones. They all help other endocrine glands to maintain their activity.

## Thyroid Hormones

The thyroid hormones are secreted by the thyroid gland, located in the anterior neck region. Although thyroxine and triiodothyronine influence postnatal whole-body growth, they are

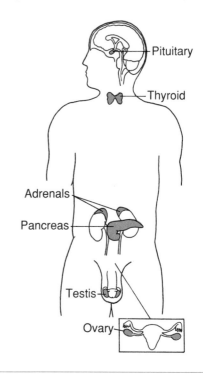

**Figure 2.26**  Location of the various endocrine glands.

particularly influential in the development of certain tissues by increasing oxygen consumption in these tissues. The level of pituitary thyrotropic or thyroid-stimulating hormone (TSH) regulates secretion of the thyroid hormones. TSH excretion is, in turn, increased by a releasing factor found in the brain's hypothalamus. Thus, two systems appear to be acting in concert: a pituitary-thyroid system, and a nervous system–thyroid system. You can see that the endocrine system is delicately balanced. In fact, a GH-thyroid relationship also exists, because thyroxine must be present for GH to be effective.

The thyroid gland also secretes thyrocalcitonin, which plays a role in growth. It decreases circulating calcium by inhibiting bone reabsorption and by promoting calcium deposition in the bones.

## Gonadal Hormones

The gonadal hormones affect growth and sexual maturation, particularly during adolescence, by stimulating development of the secondary sex characteristics and the sex organs. The androgens, specifically testosterone from the testes and androgens (dehydroepiandrosterone, androstenedione, and 11-b-hydroxyandrostenedione) from the cortex of the adrenal glands, hasten fusion of the epiphyseal growth plates in the bones. Thus, these hormones promote skeletal maturation (fusion) at the expense of linear growth; this explains why early maturers tend to be shorter in stature than later maturers.

Androgens also play a role in the adolescent growth spurt of muscle mass by increasing nitrogen retention and protein synthesis. This spurt is more significant in young men than in young women because men secrete both testosterone and adrenal androgens, whereas women produce only the adrenal androgens. In women, the ovaries and the adrenal cortex secrete estrogens. Increased estrogen secretion during adolescence, as with androgens, speeds epiphyseal closure, but estrogen also promotes fat accumulation, primarily in the breasts and hips. Androstenedione is converted to estrogen in males, and dehydroepiandrosterone is converted to testosterone in females. As a result, men and women have both estrogen and testosterone, but in very different proportions.

## Insulin

The hormones we have discussed up to this point all play a major and direct role in growth and development. Another familiar hormone, insulin, has an indirect role in growth. Produced in the pancreas, insulin is vital to carbohydrate metabolism, stimulating the transportation of glucose and amino acids through membranes. Its presence also is necessary for the full functioning of GH. A deficiency of insulin can decrease protein synthesis, too. This is detrimental at any time in life, but especially during growth.

## Feedback Loops

Much interdependence exists among hormones and between the endocrine glands and the central nervous system. Some of these relationships take the form of feedback loops that allow for a delicate balance in the amounts of hormones circulating in the body. Though a discussion of all the body's regulatory feedback loops is beyond the scope of this text, the general format of a feedback loop for the anterior pituitary gland is shown in Figure 2.27. In this loop the hypothalamus of the central nervous system secretes a releasing factor that stimulates the anterior pituitary to secrete the tropic hormone of a particular gland, referred to as the target gland. The target gland then releases its hormone. This hormone circulates to its target tissues and to the hypothalamus and anterior pituitary. The hypothalamus then inhibits output of the releasing factor, ultimately causing the hormone level to drop. When this level falls too low, the hypothalamus secretes the releasing factor. In this way the amount of hormone circulating is regulated.

## The Endocrine System in Older Adults

In adults, hormones play a role in three areas that relate to physical activity:

1. Regulation of cardiovascular performance
2. Mobilization of fuel
3. Synthesis of new protein (Shephard, 1978b)

Information about age-related hormonal changes is limited, but we are aware of several features of hormonal function in aging. Basal

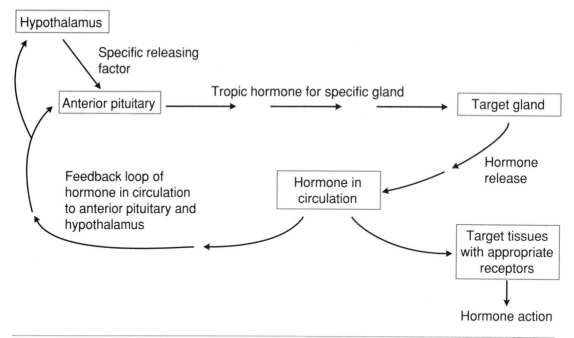

**Figure 2.27**    The hypothalamus-anterior pituitary-endocrine (target) glands loop plays a role in regulating the amount of hormone in circulation.
(Reprinted by permission from Malina & Bouchard, 1991.)

levels of GH seem to be stable throughout life, but during exercise, older adults can have a more pronounced increase in GH levels than younger exercisers. This increase may be an attempt by the body's metabolism to conserve glycogen (the form in which the body stores glucose, a sugar) and reduce protein breakdown through the release of stored fat.

Thyroid function also declines with aging, and thyroid disorders become more prevalent in older adults. Researchers do not completely understand the exact role of changing thyroid function in aging. One reason for this is the close relationship of thyroid hormone levels to nutrition and illness. It is difficult to isolate age-related changes that occur independently of these factors (Korenman, 1982). A long-term increase in thyroid hormone levels can be re-lated to congestive heart failure. It is therefore important for older adults to be screened for hyperthyroidism.

Gonadal hormone levels decrease with age. Though we lack information on this aspect of aging, prescribing androgen supplements has been successful in countering muscle wasting and osteoporosis. Women with osteoporosis sometimes undergo estrogen replacement therapy. We know that older adults maintain the secretion level of insulin, but the incidence of Type II diabetes (non-insulin-dependent diabetes mellitus, which is caused by insulin deficiency) increases markedly with age. It is possible that older adults do not utilize insulin as effectively as younger adults to promote glycogen storage, thus retarding the mobilization of fuel for exercise.

## The Nervous System

Growth and development of the nervous system provides a prime example of the interplay of genetic and environmental factors. The precise and predictable course of early nervous system development is genetically directed. Immature neurons are generated, differentiate in their general type, and migrate to a final position. Formation of cell processes (dendrites and axons) occurs next with arborization (branching) of the processes and further differentiation (see Figure 2.28). Finally, *myelination* (an insulating process) of the processes takes place (Williams, 1983). For the most part, proliferation and migration of cells occur prenatally, and cell arborization and myelination take place postnatally.

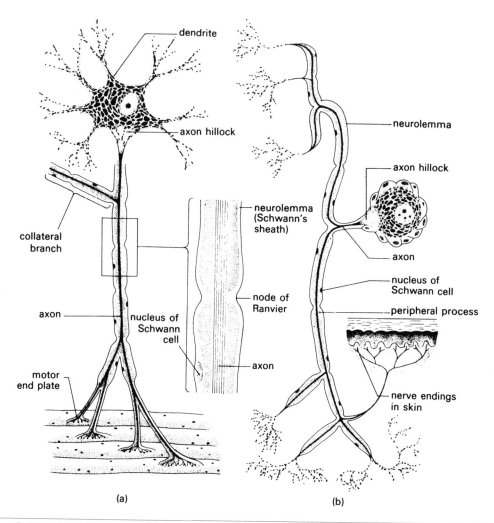

(a)     (b)

**Figure 2.28**   A myelinated (a) motor neuron and (b) sensory neuron. (Reprinted by permission from Crouch, 1985.)

## Early Development

Despite its plasticity—that is, the ability of neural cells to take on a new function in the event of trauma—the nervous system is vulnerable to environmental factors as it grows and develops. This is particularly true during several critical periods of rapid development. These critical periods occur early in life—prenatally and during the first year after birth—but nervous system development continues through puberty (some myelination may occur as late as young adulthood) and is susceptible to environmental influence until this time. To help you understand how and when nervous system development is subject to genetic and environmental influence, here is a brief outline of its structural development.

### The Brain

Because neurons of the brain are formed prenatally, the rapid gains in brain weight during the first postnatal year (when the brain reaches half of its adult weight) primarily reflect two processes:

1. An increase of myelin and glial cells (which support and nourish the neuron)
2. An increase in the size of neurons and their arborization, or branching

In arborization, each neuron establishes 1,000 to 100,000 connections with other neurons during the first year after birth. The processes of neurons reach specific locations by growing along a chemical trail, probably under genetic control. Once there, axons proliferate branches with a bulbous terminal that forms a connection or synapse with the dendritic process or cell body of another neuron. Recent animal research demonstrates that the firing of impulses along neural pathways is critical to further brain development. Environmental stimuli cause impulses to fire (Kalil, 1989).

### Lower Brain Centers

The spinal cord and lower brain structures are more advanced at birth than the higher brain structures. Those lower brain centers involved in vital tasks, such as respiration and food intake, are relatively mature. Lower brain centers also mediate many reflexes and reactions. These automatic movement responses dominate the fetus's and newborn's movements. This, too, indicates that lower brain centers are relatively more advanced than higher brain centers.

For many years, researchers have interpreted the onset of goal-directed movements in infants as evidence that higher brain centers are maturing. The cortex, or outer layer, of the cerebral hemispheres (the two large lobes of the brain; see Figure 2.29) is involved in purposeful, goal-directed movement. The first clear evidence of successful, intentional movement (reaching) occurs at 4 to 5 postnatal months (Bushnell, 1982; McDonnell, 1979). Hence, researchers assumed that this behavior signaled the functioning of the cortex at about 4 months of age, even though the cerebral hemispheres are formed at birth. You will recall from our discussion in chapter 1 that maturationists often inferred neurologic development from the onset of new skills. From the dynamic multiple-systems perspective, one or more other systems could be the slower developing, or rate-controlling, system. Hence, we must use caution in continuing to relate behavior only to neurologic advancements that could in fact precede overt behaviors.

In general, though, phylogenetically older lower brain centers are the most mature at birth. The early postnatal months are an important time in brain maturation. The cells of the cortex continue to differentiate in the early postnatal years, as do the cortical cells of the cerebellum, the two smaller lobes at the base of the brain.

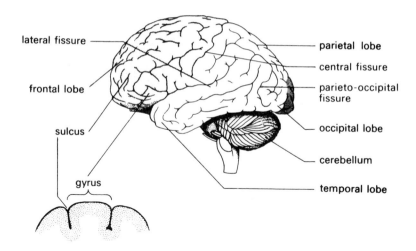

**Figure 2.29** The cerebrum and a cross section of the cerebral cortex.
(Reprinted by permission from Langley, Telford, & Christensen, 1980.)

## Myelin

The development of myelin in the nervous system contributes to speedy conduction of nerve impulses. Myelin cells, composed mostly of fat, wrap themselves around the outgoing neuron cell process, or axon (see Figure 2.30). The myelin sheath is interrupted periodically by nodes (called nodes of Ranvier). The neuron cell membrane is involved in nerve impulse conduction only at the nodes, so the impulse jumps from node to node. This type of nerve impulse conduction is known as saltatory conduction, and it is much faster than conduction in non-myelinated axons. Saltatory conduction also requires less metabolic energy so that myelinated axons can fire nerve impulses at higher frequencies for longer periods (Kuffler, Nicholls, & Martin, 1984).

Axons that are as yet unmyelinated in the newborn are probably functional, but myelination improves the speed and frequency of firing. The function of the nervous system in movements requiring or benefiting from speedy conduction of nerve impulses, such as

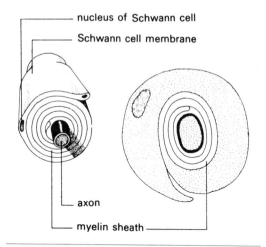

**Figure 2.30** A myelinated axon.
(Reprinted by permission from DeCoursey & Renfro, 1980.)

a series of rapid movements or postural responses, might be related to the myelination process during development. Multiple sclerosis, a disease that strikes young adults and breaks down the myelin sheath, results in tremor, loss of coordination, and possibly paralysis.

## The Spinal Cord

The spinal cord is relatively small and short at birth. A cross-sectional view of the spinal cord, as seen in Figure 2.31, shows a central horn-shaped area of gray matter and a surrounding area of white matter. This central area contains tightly packed neuron cell bodies. Note the roots that lie just outside the cord and contain the axons of the cord's neurons and, in the case of the sensory roots, nerve cell bodies as well. Fibers from the dorsal and ventral roots merge to form the peripheral (spinal) nerves outside the cord. A marked increase in the myelination of these peripheral nerves occurs 2 to 3 weeks after birth, and this process continues through the 2nd or 3rd year of life.

The myelination pattern that the spinal cord and nerve pathways undergo might have implications for motor development. Myelination proceeds in two directions in the cord: first in the cervical portion, followed by the progressively lower portions; and then in the motor (ventral) horns, followed by the sensory (dorsal) horns. Two major motor pathways, or nerve tracts, carry impulses from the brain down the spinal cord to various parts of the body. One pathway, the extrapyramidal tract, probably is involved in delivering the commands for both random and postural movements made by the infant in the first days after birth (see Figure 2.32). The other, the pyramidal tract, myelinates after birth and is probably functional by 4 to 5 months, when the infant exhibits intentional behavior (see Figure 2.33). In studies where researchers have severed the pyramidal tracts of monkeys (Lawrence & Hopkins, 1972; Lawrence & Kuypers, 1968), the effect has been a loss of individual finger movement with an accompanying decrease in the speed and agility of movement.

The direction of myelination tends to be away from the brain in both of these motor tracts. In contrast, the direction of myelination is toward the brain in sensory tracts, occurring first in the tactile and olfactory pathways, then in the visual pathways, and finally in the audi-

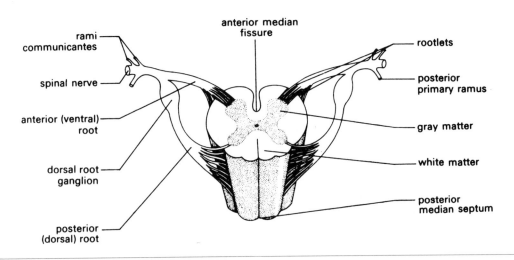

**Figure 2.31** A cross section of the spinal cord.
(Reprinted by permission from Langley, Telford, & Christensen, 1969.)

tory pathways. Sensory pathways mature slightly faster than motor pathways, except in the motor roots and cerebral hemispheres.

## The Nervous System in Older Adults

As an individual ages, the number of neurons in the nervous system, including the cerebral cortex, decreases, but the number of glial cells increases. Overall, this results in decreased brain weight by old age. This decrease might be related to a gradual reduction in circulation and in oxygen utilization in the brain after adolescence. The electrophysiologic effects of aging seem to be lower nerve signal strength, an increase in "neural noise" (random background activity in the central nervous system), fewer neural connections to integrate and smooth neural signals, and longer lasting aftereffects (prolonged electrical activity after stimulus cessation). An older adult can experience these effects as a general slowing of sensory and motor function.

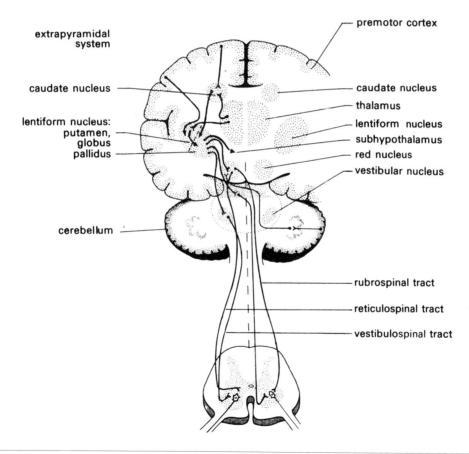

**Figure 2.32** The extrapyramidal motor pathways.
(Reprinted by permission from McNaught & Callander, 1983.)

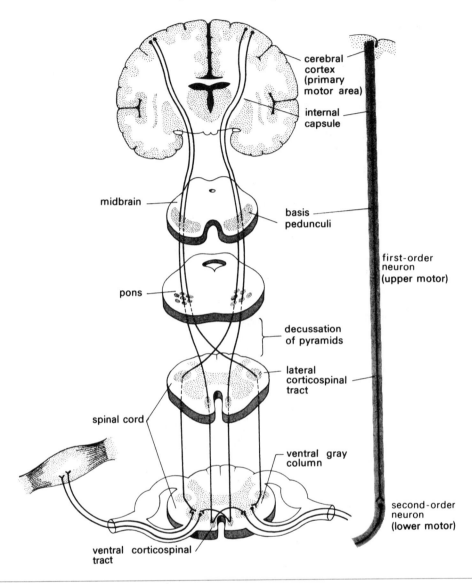

**Figure 2.33** The pyramidal motor pathways.
(Reprinted by permission from Langley, Telford, & Christensen, 1969.)

## REVIEW 2.4

Professionals who work with individuals need to understand normal growth and maturation of the body and its tissues. Whole-body growth proceeds in a characteristic pattern known as sigmoid growth, but the rate of maturation varies between the sexes and among individuals. Allowing for these individual differences, we can detect abnormal or retarded growth by comparing an individual child to average growth curves.

The various body tissues and systems can have unique growth patterns. Educators should be aware of these patterns, because growth is more susceptible to external influence during periods of rapid change. Some external or environmental influences can be positive and help persons attain their full growth potential. Others can retard growth or permanently affect growth and maturation. Next, we will review many of the environmental factors that can affect growth, development, and maturation.

## FACTORS INFLUENCING POSTNATAL DEVELOPMENT

Educators must recognize the influence of environmental factors on postnatal growth, development, and aging. These environmental influences become increasingly important, relative to genetic factors, as a person matures. In fact, critical or sensitive periods might exist for some aspects of postnatal growth because vulnerability to environmental influence is greatest during periods of rapid development. The presence or absence of an environmental factor at a given time might affect an individual's potential for skilled performance during the rest of his or her life. What are these environmental factors, and how might they affect a person's physical growth and lifelong development?

---

**CONCEPT 2.5**
Environmental factors become more important as postnatal growth and maturation proceed.

---

## The Birth Process

The birth process (see Figure 2.34), as the transition from a prenatal, internal environment to a postnatal, external environment, has the potential to affect growth and development. Even normal birth is somewhat traumatic for the fetus; abnormal labor or delivery can be harmful. Recall from our earlier discussion of

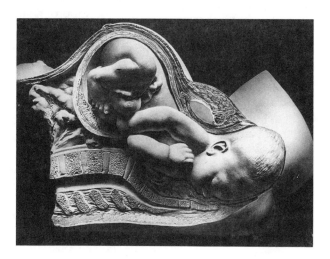

**Figure 2.34** The second stage of labor. The baby's head is now showing. (Reprinted by permission from the Maternity Center Association.)

prenatal growth that the fetus's oxygen supply passes through the placenta via the umbilical cord, and that *hypoxia* (oxygen deficiency) can impair normal brain development. Circumstances that put pressure on the cord, such as breech birth, where the infant emerges feet, knees, or buttocks first rather than headfirst, can reduce or block the infant's oxygen and blood supply, causing brain damage. Abnormal pressure on the infant's head, as might occur in breech birth or with the use of forceps during delivery, can also affect brain development. The use of forceps can cause other injuries, too, especially to the epiphyseal growth plates of the bones.

Low birth weight (under 2,500 g) is associated with increased health risks during early postnatal growth and development (Brandt, 1978). Low birth weight also increases the risk of infant mortality. It is important to distinguish between low-birth-weight infants who are born prematurely and those born full-term. Medical personnel expect a premature infant to be small at birth and small for age when compared with average growth charts. In fact, the premature child often compares favorably to growth charts if his or her age is adjusted downward for the early birth date. In contrast, the small but full-term infant has grown slowly during the prenatal period, probably as a result of negative factors in the prenatal environment. These environmental factors during prenatal growth have jeopardized normal growth after birth. A mother's cigarette smoking during pregnancy is a common example of an adverse prenatal factor strongly associated with low birth weight. Maternal malnutrition is another. Fortunately, improving environmental factors in the early postnatal months can bring about a period of catch-up growth, so it is difficult to predict the effect of low birth weight on adult size.

The long-term effect of low birth weight depends on the timing, duration, and severity of the adverse factor as well as on postnatal nutrition and care (Brandt, 1978).

## Postnatal Nutrition

Nutrition is a major environmental factor affecting growth and development. The body needs the energy that food provides to grow and to maintain normal body functions. Although this need is greatest during periods when the body is growing rapidly, good nutrition is important for the maintenance and repair of body tissues throughout life. The three basic foodstuffs—proteins, carbohydrates, and fats—each play a role in growth and development. Amino acids from proteins provide the building material for different tissues and are needed for protein synthesis. Carbohydrates are the chief source of fuel the body uses to meet its energy requirements, and fats provide energy storage and insulation against heat loss. Water, vitamins, and minerals, especially calcium and magnesium, are the other essential nutrients that support growth and development.

An individual needs adequate nutrition to attain his or her growth potential, but malnutrition or overnutrition—nutrients in insufficient or excessive amounts, respectively—can affect growth adversely. These conditions can result from an inappropriate quantity or quality of nutrients, or both.

### Malnutrition

The effects of chronic malnutrition on stature alone are so severe that children suffering from prolonged malnutrition often do not attain their potential height. Puberty also may be delayed. The effects of protein malnutrition are dramatically illustrated by two diseases, kwashiorkor and marasmus, that cause growth retardation as well as muscle wasting. Malnutrition can affect the body systems differentially. Remember that the nervous system develops rapidly in early life; therefore, malnutrition during this time can limit nervous system development irreversibly. Similarly, any system developing rapidly during a period of malnutrition can be greatly affected.

Malnutrition does not occur only in under-developed nations. Even in affluent countries, there are homeless and jobless people who cannot afford to eat properly. Some individuals also may suffer from intestinal diseases that limit their assimilation of nutrients. For example, Crohn's disease is a chronic inflammatory condition that affects the small intestine and reduces its ability to absorb food. Psychological conditions can affect diet as well. For example, *anorexia nervosa* is an eating disorder characterized by aversion to food for fear of weight gain. And malnutrition can also result when people eat too much junk food. This food is high in sugar or fat and thus provides an adequate number of calories, but it does not supply the body with sufficient nutrients, vitamins, and minerals.

People who engage in heavy physical training can be undernourished if their diets do not provide sufficient fuel to meet their bodies' increased energy demands. Endurance and strength training can increase the body's daily energy requirements substantially. Adolescent athletes are particularly vulnerable to energy deficits because they experience the energy demands of rapid growth as well as those from training. An energy deficit can lead to a loss of lean body mass and permanent negative effects on growth (Lemon, 1989). Much of the dietary increase the body needs to balance consumption with need should be in the form of carbohydrates, but some increase in protein and calcium intake is also beneficial.

## Overnutrition

The dietary problem most prevalent in affluent areas is overnutrition. Obese children often experience accelerated growth and development, but they also exhibit unusually high levels of cholesterol and triglycerides. As a result, they are already at risk of coronary disease, adult obesity, diabetes, and hypertension.

Many overweight persons adopt popular fad diets in an attempt to lose excess fat weight. Many of these diets are unbalanced in nutrients,

and the dieter ends up malnourished. It is not definite that children become obese by consuming too many calories; lack of activity is another important consideration. Yet researchers are currently exploring the relationship between childhood obesity and diets high in sugar or fat because animal studies have implicated these diets as a cause of obesity (Oscai, 1989).

The influence of an environmental factor like nutrition on growth is clearly illustrated by a secular trend, a gradual change over the generations, in body size and maturity (Van Wieringen, 1978). The effect of this trend is that people today tend to be taller and heavier and to reach puberty sooner than people did in earlier generations. Whether nutrition contributes to this secular trend through an increase in total calories or in protein is unclear. Adequate nutrition is also associated with increased life span, because malnutrition predisposes an individual to disease. At the other extreme, obesity is correlated with a higher death rate in middle and old age.

## The Physical Environment

Several characteristics of the physical environment in which children grow can potentially affect growth patterns: climate, seasons of the year, and altitude.

### Climate

Researchers have observed a relationship between climate and body physique. Tall, thin physiques are more common in hot climates where more body surface area helps dissipate body heat. Short, stocky physiques are indigenous to cold climates where minimal body surface area is advantageous in preserving body heat. These trends imply that the growth period is longer and maturity is delayed in tropical climates. The reverse would be true in cold climates.

The data available on maturation, however, are not consistent with this hypothesis. Eskimo children living in extremely cold zones grow over a prolonged period and attain their adult height at an older age than average. This suggests that some energy is diverted from growth into producing heat and maintaining body temperature (Little & Hochner, 1973). It is obvious that a variety of environmental and genetic factors influence physique, including nutrition, exercise patterns, exposure to disease, and race. Because of the number of factors that overlap to influence body physique, it is difficult to assess the influence of climate alone on growth.

## Seasons of the Year

Seasonal cycles may also influence patterns of growth. Researchers in at least one early study recorded greater weight gains in fall than in spring, and greater height gains in spring than in fall (Tanner, 1961). Nutrition and exercise patterns may act in concert with seasonal cycles to produce this pattern of growth. People tend to consume heavier, richer foods in the winter and lighter foods in the summer. Cold weather and fewer hours of daylight also can make it more difficult for people to participate in recreational activities in the winter.

## Altitude

Living at high altitudes can affect growth, too. Children reared high in the Andes Mountains in South America and the Himalayas in Asia have smaller bodies and a slower growth rate than children living at lower altitudes. Adequate oxygen is important for normal growth and development. Because the barometric pressure at high altitudes is lower, less oxygen is diffused into the blood. Children living at very high altitudes over a long period can therefore suffer hypoxia, possibly resulting in retarded growth and development. It is also possible that the cold climate at high altitudes and the nutritional status of these children simultaneously affect growth patterns. Another aspect of growth demonstrates the body's adaptability to environmental factors: Children living at high altitudes develop greater lung capacities than their peers at sea level. This allows individuals living at high altitudes to offset hypoxia, at least in part, by extracting oxygen from a larger quantity of air in their lungs.

## Other Environmental Factors

Radiation can have a harmful effect on growth. Children can be exposed to radiation from natural sources, such as cosmic rays and radon from soil, rocks, and building materials; or from artificial sources, such as therapeutic radiation or accidents at nuclear power plants. High dosages of radiation produce a variety of devastating effects on any growing organism, especially if they occur early in life. Among these effects are cell mutations, damage to the nervous system, growth retardation, and leukemia.

Substances present in the environment can affect growing children. For example, children exposed to old paint that contains lead are at risk. The paint peels and becomes a part of household dust. Young children get the dust on their hands and often put their hands in their mouths. Lower IQ scores are associated with long-term exposure to lead. This implies that lead directly or indirectly affects neurologic growth. Other environmental hazards include toxic waste dumps and contaminated food, water, and air.

## Physical Activity and Regular Training

Of particular interest to educators is the effect of physical activity and regular training on growth, development, and aging. Experts generally agree that every individual needs some minimal amount of physical activity to support normal growth. That amount, however, is not easily determined. It is also difficult to identify the effects of regular exercise on growth and development. The effects of exercise often occur in the same direction as the changes

# Lead: Still a Problem

Lead is an environmental substance that can have very detrimental effects on individuals, especially children. This example shows us how difficult it is to identify the negative effects of an environmental substance and to remove that substance from the environment once it is identified.

Lead poisoning was recognized for centuries, but not until the 1940s did anyone document the detrimental effects of small, frequent exposures to lead on children's development. Randolph Byers, a Boston doctor, and Elizabeth Lord, a Harvard psychologist, identified 20 toddlers who cut their teeth on painted crib rails or windowsills and subsequently displayed the symptoms of lead poisoning. They followed these children as they entered school and found that all but two had significant academic difficulties. The children had diminished ability to recognize and manipulate shapes and patterns, a necessary skill for reading. A 1943 *Time* magazine article alerted the public to Lord and Byers's findings. Unfortunately, the lead industry denied any negative effects, and interest in the problem waned during World War II.

In the 1970s, a community psychiatrist, Herbert Needleman, discovered a new research technique that helped provide information on lead exposure. A problem in identifying children exposed to lead is that lead is cleared from the blood a couple of months after exposure, although it remains much longer in the bone and soft tissues. The simple blood tests used at the time to determine exposure to lead were inadequate. Needleman realized that he could use baby teeth to document children's cumulative lead exposure. Using baby teeth collected from schoolchildren in suburban Boston, Needleman et al. (1979) identified a high-exposure group and a low-exposure group of children. They gave all the children a battery of physical and intelligence tests. The high-exposure group scored lower on intelligence, language, and attention tests. Needleman (Needleman, Schell, Bellinger, Leviton, & Allred, 1990) was able to test approximately half these children as adolescents, 11 years later. Those in the high-exposure group still scored lower on measures of vocabulary, fine-motor skills, reaction time, and hand-eye coordination. More children from this group had dropped out of high school. Those still in high school had significantly lower grades than the low-exposure students.

Lead produces much of its damaging effects by making capillaries in the brain ooze blood into the surrounding brain tissue. Swelling results, and, because the skull encases the brain, the brain is constantly being squeezed. Recall that a large portion of brain development takes place early in life. Early exposure to lead, then, has the greatest potential to result in significant brain damage.

Many people believe that lead exposure is a problem restricted to inner cities, yet the soil in rural areas along highways contains dangerous levels of lead from automobile exhaust. The soil can contain lead around any house where layers of exterior lead paint have chalked off. Although lead has been banned from paint and gasoline for some time, plenty of old paint and contaminated soil is still around. Children can receive significant lead exposure during remodeling and renovation projects occurring in any home. The lead solder used to connect copper and steel water pipes adds lead to our drinking water. Leaded crystal and glazes on dishware contain lead. If the glazes start to disintegrate, the food stored in the dishes can absorb lead.

Though lead exposure is a significant problem for poor children living in the cities, no child is immune. Moreover, the problem has not disappeared even though paint and gasoline are no longer manufactured with lead. This substance lingers in the environment, potentially affecting the development of significant numbers of children.

accompanying growth. For example, muscle mass increases with growth but is promoted by exercise, too. This makes it difficult to distinguish normal growth from the effects of training. In addition, developmentalists prefer to use longitudinal studies so they can account for individual variation in maturation rate when distinguishing normal growth and training effects, but these are not as common as cross-sectional studies. Researchers must take many factors into account—the level of training, the emphasis of the program (strength vs. endurance), and the amount of physical activity an individual engages in outside a formal program. Because the benefits of an active lifestyle have received widespread attention in recent years, it is important to review what we know about the effects of exercise on growth and aging. We will now examine these effects more closely, but we will reserve a discussion of fitness development for a later chapter.

## Skeletal Growth

Does physical activity affect skeletal growth? To answer this question, let's consider the various aspects of bone growth—length, width, and density—separately. Physical activity does not stimulate increased bone length and therefore taller stature. You may observe that young people on sport teams look taller than others their age, but this is probably because early maturers tend to be successful in, and to be sought out for, sport participation. Regular training appears to have no detrimental effect on stature, except that prolonged, strenuous labor, such as carrying heavy loads on the shoulders, is known to be detrimental (Kato & Ishiko, 1966, cited in Rarick, 1973). On the other hand, Ivanitsky (cited in Rarick, 1973) found that the diameter of the long bones was larger in athletes than in nonathletes. He noted larger femurs (thighbones) in soccer players and larger radius bones (in the forearm) in tennis players. Activity, then, might increase bone diameter during the growing years. Bone density

increases with exercise and decreases with inactivity at any age (Nilsson & Westlin, 1971). Exercise plays a role in reducing osteoporosis in adults, especially postmenopausal women.

---

Long-term physical activity, short of strenuous labor, promotes bone density and might increase the diameter of the bones involved. Bone adapts favorably to the stimulation that physical activity provides.

---

## Body Weight

It is well established that physical activity influences body weight, often by increasing lean body mass and reducing fat weight. This apparently holds true during the growth years. Parizkova (1972) found that a regularly trained (6 hr/wk) group of boys had significantly less fat at 18 years than an untrained (2.5 hr/wk or less) group of the same age, even though the groups were similar in fat level at age 11 (see Figure 2.35). We will discuss this study and other changes in body composition that occur with growth and aging more fully in chapter 7. It is difficult to separate variations in maturity from the effects of training even in longitudinal studies, but the trend toward increased lean mass and reduced fat mass still appears to be greater than would be expected for growth and maturation alone.

## Body Physique

Regular training does not appear to influence body physique—that is, the body's build or form as a whole. For example, researchers assessed boys in three different training programs for body physique from ages 11 to 18. Although their physiques changed markedly over the adolescent years, the changes were unrelated to training (Parizkova & Carter, 1976). Postpubescent males typically respond to strength training with muscle hypertrophy in the body

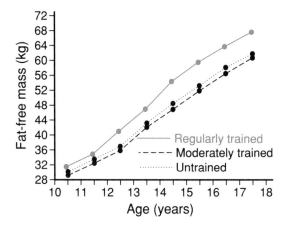

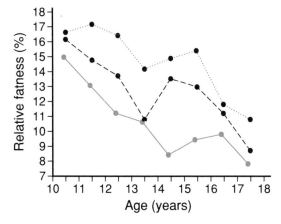

**Figure 2.35**  Fat-free mass and percent fat in boys measured longitudinally and grouped by physical activity level.
(Drawn from data reported by Parizkova, 1974, 1977; reprinted by permission from Malina & Bouchard, 1991.)

areas trained. This can give the appearance of change but does not significantly alter physique. In addition, people often associate mesomorphic (muscular) physiques with successful performance, and more people with such physiques might be chosen for sport participation.

## Maturation

Might physical training alter the timing of maturation in children? The age at which boys reach

their peak height velocity is unaffected by training (Mirwald & Bailey, 1986), and training does not accelerate or decelerate skeletal maturation (Cerney, 1970; Kotulan, Reznickova, & Placheta, 1980; Novotny, 1981). Few longitudinal studies have examined sexual maturation. Both delays and advancements are reported for young athletes in cross-sectional studies, often differing by sport.

*It is difficult to assess training effects on sexual maturation, but training does not appear to influence the overall rate of maturation.*

## Capacity for Exercise

A person's capacity for exercise decreases with age, but evidence is growing that appropriate amounts of regular activity throughout life lessen this decline. As in youth, many factors overlap regular training during adulthood. It is difficult to isolate the effects of regular training because nutrition, exposure to disease, and other factors also influence health status and performance. Yet a number of factors are associated with regular exercise in middle-aged and older adults. Those who exercise regularly have stronger skeletons, stronger muscles, more endurance, and more mobile joints than their inactive cohorts. Exercisers have less fat weight, too. They even demonstrate faster reaction times and score higher on tests of cognitive function and short-term memory than do sedentary adults. Though regular physical exercise is perhaps not the sole cause of these later effects, the improved circulation and oxygenation of tissues, including those of the brain, that accompany regular exercise could account for many of these benefits.

Extreme levels of activity harm adults; both immobility and extremely strenuous work without rest are associated with a shorter life span. Excessive training in sport, dance, and exercise can bring injury. An individual can tolerate modest anatomical imperfections and misalignments in daily activities and moderate exercise. But overuse causes injury when bones, tendons, and muscles cannot withstand the repetitive forces to which they are subjected (Stanish, 1984). Therefore, individuals of any age must learn to moderate their physical activity to achieve a healthful level of participation.

## REVIEW 2.5

After birth, the environment in which the child grows becomes increasingly important to attaining full growth potential. Body tissues and systems are more susceptible to negative environmental factors during periods of rapid growth. The effects of exposure to negative environmental influences, then, can be irreversible at one point in life but minimal at another. Those who work with children need to understand the environmental factors that can affect growth and development. Maintaining a healthy environment is critical if children are to fully attain their growth potential. Those who work with adults must understand the factors that affected growth and development in earlier years as well as those that can still affect good health.

## SUMMARY

Physical growth, maturation, and aging have implications for motor development. The development of the body and its systems potentially controls the rate of motor development. For example, if an individual needs a certain level of strength to perform a particular new skill, then the onset of this skill comes when the muscle system advances to a certain level. Physical maturation also has implications when we compare individual children's motor development to that of other children or to norms.

Early maturers are likely to reach milestones before late maturers. When assessing someone's motor development, we should be aware of that individual's rate of growth and maturation.

It is easier to measure growth than to directly measure maturation. We assess growth with size measures that also can reflect an individual's genetic potential. Maturation measures reflect advancement of the body's tissues and systems in qualitative rather than quantitative terms. Simple means of measuring maturation are not available, but a profile of growth measures can hint at maturation rate when the profile is compared to the norms for an individual's chronological age.

Growth and maturation are subject to the influence of environmental factors. This influence is present prenatally and continues throughout the life span. Environmental factors can be positive, making it likely that individuals reach their genetic potential, or negative. Negative factors can result in subtle changes or slowed growth, but they also can cause serious disorders and have irreversible consequences for development.

Even after an individual reaches adult size, the body's tissues and systems change. These changes reflect the natural aging of the tissue and the influence of environmental factors. Exercise and physical activity have so great an impact on age-related changes in the body that it is sometimes difficult to distinguish the inevitable consequences of aging from those that reflect a societal trend toward a sedentary lifestyle. With this knowledge of growth, maturation, and aging, let us turn next to the course of motor development.

## Key Terms

acceleration curve
anthropometer
anthropometry

appositional growth
catch-up growth
cephalocaudal (development)
congenital
diaphysis
differentiation
distance curve
dominant genetic disorders
epiphyseal (growth) plate
epiphyses
hyperplasia
hypertrophy
hypoxia
motor unit
peak velocity
plasticity
proximodistal (trend)
recessive genetic disorders
secondary sex characteristics
sex-linked disorders
sigmoid (s-shaped) curve
sitting height
teratogen
velocity curve

## Discussion Questions

1. Discuss the differences between measures of growth and direct measures of maturation. What does each measure? What are examples of each?
2. What is the difference between a distance curve and a velocity curve? What does each type of curve tell you about growth? Why are peaks in the velocity curves of interest?
3. In what ways do organs and tissues grow during the embryonic stage? What areas of a fetus's body advance first? In what directions does growth proceed?
4. What is the difference between a dominant genetic disorder and a recessive one?

Are sex-linked disorders dominant or recessive? Are inherited disorders the only source of genetic abnormalities?
5. Describe how teratogens reach a fetus. What are some of the factors that determine the effect a teratogen has on a fetus?
6. Describe the gender differences in the course of overall growth from infancy to adulthood. Include the average ages for entering the adolescent growth spurt, peak height velocity, puberty, and the tapering off of growth in height.
7. What is the epiphyseal growth plate? Why are injuries to growth plates a concern? What is the difference between a pressure epiphysis and a traction epiphysis?
8. What is osteoporosis? What factors contribute to it?
9. Discuss gender differences in the growth of muscle tissue. How does growth of the cardiac muscle compare to that of skeletal muscle and the rest of the body?
10. How does the distribution of fat change over the growth period? How does the amount of fat change in adulthood?
11. What are the major types of hormones involved in growth? How does the body keep the amount of hormone circulating at an appropriate level?
12. What contributes to the rapid gains in brain weight during the first year after birth? What part of the brain is most advanced at birth?
13. What are the two major motor pathways from the brain? What does each control?
14. Choose one environmental factor and describe how it influences growth.
15. What aspects of growth and maturation are affected by regular physical activity or training? How? What aspects are not affected by activity?

## Suggested Readings

Edwards, R.G. (1981). *The beginnings of human life*. Burlington, NC: Carolina Biological Supply.

Falkner, F., & Tanner, J.M. (Eds.) (1978). *Human growth* (Vols. 1-2). New York: Plenum.

Lohman, T.G., Roche, A.F., & Martorell, R. (Eds.) (1988). *Anthropometric standardization reference manual*. Champaign, IL: Human Kinetics.

Lowrey, G.H. (1973). *Growth and development of children*. Chicago: Year Book Medical.

Malina, R.M. (1975). *Growth and development: The first twenty years in man*. Minneapolis: Burgess.

Malina, R.M., & Bouchard, C. (1991). *Growth, maturation, and physical activity*. Champaign, IL: Human Kinetics.

Rarick, G.L. (1973). *Physical activity: Human growth and development*. New York: Academic Press.

Rhodes, P. (1981). *Childbirth*. Burlington, NC: Carolina Biological Supply.

Shephard, R.J. (1982). *Physical activity and growth*. Chicago: Year Book Medical.

Smith, E.L., Sempos, C.T., & Purvis, R.W. (1981). Bone mass and strength decline with age. In E.L. Smith & R.C. Serfass (Eds.), *Exercise and aging: The scientific basis* (pp. 59-87). Hillside, NJ: Enslow.

# Part II
# Change Throughout the Life Span

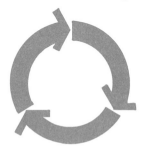

In Part II we look at motor development over the life span. We begin in chapter 3 by focusing on infancy, exploring the developments reflected in random movements and reflexive responses and examining the acquisition of voluntary motor skills. This discussion of early motor behavior concludes with a review of environmental influences on skill development.

Chapter 4 continues with motor development during childhood. The emphasis here is on qualitative changes in skill, so you will first learn about the qualitative characteristics associated with optimum performance. We then review qualitative age-related changes in specific skills—locomotor, ballistic, reception, and weight-transfer skills.

Motor development in adolescence and adulthood is the topic of chapter 5. The changes in adolescence are most often measured quantitatively, so we must consider the factors contributing to quantitative standards of performance. These, in turn, highlight gender differences. In reviewing adult motor behavior, we focus on the extent of change, especially in older adulthood, and the underlying aging processes that might affect skill performance during later life.

# Chapter 3

# Early Motor Behavior

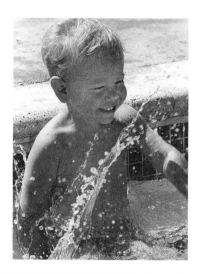

If you watch newborns, you will notice that some of their movements are undirected and without purpose and some of them are reflexive, or automatic. An example of the latter is the sucking motion that begins when a newborn's upper lip is stroked. Older infants acquire the skills to control posture, grasp objects, and move about by sitting up, reaching, crawling, standing, and walking. The process whereby the newborn's undirected movements become, over many years, the graceful and coordinated skills of a mature athlete is intriguing. At what age are children capable of the skilled movements adults take for granted? And how do children refine their skills? In this chapter we will first examine the sequence of motor development, beginning with a discussion of the ways we can assess motor development. Then we will consider reflexive movements, followed by the voluntary, basic skills children acquire during the first 2 years of life.

## ACQUISITION AND REFINEMENT OF NEW SKILLS

The first 3 to 4 months of an infant's life are characterized by involuntary, reflexive movements and by spontaneous movements of the arms and legs. During the 1st year, many of the *reflexes* gradually disappear while the infant acquires the basic rudimentary, but voluntary, movements that lead to grasping with the hands (prehension), upright posture, and locomotion. We could describe motor development, then, in terms of the new skills the infant learns. These skills appear in a sequence that is relatively consistent from child to child, even though the time of their appearance varies. But consider motor development in early childhood. Children acquire new skills—additional locomotor skills such as running and skipping; stationary movements such as turning and twisting; and manipulative skills such as throwing, catching, and kicking. Yet children at-

tempting any of these skills for the first time can only approximate the perfected skills seen in elite performances. Children must repeat these skills again and again to perfect them. Therefore, motor development in early childhood is not just the acquisition of new skills but the refinement of new skills as well.

---

**CONCEPT 3.1**

Motor development is reflected in the appearance of new skills and their refinement in movement process and product.

---

### Skill Refinement: Movement Process and Product

We can gauge skill refinement in several ways. Two methods are important in assessing children's motor skills. One gauge is the *move-*

ment process. This means the movement pattern, or what some might call technique. For example, a right-handed boy who steps forward with his right foot, lifts his elbow up by his ear, and throws by extending his forearm has not mastered the skill of throwing. He could refine his throw by performing it in a more mechanically efficient manner. This gradual transition is termed skill refinement by movement process.

The second gauge of skill refinement is movement product. This means the outcome or result of the movement. For example, as children refine their throwing skills, they throw faster, more accurately, and for longer distances.

---

Process and product are not independent of one another.

---

Refinements in the skill process tend to yield improvements in the product because the individual uses energy more efficiently. Once individuals master an advanced movement pattern, they can still improve the movement product. We can attribute some of this improvement to physical growth and maturation and some to increased strength and endurance. During the preadolescent and adolescent years, individuals typically improve the product of their skills. They may continue to refine the process of skill performance, as well as improve their ability to combine single skills into complex sequences. People in this age group also increase their ability to match or adapt a movement to specific environmental situations and goals. For example, they learn that a forceful throw is appropriate when the person catching the ball is some distance away but is inappropriate when the catcher is close.

## Progress in Motor Development

Thus, we see that progress in motor development can be gauged in several ways:

1. Appearance of new skills
2. Refinements in the movement process
3. Improvements in the movement product
4. Acquisition of skill combinations
5. Improved adaptation to the environment

We can often characterize an age period by advancement in one of these areas (new skills, refinement, etc.), but improvement in different areas can take place simultaneously. That does not mean that all children and adolescents automatically improve just like others in their particular age group or reach the optimal level of motor performance. Individuals may experience slowed or arrested motor development during the growing years. On the other hand, in some children motor development may be rapid. The improvements we describe as characteristic of a given age range are achieved by most, but not necessarily all, children. Often children of the same chronological age exhibit a wide range of skill levels. Think of the difference between a high school student who is just learning basic tennis strokes and an adolescent who is already a successful professional tennis player!

In chapter 2 we stressed the importance of physical maturity to motor development. Because children mature physically at different rates, they acquire new skills and achieve specific levels of movement products (such as the distance of a throw) at different rates. We can attribute some of the variability in skill level at a given chronological age to the variability in physical maturity. Experience and environmental settings also influence motor development. A child who has plenty of practice opportunities is likely to refine a skill at an earlier age than one who does not. This means that individual children might be relatively advanced in some skills but unskilled in others. We can expect, then, skill acquisition and refinement to vary among different children as well as with each individual child.

We can describe motor development in terms of the appearance of new skills, the refinement of the movement pattern used to execute a skill, or the outcome of a movement. We often gauge infants' motor development by the appearance of new basic skills, whereas children's motor development is often measured by refinements in the skill process and product. All of these processes occur throughout infancy and childhood, although the rate of individual skill acquisition and refinement varies. This variability is attributable in large part to differing rates of physical growth and maturation among children and to movement experiences unique to each child. Keeping the extent of this variability in mind, we will next examine the motor development process characteristic of the various age periods, beginning with infancy.

# RANDOM MOVEMENT AND INFANTILE REFLEXES

You may have seen how hungry newborns kick and thrash their arms about. These movements are random, not purposeful, and very common in infants. Or perhaps you have placed your finger in an infant's palm and felt the baby grasp it tightly. This involuntary response is known as the palmar grasping reflex. Many fetal movements and some of an infant's movements in the early postnatal months are reflexive; that is, they are automatic movements triggered by specific stimuli. Later, other reflexes appear that help an infant to maintain posture in changing environmental conditions.

The exact role of *random movement* and the *infantile reflexes* in motor development is still a subject of debate among developmentalists, and considerable controversy exists regarding the relationship of reflexes to later vol-

untary responses. For example, can you accelerate an individual's learning of voluntary skills by repeatedly stimulating his or her reflexes in early life? Developmentalists are taking a new perspective on the relationship of both spontaneous and reflexive movement to later motor development. We will describe in more detail those movements that are characteristic of infants in the early months. Then we will explore their possible relationship to the voluntary skills that emerge later.

## Random Movement

When newborn infants are awake and alert, they move their heads, arms, and legs. The movements are spontaneous and have no goal; they may appear disorganized but are actually coordinated.

### Supine Kicking

Thelen and her colleagues (Thelen, 1985; Thelen & Fisher, 1983; Thelen, Ridley-Johnson, & Fisher, 1983) analyzed the positioning and timing of infants' kicks as they lay on their backs (the supine position). They also recorded the muscular activity in the leg muscles during *supine kicking*. Thelen found that the kicks were rhythmical and had a coordinated pattern. The hip, ankle, and knee joints moved cooperatively, not independently of one another. The kicks had four phases:

1. A flexion phase
2. A pause
3. A forward extension phase
4. A between-kick interval

This is similar in positioning and timing to an adult walking step, with the between-kick interval similar to the stance phase in walking (see Figure 3.1a and b). When an infant kicks faster, the between-kick interval decreases while the other phases keep their timing. When an adult walks, the stance phase decreases as walking speed increases and the leg-swing phase remains constant. The pattern of muscle use in infant supine kicking is also coordinated.

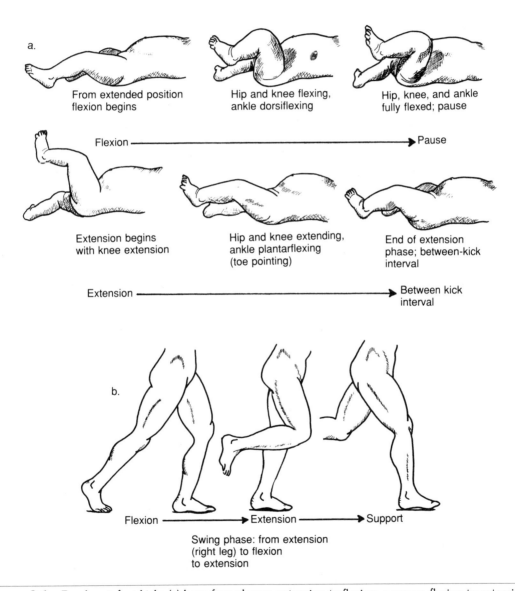

**Figure 3.1** Random infant kicks (a) have four phases: extension to flexion; a pause; flexion to extension; and a between-kick interval. These phases are similar to the adult walking step (b): a swing phase (extension to flexion to extension); and a between-step support phase, similar to the between-kick interval. (a is adapted by permission from Thelen, Bradshaw, & Ward, 1981.)

Sometimes an infant kicks only one leg, but at other times an infant will kick both legs alternately, just as an adult alternates legs in walking. Even premature infants perform coordinated supine kicks (Heriza, 1986).

An infant's supine kicks are similar to an adult's walking steps, but they are not identical. Infants' timing is more variable from kick to kick, and they tend to move the joints more in unison than in sequence. Infants also tend to activate both the muscles for flexing the limb (flexors) and the muscles for extending the limb (extensors), termed *co-contraction*. The flexion is stronger and the limb moves. In contrast, adults activate the flexors but relax the extensors through reciprocal innervation, which allows antagonistic muscles to act in this coordinated manner, and the joints move sequentially. So infants' kicks are coordinated but not identical to adult movement. By the end of their 1st year, however, infants begin to move the hip, knee, and ankle joints sequentially rather than in tight unison. Both alternating and synchronous (both legs in unison) kicks are evident after 6 months, indicating that infants are developing more ways to coordinate the two limbs (Thelen, 1985; Thelen & Fisher, 1983; Thelen et al., 1983).

### Spontaneous Arm Movements

The *spontaneous arm movements* of newborns also show well-coordinated extensions of the elbow, wrist, and finger joints; that is, the joints do not extend independently, or one at a time, but at the same time. Arm movements are not as rhythmical and repetitious as leg kicks (Thelen, 1981; Thelen, Kelso, & Fogel, 1987). Early arm thrusts are not identical to adults' reaching movements. It takes infants several months to begin opening their fingers independently of the other joints in anticipation of grasping objects, as adults do (Trevarthan, 1984; von Hofsten, 1982, 1984).

---

Arm reaches and leg kicks in the newborn are coordinated movements. These movements undergo change such that by the end of the 1st year or so, infants can walk upright, grasp objects, and feed themselves.

---

Later, we will discuss the role of arm reaches and leg kicks in motor development and their relation to complex voluntary skills.

## Infantile Reflexes

Unlike random movements, reflexes are involuntary movements that a person makes in response to specific stimuli, sometimes only when the body is positioned in a particular way. A person does not have to think about making reflexive responses; they are automatic. Some reflexes, like eye blinking, are present throughout the life span, but others are present only in infancy. Table 3.1 categorizes many of the infantile reflexes and reactions into three types:

1. Primitive reflexes
2. Postural reactions
3. Locomotor reflexes (see also Figure 3.2a-d).

### Primitive Reflexes

*Primitive reflexes*, the first group, are involuntary responses, many of which are mediated by the lower brain centers (Peiper, 1963). Many of these reflexes function prenatally and can be elicited in utero or in premature infants. One of their prenatal functions might be to help the fetus move around in the uterine cavity to position itself for birth (Milani-Comparetti, 1981). At birth and in the first days afterward, some primitive reflexes are necessary for survival. For example, the Moro reflex assists with the first inspiration, and the sucking and

**Table 3.1   The Reflexes**

| Reflex/reaction | Starting position (if important) | Stimulus | Response | Time | Warning signs |
|---|---|---|---|---|---|
| *Primitive reflexes* | | | | | |
| Asymmetrical tonic neck reflex | Supine | Turn head to one side | Same-side arm and leg extend | Prenatal to 4 mo | Persistence after 6 mo |
| Symmetrical tonic neck reflex | Supported sitting | Extend head and neck<br>Flex head and neck | Arms extend, legs flex<br>Arms flex, legs extend | 6 mo to 7 mo | |
| Doll-eye | | Flex head<br>Extend head | Eyes look up<br>Eyes look down | Prenatal to 2 wk | Persistence after first days of life |
| Palmar grasping | | Touch palm with finger or object | Hand closes tightly around object | Prenatal to 4 mo | Persistence after 1 yr; asymmetrical reflex |
| Moro | Supine | Shake head, as by tapping pillow | Arms and legs extend, fingers spread; then arms and legs flex | Prenatal to 3 mo | Presence after 6 mo; asymmetrical reflex |
| Sucking | | Touch face above or below lips | Sucking motion begins | B to 3 mo | |
| Babinski | | Stroke sole of foot from heel to toes | Toes extend | B to 4 mo | Persistence after 6 mo |
| Searching or rooting | | Touch cheek with smooth object | Head turns to side stimulated | B to 1 yr | Absence of reflex; persistence after 1 yr |
| Palmar-mandibular (Babkin) | | Apply pressure to both palms | Mouth opens; eyes close; head flexes | 1 to 3 mo | |
| Plantar grasping | | Stroke ball of foot | Toes contract around object stroking foot | B to 12 mo | |

*(continued)*

**Table 3.1**  *(continued)*

| Reflex/reaction | Starting position (if important) | Stimulus | Response | Time | Warning signs |
|---|---|---|---|---|---|
| Startle | Supine | Tap abdomen or startle infant | Arms and legs flex | 7 to 12 mo | |
| *Postural reactions* | | | | | |
| Derotative righting | Supine | Turn legs and pelvis to other side | Trunk and head follow rotation | From 4 mo | |
| | Supine | Turn head sideways | Body follows head in rotation | From 4 mo | |
| Labyrinthine righting reflex | Supported upright | Tilt infant | Head moves to stay upright | 2 to 12 mo | |
| Pull-up | Sitting upright, held by 1 or 2 hands | Tip infant backward or forward | Arms flex | 3 to 12 mo | |
| Parachute | Held upright | Lower infant toward ground rapidly | Legs extend | From 4 mo | |
| | Held upright | Tilt forward | Arms extend | From 7 mo | |
| | Held upright | Tilt sideways | Arms extend | From 6 mo | |
| | Held upright | Tilt backwards | Arms extend | From 9 mo | |
| *Locomotor reflexes* | | | | | |
| Crawling | Prone | Apply pressure to sole of one foot or both feet alternately | Crawling pattern in arms and legs | B to 4 mo | |
| Walking | Held upright | Place infant on flat surface | Walking pattern in legs | B to 5 mo | |
| Swimming | Prone | Place infant in or over water | Swimming movement of arms and legs | 11 days to 5 mo | |

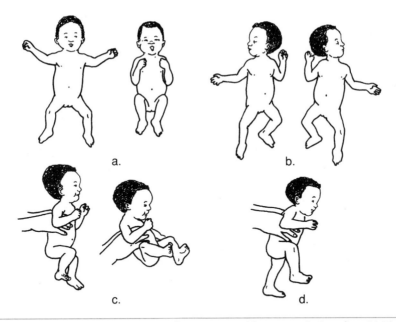

**Figure 3.2** Selected reflexes. (a) The Moro reflex. Arms and legs extend, then flex. (b) The asymmetrical tonic neck reflex. Note the fencer's position. (c) The labyrinthine righting reflex. The infant rights the head when tipped backward. (d) The walking reflex.

rooting reflexes enable the newborn to feed (Milani-Comparetti, 1981). Some of the primitive reflexes, such as the asymmetric tonic neck reflex, must disappear before the infant can attain the postures required for voluntary motor acts (Milani-Comparetti, 1967).

## Postural Reactions

As their name implies, *postural reactions* (or gravity reflexes) help the infant to automatically maintain posture in a changing environment (Peiper, 1963). Some of these responses keep the head upright, thereby keeping the breathing passages open. Others help the infant roll over and eventually attain a vertical position. They generally appear after the infant is 2 months old. For example, an infant can roll

over only after derotative righting appears after 4 months of age. By late in the 1st year or early in the 2nd year of life, the postural reactions drop out of the infant's repertoire of movements as isolated reactions requiring specific postures and stimuli. Children and adults, of course, react to being thrown off balance with specific muscle responses intended to bring the body back into balance. We will discuss this topic in chapter 6.

## Locomotor Reflexes

The last category is the *locomotor reflexes* These actions appear to be related to the voluntary behaviors from which they take their individual names, such as the walking reflex. The locomotor reflexes appear much earlier than the corresponding voluntary behaviors and typically disappear months before the infant attempts the voluntary locomotor skills.

## Appearance and Disappearance of Reflexes

Infantile reflexes gradually weaken as the infant matures until they can no longer be stimulated. Those who work with infants sometimes use the pattern of reflex appearance and disappearance to assess an individual infant's development. If the reflexes appear and disappear at an age close to the average, development is considered normal. Deviation from the normal pattern and execution of the response may signal a problem. A reflex that persists well after the average age of disappearance could possibly indicate a pathological cerebral condition (Peiper, 1963). A nonexistent or very weak response on one side of the body compared to the other also could reflect a pathological condition.

---

The reappearance of an infantile reflex later in life is associated with neuropathology.

---

Remember that individuals develop on their own time schedules and can be ahead of or behind these average ages. In addition, the exact time a reflex disappears is often difficult to establish. Only when the reflex persists for several months past the average might it constitute a warning sign of a pathological condition. Reflexive responses are very sensitive to environmental conditions. The infant's body position and the stimulus must be as indicated in Table 3.1 or there will be no response. An untrained person might overlook some aspect of the environment, fail to elicit a response, and incorrectly conclude that a pathological condition exists. Therefore, it is best to rely on trained professionals for such assessments.

## Views on the Role of Reflexes

The role of reflexes in motor development is unclear. Some theorists believe that reflexes merely reflect the structure of the nervous system—in other words, the way humans are "wired." Others take the view that reflexive movements lead to coordinated limb movements (Peiper, 1963), giving the infant the opportunity to practice coordinated movements before the higher brain centers are ready to mediate such actions. Still others (Molnar, 1978) suggest that certain primitive reflexes must disappear and posture reactions appear before an infant can undertake some of the basic voluntary motor skills such as rolling, sitting, and walking. Consider the asymmetrical tonic neck reflex, a primitive reflex elicited when an infant is lying supine. If the head is turned to one side, the arm and leg on that side of the body extend. This reflex must be inhibited so that the infant can perform the body and neck righting reactions (described in Table 3.1) without the extended arm getting in the way of a roll. The body and neck righting reactions are necessary because the upper and lower trunk must turn sequentially in voluntary rolling (Roberton, 1984). We can detect similar transitions for other voluntary skills.

Many of the traditional views on reflexive movements reflect the maturation perspective. Now, developmentalists who work from the dynamic systems perspective offer a different idea of the role reflexes play in motor development. Next, we will consider these two perspectives on reflexes in more detail.

### Maturation Perspective

Maturationists consider the existence and disappearance of reflexes as evidence of nervous system growth and development. Recall that the maturationists of the 1930s and 1940s tended to link behavior to the development of just one system, the nervous system, and that this perspective tended to dominate explanations of development for decades thereafter.

---

*Maturationists interpret the high level of reflex activity in prenatal and early postnatal life as an indication of cerebral cortex (higher brain) immaturity.*

---

As maturation of the cortex and the spinal motor nerve pathways proceeds, the cortical centers assume control of the lower brain and spinal cord centers. This is thought to take place at about 3 to 4 months after birth, the time when many primitive reflexes either disappear (that is, are inhibited by the cortical centers) or become localized (specific to a particular part of the nervous system) (Peiper, 1963). This transition occurs in a fairly predictable but gradual time sequence.

As more research emerged, developmentalists began to question the maturation explanation. Zelazo and his co-workers (Zelazo, Konner, Kolb, & Zelazo, 1974; Zelazo, Zelazo, & Kolb, 1972a, 1972b) elicited the walking reflex daily in a small number of infants during their first 8 weeks. This daily practice actually increased the walking reflex in these infants. It also resulted in the earlier onset of voluntary walking compared to infants who did not practice the reflex. The investigators concluded that the involuntary walking reflex could be transformed to voluntary walking (see also Zelazo, 1983). They proposed that the disappearance of the reflex was due to disuse, that the period of reflex inhibition before onset of the voluntary skill was unnecessary, and that systematic stimulation of a locomotor reflex could enhance infants' acquisition of voluntary locomotion.

## Dynamic Systems Perspective

Thelen (1983) also questioned whether the reflex inhibition period was a necessary consequence of nervous system maturation. She proposed a different explanation for the walking reflex's disappearance. Thelen observed that 4- to 6-week-old infants who normally performed the reflex reduced their responses when small weights were added to their ankles, mimicking the dramatic increase in leg mass (skeletal weight, muscle weight, and especially fat weight) during the 2 months after birth. Hence, the walking reflex may disappear because the infant has insufficient strength to lift the now-heavier legs.

Change in strength could explain Zelazo's finding of increased stepping responses as well: Perhaps the "walking" practice that Zelazo provided served as training to increase leg strength so that the growing infants could continue to step even with heavier limbs. Thelen also observed an increase in stepping when she submerged the infants in water to their chests, the water buoying the legs. Finally, Thelen (1986) found that infants at 7 months who otherwise inhibited the stepping reflex did "step" when held over the moving belt of a motorized treadmill (see Figure 3.3).

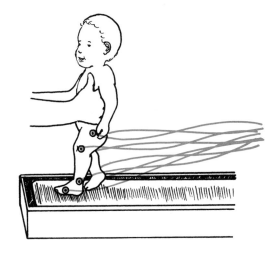

**Figure 3.3** The moving belt of a motorized treadmill elicits stepping in infants who otherwise inhibit the stepping reflex.
(Drawn from a photograph provided by Esther Thelen, Indiana University.)

> The increase and decrease of stepping with changes in the environmental context (moving treadmill belt and manipulation of leg weight) indicate that systems other than the nervous system must be involved in this aspect of motor development. If inhibition of the locomotor reflexes is connected only to nervous system maturation, such manipulations could not increase the stepping response.

Thelen and her colleagues (Thelen, Bradshaw, & Ward, 1981; Thelen & Fisher, 1982) further compared the steps of the walking reflex to the kicks infants perform while lying on their backs. The steps and kicks were identical in the positioning and timing of joint movements. This has implications for our understanding of the role of the nervous system in such movements. The similarity of supine kicks and upright steps in an infant with an immature cerebral cortex can mean that such fundamental movements are mediated by lower centers, even in the spinal cord, called *movement pattern generators* (Grillner, 1975). The many muscles, crossing several joints, share a systematic relationship mediated at the spinal cord so that the higher brain centers are not necessarily involved in directing the details of movements such as reaching or stepping (Kelso, Holt, Kugler, & Turvey, 1980; Kugler et al., 1980). Most likely, a generator exists for each limb (Forssberg, 1982). Such generators account for the execution of steps in research animals deprived of their cerebral cortex. The movement pattern generator then mediates the reflexive movement that is shaped by the infant's environment. We will discuss pattern generators again as we consider the development of voluntary motor skills.

**REVIEW 3.2**

Some of an infant's movements in the early months are primitive, involuntary reflexes pre-sumably mediated by lower brain centers. These reflexes soon disappear and postural reactions appear. Locomotor reflexes also appear during an infant's 1st year. They tend to disappear months before voluntary locomotion occurs, but whether this is linked only to neurologic maturation is doubtful. Though developmentalists still do not completely understand the role of reflexes in motor development, the dynamic systems perspective has provided some clues. Moreover, the similarity between random supine kicks and the steps of the walking reflex adds to our knowledge of the nervous system's role in such movements. Systematic relationships of limb muscles, called pattern generators, are established at the spinal cord level so that an infant can perform a step or kick without the higher brain centers specifically directing every aspect of the movement. The environment, especially gravity, affects the movement outcome as well.

Reflexes may disappear or become localized as the body's systems mature. These include the nervous system, muscular system, skeletal system, and adipose tissue system. As the infant continues to develop, the higher brain centers begin to use the pattern generators in directing more complex and voluntary movements. We will turn now to the voluntary skills that the infant acquires early in life.

## MOTOR MILESTONES

In the 1st year of life, children acquire locomotion and visually guided reaching through a series of new motor skills. We often refer to these new skills as *motor milestones* because they are fundamental to skilled performances and because the acquisition of each skill is a landmark in the individual's motor development. For example, infants first learn to hold their heads erect, then to sit, then to stand,

and then to walk. Individual infants vary in the time they reach a motor milestone, but they acquire these different rudimentary skills in a relatively consistent sequence. The average ages at which infants achieve these various skills are well documented (Bayley, 1935; Shirley, 1963). This progressive pattern of skill acquisition is related in part to physical maturation, especially

- maturation of the central nervous system,
- development of muscular strength and endurance,
- development of posture and balance, and
- improvement in sensory processing.

The onset of a certain skill can require that a certain system be developed to a particular level. Thus, partly because these systems advance earlier in some infants than in others, the rate of appearance of the motor milestones varies. Environmental factors also play a role in individual variability. The orderly, sequential acquisition of rudimentary skills is the beginning of the process that leads to the amazingly complex movements of mature performers. We will examine this process in more detail to better understand the development of motor skills. Let us consider first the acquisition of locomotor skills, and then the achievement of reaching and grasping.

---

**CONCEPT 3.3**
Infants achieve control of their environment by acquiring the motor milestone skills in an identified sequence.

---

## Locomotor Milestones

Five developmentalists provided us with information about the appearance of the motor milestones: Mary Shirley (1931, 1933), Nancy Bayley (1935), Louise Ames (1937), Arnold Gesell (1939, 1946; Gesell & Ames, 1940),

and Myrtle McGraw (1940, 1943). All reflect the maturation perspective. The authors basically agree on the sequential appearance of the motor milestones but have found minor variations in the age at onset of some milestone skills. The variations probably reflect several factors that differentially affect the infant groups each author studied: differences in growth and maturation rate, in environmental factors (such as climate, number of siblings, and child-rearing practices), and in the author's scoring criteria. The researchers also approached motor development from slightly different viewpoints. Each made a unique contribution to our knowledge of locomotor development in early postnatal life.

### The Work of Mary Shirley and Nancy Bayley

The studies by Shirley and Bayley are largely descriptive. They determined the sequence and average age at onset of the motor milestones by carefully observing groups of infants. Selected milestone skills from Shirley's early work and from the Bayley Scale of Infant Development (Bayley, 1969), based on Bayley's 1935 work, are displayed in Table 3.2. Note that due to a secular trend, infants born in recent years reach the milestones at slightly earlier ages than did infants of earlier generations. Age at onset is generally younger on the Bayley Scale from 1969 than on the Shirley Sequence from the 1930s. Children observed in the 1980s reached milestone skills at average ages similar to those given on the Bayley Scale and much younger than those on the Shirley Sequence or reported by Gesell in 1934 (Capute, Shapiro, Palmer, Ross, & Wachtel, 1985; Gesell & Thompson, 1934).

Infants generally achieve postural control of the upper body by about 5 months, according to the scales, then control of the entire trunk during the next 3 months. Rolling from back to front is an important milestone skill. Infants, even if placed on their backs, can get to the

**Table 3.2  Selected Motor Milestones**

| Average age (mo) | Age range (mo) | Milestone (Bayley Scale of Infant Development) | Milestone (Shirley Sequence) |
|---|---|---|---|
| 0.1 | | Lifts head when held at shoulder | |
| 0.1 | | Lateral head movements | |
| 0.8 | 0.3- 3.0 | Retains red ring | |
| 0.8 | 0.3- 2.0 | Arm thrusts in play | |
| 0.8 | 0.3- 2.0 | Leg thrusts in play | Chin up |
| 1.6 | 0.7- 4.0 | Head erect and steady | |
| 1.8 | 0.7- 5.0 | Turns from side to back | |
| 2.0 | | | Chest up |
| 2.3 | 1.0- 5.0 | Sits with slight support | |
| 4.0 | | | Sits with support |
| 4.4 | 2.0- 7.0 | Turns from back to side | |
| 4.9 | 4.0- 8.0 | Partial thumb opposition | |
| 5.0 | | | Sits on lap |
| | | | Grasps object |
| 5.3 | 4.0- 8.0 | Sits alone momentarily | |
| 5.4 | 4.0- 8.0 | Unilateral reaching | |
| 5.7 | 4.0- 8.0 | Rotates wrist | |
| 6.0 | | | Sits in chair |
| | | | Grasps dangling object |
| 6.4 | 4.0-10.0 | Rolls from back to front | |
| 6.6 | 5.0- 9.0 | Sits alone steadily | |
| 6.9 | 5.0- 9.0 | Complete thumb opposition | |
| 7.0 | | | Sits alone |
| 7.1 | 5.0-11.0 | Prewalking progression | |
| 7.4 | 6.0-10.0 | Partial finger prehension | |
| 8.0 | | | Stands with help |
| 8.1 | 5.0-12.0 | Pulls to standing | |
| 8.6 | 6.0-12.0 | Stands up by furniture | |
| 8.8 | 6.0-12.0 | Stepping movements | |
| 9.0 | | | Stands holding furniture |
| 9.6 | 7.0-12.0 | Walks with help | |
| 10.0 | | | Creeps |
| 11.0 | 9.0-16.0 | Stands alone | Walks when led |
| 11.7 | 9.0-17.0 | Walks alone | |
| 12.0 | | | Pulls to stand |
| 14.0 | | | Stands alone |
| 14.6 | 11.0-20.0 | Walks backward | |
| 15.0 | | | Walks alone |
| 16.1 | 12.0-23.0 | Walks up stairs with help | |
| 16.4 | 13.0-23.0 | Walks down stairs with help | |
| 23.4 | 17.0-30.0+ | Jumps off floor, both feet | |
| 24.8 | 19.0-30.0+ | Jumps from bottom step | |

prone position by 8 months of age. By about the 9th month, infants attempt locomotion from the prone position through a sequence of achievements leading to creeping. In everyday terms we often call moving on hands and knees *crawling* In the developmental literature, *crawling* often indicates movement with the abdomen still on the floor, whereas *creeping* describes movement on hands and knees with the stomach off the floor. As students, you must read sources closely to determine the definition of crawling each author uses. Here we will use the terms as they are used in the developmental literature.

The work of Ames (1937) focused on the sequential pattern of development leading to creeping. This progression begins at about 7 months with the infant drawing the knee and

thigh forward beside the body. Within a few weeks the infant can assume a low creeping position and several weeks later creep about the floor. Once infants can assume the high creeping position, they may rock back and forth on their hands and knees or creep backward before learning to creep forward.

The milestone skills identified by Bayley in Table 3.2 (see also Figure 3.4) also point out that infants achieve coordination for walking at approximately 11 to 12 months. The child initially learns to stand with adult help or supported by furniture, then begins to walk along the furniture or when led by an adult. Eventually the child is able to stand and then walk alone. In the next few months the child masters walking in different directions and on steps. A child usually begins negotiating steps

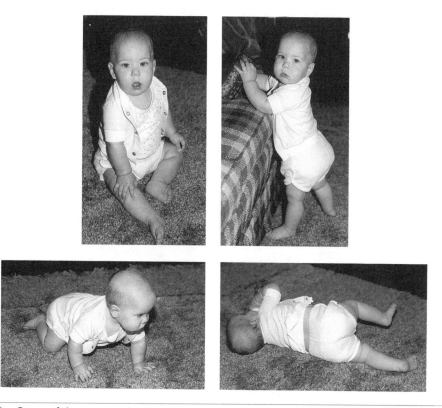

**Figure 3.4**   Some of the motor milestone skills.

with a *mark-time pattern*: He or she places one foot on a step, then places the other foot on the same step rather than on the next higher one. Eventually the child masters the mature, alternate-stepping pattern.

---

Attaining locomotion is a significant achievement for infants. No longer must they be relegated to the role of spectator—now they can move independently to the places in their environment they wish to explore.

---

## Gender Differences

Neither of the published motor milestone charts lists separate ages of skill acquisition for boys and girls, simply because no significant gender differences exist in the sequence of skill acquisition or in the average ages for skill onset. As we noted in chapter 2, girls mature physically a bit faster than boys on the average, so the average girl may acquire the milestones slightly earlier than the average boy. But for all practical purposes, individual differences in the rate of development overshadow these small average gender differences.

## Views on Locomotor Milestones

A description of what locomotor skills infants acquire and when they acquire them is valuable and interesting. Even more interesting is knowing what brings about these remarkable changes. How is it that an infant executes a completely new skill? Why does the infant first execute it at that time? Why not sooner? These questions have intrigued developmentalists for decades. In fact, questioning the source of new behavior is fundamental to many areas of study (Thelen, 1989). Let us consider from two differing perspectives some of the factors that might bring about new skills.

## Maturation Perspective

The maturationists of the 1930s and 1940s are best known for their descriptive research of what skills infants acquire and when they acquire them, but these researchers also attempted to explain why new skills emerged (Clark & Whitall, 1989a). Neuroanatomists of the era were making advances in identifying structural changes in the infant brain (e.g., Conel, 1939). Perhaps this led developmentalists to emphasize the relationship between new skill emergence and neuromuscular maturation alone.

### The Work of Myrtle McGraw

Myrtle McGraw (1940, 1943) attempted to link the progression from lying prone to creeping and eventually to upright locomotion to the development of cortical (cerebral cortex) control over muscle function. She noted that infants acquire muscle function in a cephalocaudal direction. McGraw used seven phases to describe the progression to erect locomotion:

*Phase I:* Walking reflex (birth to 5 months)
- Child makes reflexive stepping movements when held over a surface.
- The lower brain centers control the movement.

*Phase II:* Inhibition (4 to 5 months)
- The walking reflex diminishes.
- Higher brain centers inhibit subcortical control.
- Child achieves control of head movement.

*Phase III:* Transition (4 to 7.5 months)
- A child held upright over a surface makes stepping or bouncing movements.
- Advancing cortical maturation is evident.
- Child displays better trunk control.

*Phase IV:* Deliberate stepping (7.5 to 9 months)

- Child walks when led by an adult.
- Child displays better foot control.

*Phase V:* Independent stepping phase (9 to 15 months)

- Child takes flat-footed steps.
- Movement demands less conscious attention from the cortex.
- Walking movements become more and more automatic.

*Phase VI:* Heel-toe progression (after 18 months)

- Child transfers weight from heel to toe.
- Trend toward automaticity continues.

*Phase VII:* Maturity (at approximately 2.5 years)

- Child swings opposite arm and leg simultaneously.
- Muscular control is optimal.
- Little attention is required to execute walking steps.

Hence, the child achieves cortical control, which leads to the establishment of muscle action patterns that can be carried out without conscious control.

## The Work of Arnold Gesell and Louise Ames

Gesell and Ames (1940) described early motor development by emphasizing the alternation between dominance of extension (straightening) and dominance of flexion (bending) movements of the limbs as children achieve upright locomotion. These researchers noted the prevalence of extension or flexion for unilateral (one side of the body), bilateral (both sides), and cross-lateral (opposite hand and foot) movements as well.

For example, the newborn's dominant pattern of limb movement is bilateral flexion, as in bending both arms. Over the first 7 months unilateral flexion of the limbs gradually replaces bilateral flexion. But an infant reverts to bilateral flexion when he or she first attempts to lift the trunk from the floor. As an infant attempts locomotor skills (backward crawling, rocking on hands and knees, creeping), he or she displays bilateral arm extension and bilateral leg flexion and extension. The infant must learn to move the opposite limbs alternately—that is, to use cross-lateral patterns of movement in order to creep. This alternation is repeated with standing and walking. The infant again reverts to bilateral extension when learning to stand at 10 to 14 months but eventually masters alternate arm and leg movements in attempting his or her first walking steps.

Gesell and Ames noted that the direction of progress in locomotion is cephalocaudal and proximodistal, the pattern reflecting advancement in neuromotor coordination. Again, it is evident that maturationists link the onset of the locomotor milestones to nervous system development.

### Reversion

The type of analysis of early motor development that Gesell and Ames used highlights an interesting facet of skill development: *reversion*, or *regression*. An infant reverts to a pattern of movement he or she has previously "outgrown" when faced with learning a new skill in a new posture. After all, this new skill requires a higher center of gravity and a smaller base of support than previously learned skills. An infant initially meets the challenge of this more difficult skill by using a simple bilateral limb movement to assume a stationary position. As the infant gains skill and confidence, he or she progresses to alternate-limb actions.

## Dynamic Systems Perspective

From the dynamic systems perspective, locomotor development is a consequence of the development of various body systems, the task to be undertaken, and the environmental context in which the task is done. This is in contrast to the maturation perspective.

## Rate Controllers

Consideration of multiple systems provides developmentalists the opportunity to identify which of the many systems is important to the onset of new skills. It is possible that many of the body's systems have developed to the point where a new skill is possible but that one or more other systems are slower in developing. The new behavior cannot start until these slower developing systems reach a critical point. As we saw in chapter 1, dynamic systems developmentalists call these systems *rate controllers*, or rate limiters, for that particular behavior—that is, these systems limit the rate of development.

---

For maturationists, the nervous system is always the rate controller. Dynamic systems developmentalists consider many systems in determining the rate-controlling factors in development.

---

Let us consider two locomotor milestones, creeping and walking, and the systems that might be rate controllers for these two skills.

## Creeping

Recall the milestone skills that make up the progression leading to creeping:

1. Crawling with the chest and stomach on the floor
2. Low creeping with the stomach off the floor but the legs working together (symmetrically)
3. Rocking back and forth in the high-creep position
4. Creeping with the legs and arms working alternately

Notice that in making the transition from rocking to creeping, infants must progress from a bilateral to a cross-lateral movement pattern. What might initiate this transition? Goldfield (1989) proposed that head orientation, hand preference, and kicking play a role in the transition. He videotaped the crawling and rocking movements of infants until they began to creep and also noted whether the infants used either hand or one hand in particular to reach for a toy placed directly in front of them. Before infants were able to raise the trunk off the floor, they tended to link leg activity and arm position to head orientation. If the head turned to the left, for example, the left arm likely extended and the right leg kicked. So infants demonstrate a cross-lateral link but lack the strength to push against the surface and raise the trunk from the floor. When arm strength increases, infants can push to the high-creep position, but they need both arms for support. The symmetrical, bilateral movement pattern still dominates.

Goldfield noted that during the crawling and rocking periods of locomotor development, infants use either hand to reach. As they spend more and more time rocking in the high-creep position, infants develop the strength and balance to support themselves in a tripod with one arm off the ground. At about the same time, they develop a preference for using one hand, and this is the hand they use to begin creeping forward.

The onset of creeping on hands and knees, then, occurs when the infant's balance and muscular systems advance to permit a tripod stance and when the infant demonstrates strong hand preference. The progression to creeping in steps may reflect the development of these systems and related functions (see Table 3.3 and Figure 3.5). Eventually, the infant develops the strength and balance to support the body's weight on one arm and the opposite leg while the other two limbs move forward (Benson, 1985, 1987, 1990). Hence, the alternating, cross-lateral pattern is firmly established.

**Table 3.3   Development of Three Independent Functions Contributing to Crawling Development**

| Stage | Orienting | Reaching | Kicking |
|---|---|---|---|
| Early | Achieves head control | Uses hands to reach, not support weight | Kicks but doesn't plant feet on surface |
| Middle | Orients head away from body midline | Uses hand to reach and support but not at the same time | Creates friction with feet and legs to push forward |
| Late | Raises head, shifts weight backward | Prefers to reach with one hand | Kicks leg opposite reaching arm |

Adapted by permission from Goldfield, 1989.

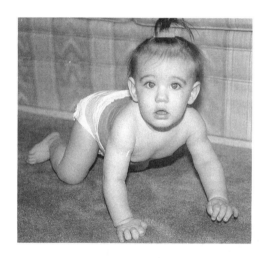

**Figure 3.5**   Balance and strength must be sufficient for infants to support themselves, first on three limbs and eventually on one arm and the opposite leg in creeping.

## Walking

Recall that Thelen (1986) observed alternate-leg stepping in 7-month-old infants held over a moving treadmill belt and that creeping 9-month-olds use an alternate, cross-lateral movement pattern. By the time they creep, infants have the elements of limb coordination needed for walking. What then do they lack

for independent walking? Thelen et al. (1989) suggest that the rate-controlling factors for walking are (a) muscle strength in the trunk and leg extensor muscles to allow the infant to maintain an upright posture on a small base of support, and (b) the development of balance to the point that the infant can compensate for a shift of weight from one leg to the other. The characteristics of infants' early walking are consistent with this suggestion. Early walking is characterized by a short stride, a flat-footed step, little coordinated arm action, and more variable timing between the two legs (Burnett & Johnson, 1971; Clark, Whitall, & Phillips, 1988; Sutherland, Olshen, Cooper, & Woo, 1980). All of these factors are consistent with just-adequate strength and dynamic balance. In fact, for children new to walking, the timing of their steps is more adultlike when adults hold their hands as they walk, thus assisting their strength and balance (Clark et al., 1988).

From the dynamic systems perspective, then, the onset of locomotor milestones is a consequence of the development of many systems. The rate-controlling system is not necessarily the nervous system alone. In fact, for two key locomotor milestones, creeping and walking, muscle strength, posture, and balance appear to be important limiting factors.

## Reaching and Grasping Milestones

Reaching for, grasping, and manipulating objects is important in a variety of endeavors ranging from eating to typing to playing the piano. These motor skills are also important in skilled sport performance—think about the skills an athlete needs to field a baseball, rebound a basketball, or swing a racket.

### Prehension

In 1931, H.M. Halverson published a classic description of grasping development, the 10 phases of which are summarized in Figure 3.6. In early grasping, the infant squeezes an object against the palm. Soon he or she can place the object in the thumb side of the palm and eventually use the thumb in a pincer movement opposing the forefinger. Early arm reaches are imprecise; the infant tends to thrust the hand forward, then lower it onto the object. Later the infant might reach for even a small object with both hands, because an error with one hand still pushes the object into the other hand so the infant can squeeze it between the two. At about 10 months the infant begins to master a continuous, direct reach and grasp with one hand.

Hence, this early research established the development of prehension as a sequence of steps or phases. Halverson's work was published in the 1930s, and maturationists of the era viewed the age-related changes in prehension much as they did the locomotor milestones. They linked the onset of a new grip configuration to neuromotor maturation. Later, developmentalists with an information processing perspective linked Halverson's steps of grip development to infants' advancing cognitive capacity. As they saw it, new grip configurations emerged as infants acquired more motor programs for prehension. Consider, though, that Halverson's phases reflect a single set of environment and task characteristics. For example, he used a 1-in. cube as the

| Type of Grasp | Weeks of Age | |
|---|---|---|
| No Contact | 16 | |
| Contact Only | 20 | |
| Primitive Squeeze | 20 | |
| Squeeze Grasp | 24 | |
| Hand Grasp | 28 | |
| Palm Grasp | 28 | |
| Superior-Palm Grasp | 32 | |
| Inferior-Forefinger Grasp | 36 | |
| Forefinger Grasp | 52 | |
| Superior-Forefinger Grasp | 52 | |

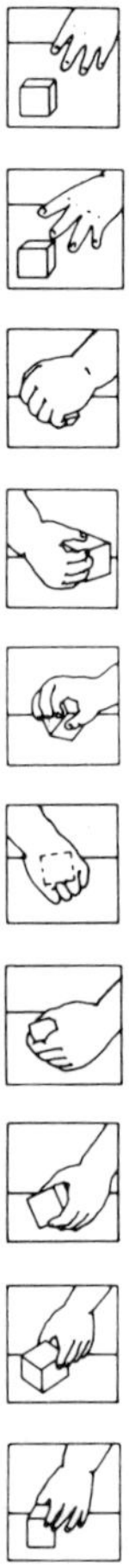

Figure 3.6　A developmental grasping progression.
(Reprinted by permission from Halverson, 1931.)

object for the infants to grasp. What grip would infants use if an object of a different size or shape was placed in front of them? What if the infant is positioned differently? In fact, when researchers vary these task characteristics, "new" grip configurations appear (Newell, Scully, McDonald, & Baillargeon, 1989; see Figure 3.7). For example, 4- to 8-month-old infants use fewer fingers to grasp small objects than to grasp large objects.

Evidence that infants adapt their grips to different environments and tasks presents the

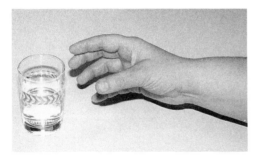
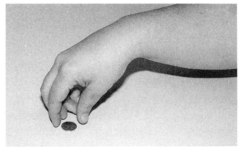
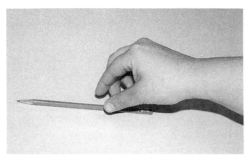

Figure 3.7 The type of grip one uses to pick up an object depends in part on the size and shape of the object. An adult configures or shapes the hand for the object to be grasped before making contact.

same problem in the maturational and cognitive perspectives on development as did evidence of stepping in new environments (buoyed by water or supported on a treadmill). If we can elicit a behavior at an earlier age by changing the environment or task, then the nervous system must be capable of controlling that movement. Again, it seems that nervous system development alone cannot account for the onset of new skills. From the dynamic systems perspective, the environmental context may bring out different movement behaviors.

## Reaching

Recent research also focuses on the nature of reaching in the newborn. During their 1st year, infants exhibit three types of reaching:

1. Prereaching (birth to 4 months)
2. Visually guided reaching (4 to 8 months)
3. Visually elicited reaching (9+ months) (Bushnell, 1985)

Let us examine each type.

### Prereaching

Contradictory hypotheses have prompted research on prereaching (see Whitall, 1988a, for a review). The traditional viewpoint is that in newborns, reaching is limited to excited thrashing of the limbs and reflexive movements (White, Castle, & Held, 1964). But Bower and his colleagues (Bower, 1972, 1977; Bower, Broughton, & Moore, 1970a, 1970b, 1970c) contend that newborns demonstrate eye-hand coordination. They observed newborns reaching toward objects and making grasping motions, although actual contact with the objects was sporadic. These extension movements in the newborn are called *prereaching* Moving objects trigger prereaching better than stationary ones, and infants prereach more often when they fix their gaze on an object (von Hofsten, 1982).

The controversy over the degree of eye-hand coordination in newborns is fueled by researchers who failed to replicate Bower's results (Dodwell, Muir, & DiFranco, 1976; Ruff & Halton, 1978). A variable that influences results is the infant's posture. The researcher observing prereaching movements typically supports the infant in an upright sitting position with the arms free to move. So posture is a rate controller for prereaching, and typically it occurs only when an infant's trunk is supported. Even if some degree of eye-hand coordination is present in newborns, important differences still exist between prereaching and the reaching that older children demonstrate:

- Newborns do not use visual information to guide their hands to objects.
- Infants do not correct their movements midcourse, as older children do.
- Newborns also do not shape or configure their hands to correspond to the properties and shapes of the objects for which they are reaching.
- Infants who prereach rarely contact the target objects (Bushnell, 1985).

### Visually Guided Reaching

Success in reaching for and grasping objects increases greatly when an infant reaches approximately 4 months of age. Between 4 and 7 months, infants increasingly use vision to guide their hands to an object (*visually guided reaching*), typically making several corrections in their reach before making contact (Hofsten, 1979). Infants at this age adapt their reach when their view of an object is distorted by prisms that displace the apparent location of the object (McDonnell, 1975), and their reaching is disrupted when they are not allowed to see their hands (Lasky, 1977). As shown in Figure 3.8, placing a prism over a person's eyes causes the apparent or virtual position of an object to shift. An adult would grasp directly

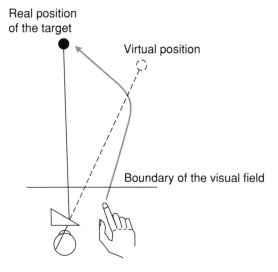

**Figure 3.8** An infant's reliance on visual guidance in reaching is demonstrated in a displaced vision task. Prisms placed in front of the eyes shift the apparent location of an object from its real position. An individual relying on visual guidance begins to adapt the hand position as the hand comes into sight after initially moving toward the object's apparent or virtual position. (Reprinted by permission from Hay, 1990.)

at the virtual location of the object, not needing to see the hand (a visually elicited or triggered reach). An infant, however, would adjust the position of the hand as it came into view, using the apparent location of the hand and the apparent location of the object to close the gap between the two and obtain the object. An infant uses vision to guide the hand to the object. In addition, starting at about 4 months of age, infants shape their hands according to the shape, location, and orientation of the object they are reaching for. Visually guided reaching predominates around 7 months of age, then gives way to a more thrusting, ballistic type of reach that is visually elicited.

### Visually Elicited Reaching

Toward the end of the 1st year, the initial part of an infant's reach becomes so accurate that he or she needs to make few, if any, corrections (McDonnell, 1979). Presumably, complete and fast arm movements result from the initial information of an object's position (*visually elicited reaching*) rather than the slower method of comparing arm and object position (visually guided) (McDonnell, 1979). The infant no longer needs to see the hand to complete a successful reach (Bushnell, 1982)—that is, less attention to the hand is required (Bushnell, 1985). Further improvements in prehension appear by the end of the 1st year. The infant shapes the hand very early in the reach, and the shape is more likely to be appropriate for the object.

## Bimanual Reaching

The reaching and grasping we've discussed thus far is unimanual (one-handed or unilateral). Infants also acquire *bimanual reaching* and grasping (two-handed or bilateral) (Corbetta & Mounoud, 1990; Fagard, 1990). Skilled performers know to grasp objects that are too large for one hand with two hands, and they use one hand to complement the other. For example, a child might use one hand to hold a container still and the other to open the lid. Newborns' random arm movements are asymmetrical (Cobb, Goodwin, & Saelens, 1966). The first bilateral movements are extending and raising the arms, observed at approximately 2 months of age (White et al., 1964). Within a few months, infants can clasp their hands at the body midline. At approximately 4.5 months, infants often reach for objects with both arms (Fagard, 1990). Reaches begun with two hands usually result in one hand reaching and grasping the object first, so that after 5 months, bimanual reaching declines (Ramsay & Willis, 1984). After 7 months, infants use a unimanual or a bimanual reach depending on their position and the size, weight, and shape of the object they wish to grasp (Fagard, 1990; see Figure 3.9). Bimanual reaches at this age are simultaneous in time and space. Both hands start for the object at the same time and arrive

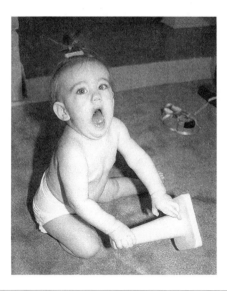

**Figure 3.9**  Obtaining large objects necessitates bimanual reaching. In young infants, one hand might reach the object before the other. Infants older than 7 months reach either unimanually or bimanually, depending on the object's characteristics.

at the object at the same time (Goldfield & Michel, 1986a).

After 8 months, infants start to dissociate simultaneous arm activity so they can manipulate an object cooperatively with both hands (Goldfield & Michel, 1986b; Ruff, 1984). Late in the 1st year, infants learn to hold two objects, one in each hand, and often bang them together (Ramsay, 1985). By 12 months, they can pull things apart and insert one object into another. Soon infants can reach for two objects simultaneously.

Not until the end of the 2nd year can infants perform complementary activities with the hands, such as holding a lid open with one hand while withdrawing an object with the other (Bruner, 1970).

## Views on Reaching and Grasping Milestones

The onset of new reaching and grasping skills intrigues developmentalists as much as the onset of locomotor skills. Just as with locomotion, explanations for the source of these new behaviors depend on the perspective one adopts. Let us again look at these skills from the maturation and dynamic systems perspectives.

### Maturation Perspective

As they did with locomotion, maturationists interpreted these reaching and grasping developments as reflecting neurologic development. The area of the motor cortex associated with the hand undergoes rapid maturation in early postnatal life. When an infant is about 3 months old, the cerebral cortex begins to develop rapidly, and soon thereafter the infant demonstrates visually guided reaching. So prereaching might reflect the nervous system's early subcortical control of the arms while visually guided reaching reflects an emerging integration of subcortical and cortical modes of control (Bushnell, 1985). The eye-hand coordination of accurate reaching achieves an adult pattern around age 9, while continued maturation of the cerebral cortex is noted over the first decade (Woollacott, 1983).

### Dynamic Systems Perspective

Although reaching and grasping development can be associated with neurologic development, it also might be associated with changing mechanical factors. A dynamic systems developmentalist (Kugler et al., 1982) would predict that continuous changes in factors such as arm length and weight that occur with physical growth could bring about sudden qualitative changes in an infant's control of arm reaches. More research is needed on the transitions in these motor behaviors and their associations with mechanical and neurologic factors (Wool-

lacott, 1983). It is clear that the current perspectives will better account for the influence of the environment and how infants are positioned in it than did the early descriptive accounts of reaching and grasping.

## Motor Scales

The early descriptive studies were instrumental in identifying the sequence and direction of locomotor development. They were also helpful in establishing the average rate of skill development during the early months. Although developmentalists traditionally accepted this regular progress toward locomotion as evidence of development by maturation alone (rather than environmental experience), recent research has countered this one-sided view. We still have much to learn about the processes underlying the onset of new skills. Nevertheless, these early works still reflect the order in which an individual acquires the motor milestones.

Developmentalists still use the *motor scale* developed by Bayley (1969) to assess an individual's rate of motor development by comparing the individual's age at acquisition of a given skill to the average age provided by the scale. This process is particularly valuable in identifying infants who lag behind the majority of children in acquiring locomotor skills. It is possible that some of these infants are growing and maturing normally but a bit more slowly than other children. They may eventually catch up with the average scores. However, it is also possible that the developmental lag indicates a neurologic impairment. In this case, comparing a child's performance to a motor scale may help medical professionals detect the problem early.

Remember that the average age at which a motor skill appears is really the middle of the age span when most children acquire the skill. This age span typically widens as we deal with skills individuals acquire when they are older, as is evident in Table 3.2. The increasing variation in age at onset relates in part to the environment in which the child develops and in part to individual maturation rates.

Only those lags in motor development that are so large as to fall outside the normal age span for acquisition of a skill may indicate a neurologic impairment. We must also use caution in evaluating individual children because it is not unusual for an infant to skip a milestone skill. For example, some infants never crawl, but they do acquire subsequent upright skills

## Norm-Referenced Versus Criterion-Referenced Scales

It is obviously necessary and beneficial to assess individual children and groups of children. Assessment can help professionals identify children who need special attention, chart individual and group progress, choose appropriate educational tasks, and so on. Professionals must recognize, though, that testing instruments have specific purposes and are best used when the purpose matches a particular need. For example, we can broadly classify testing instruments as *norm-referenced* or *criterion-referenced*.

The purpose of *norm-referenced scales* is to compare an individual or group to previously established norms. This comparison indicates where a person falls within a group of like individuals matched on relevant factors, such as age, gender, and race. The value of norm-referenced scales in identifying slowly developing children is obvious. On the other hand, such scales give professionals no information about the nature or cause of a delay, or about what educational experiences to prescribe to facilitate future development.

*Criterion-referenced scales* are designed to indicate where a child falls on a continuum of skills that we know are acquired in sequence. The developmentalist administers the criterion-referenced scale periodically, comparing individuals to their own previous performances rather than to a population norm. Often, criterion-referenced scales indicate what skills the individual has mastered and what skills are just emerging. Educators can prescribe educational and practice activities

based on those emerging skills, guaranteeing that the educational task is developmentally appropriate for the individual.

Most of the scales developed for infants are the norm-referenced type. Typically, more expertise is needed to administer a criterion-referenced scale than a norm-referenced scale. The Bayley Scales of Infant Development, discussed in this chapter, are norm-referenced (Bayley, 1969). The complete Bayley Scales consist of a mental scale (163 items), a motor scale (81 items), and a behavior record for social and attentional behaviors. Those using these scales can compare infants and toddlers from 2 months to 2.5 years to mental and motor norms.

Another well-known norm-referenced scale is the Denver Developmental Screening Test (Frankenburg & Dodds, 1967). This test can be used from birth to 6 years of age and assesses four areas:

1. Gross-motor performance (31 items)
2. Fine-motor performance (30 items)
3. Language development (21 items)
4. Personal-social skills (22 items)

A third well-known norm-referenced scale is the Gesell Developmental Schedules (Gesell & Amatruda, 1949). All these instruments are well standardized, but their motor scales are less reliable and valid than is desirable. In this sense they are useful but limited in the information they provide about motor development.

in the normal time frame. Other more slowly developing children might learn to crawl at a relatively late age, and their subsequent skills are also remarkably delayed.

---

*The longer an environmental factor influences both a child's growth and his or her experiences with motor skills, the greater the effect on age of acquisition.*

---

## REVIEW 3.3

Infants acquire upright locomotion and visually guided reaching through a relatively consistent set of steps or motor milestones. The onset of new skills might be linked to the development of one or more systems. For example, a child logically needs certain levels of neurologic, postural, and musculoskeletal development to execute many milestone skills. Motor skills are shaped, though, not just by the development of body systems, but also by the child's environment and the task itself. Neither adults nor children necessarily use the same grasp to pick up objects of various sizes and weights. Rather, they adapt their grasp to the particular object. One way to see the influence of environment on motor development is to consider information on environments that are either deprived or enriched. We can then determine if motor development was sensitive to the prevailing environment. This is the topic we will address next.

## SENSITIVE PERIODS

We have identified the sequence of infants' motor skill acquisition and the normal age span during which each skill appears. Can environmental factors alter this normal progression?

Might a deprived environment retard motor development and an enriched environment accelerate it? We could answer these questions if we knew whether or not sensitive periods exist for motor skills. Remember that sensitive periods are a finite time during which a child is most sensitive to learning a particular skill. These periods are important because children who do not learn a skill during its sensitive period might find it difficult or even impossible to learn the skill when they are older.

There is strong evidence for the existence of sensitive and even critical periods in the development of many animals. It also appears that sensitive periods exist for certain aspects of human development, such as language acquisition (Dennis, 1963; Hecaen, 1976; Lenneberg, 1967) and binocular vision (Banks, Aslin, & Letson, 1975; Hohmann & Creutzfeldt, 1975; see chapter 6). Unfortunately, the information on sensitive periods for motor development is not plentiful. Let us review the evidence available on this topic.

---

**CONCEPT 3.4**
The environment in which the child is placed can facilitate or delay motor development.

---

## Deprived Environments

For obvious ethical reasons, researchers today cannot place human infants in deprived living conditions. Some information about humans is available, though, from studies of institutionalized infants, of varying cultures, and from a few studies conducted before researchers realized the repercussions of such deprivation.

### Institutionalized Children

The institutional environment typically cannot provide the same degree of parental care and interaction as occurs in the home. Infants may not be given an adequate amount of space in an institution or the freedom to attempt and practice motor skills, because one adult must supervise many babies. Hence, we may consider some institutions deprived environments for development.

Dennis (1963) reported that institutionalized children in Iran demonstrated retarded loco-motor development in four areas:

1. Sitting alone
2. Creeping
3. Standing
4. Walking alone

In one institution, only 15% of the children could walk alone when tested between their third and fourth birthdays. Dennis noted that infants at the institution spent most of their time supine. Their caretakers rarely placed them in sitting and prone positions from which they could more easily attempt locomotion. Bowlby (1978) concluded from a review of four studies that institutionalized children lag behind those raised in homes in physical, intellectual, emotional, social, and speech development.

---

At the very least, deprived institutional environments are associated with retarded motor development, although they obviously have a more widespread detrimental effect on development.

---

## Cradle-Bound Infants

A unique child-rearing practice of the Hopi Indians many years ago also attracted Dennis's attention. The Hopi bound or swaddled their infants to cradle boards for most of the day until they were approximately 9 months old. Infants could not move their arms or legs when bound and typically were laid on their backs, not strapped upright on their mother's backs as often pictured. The average age of the onset of walking among these cradle-bound infants was nearly the same as that of a group of Hopi infants not cradle-bound (Dennis, 1940). Developmentalists often interpreted this as a demonstration that restricting movement does not alter acquisition of the milestone skills. However, the very late average age at which both groups of Hopi infants began walking, about 15 months, precludes a definitive conclusion. This is approximately 3 months later than the average given by Bayley (1969). Razel (1985, 1988) suggested that the infant group not bound to cradle boards might still have been raised in a similar way to the bound group—that is, mothers might have consistently placed those infants on their backs as well. No such information about the unbound group is available, but considering the slow development of walking, we cannot rule out a negative effect of child-rearing practices that restrict movement.

## Del and Rey

Dennis (1935, 1938, 1941; Dennis & Dennis, 1951) also conducted an experimental study on deprivation effects. He and his wife raised two fraternal twins, Del and Rey, from age 36 days to 14 months. During this time they left the infants alone in a room, lying on their backs in two cribs separated by a screen. They were given no toys. The experimenters removed the infants only for feeding and cleaning and did not talk to or interact with them. Dennis (1938) reported that Del and Rey acquired 45 typical behaviors for infants up to 7 months of age within the normal age range. Razel (1985) reanalyzed Dennis's data and noted that Rey reached 20 of the first 28 landmarks at a later age than the median and Del reached 19 landmarks at a later age. Toward the end of the experimental period, the twins were reaching almost all of the assessment items at a later age than the median. Whereas Dennis interpreted assessments of the twins' development as normal, Razel concluded the infants developed at a slower pace than normal.

Dennis (1935) provided the twins some training at 8 months. For example, he placed the infants prone on the floor 5 to 30 minutes a day (Dennis, 1941). Rey began creeping 5 months later at 13 months, but Del never achieved this motor milestone (Dennis, 1938). Rey and Del stood alone at 15 and 25 months, respectively, and walked at 17 and 25 months. Hence, the twins reached these milestones very late. Despite Dennis's early belief that training at 8 months would accelerate the twins' delayed motor development (Dennis, 1935), it eventually became apparent that the extreme deprivation the twins experienced had significant effects that training could not erase (Dennis, 1941; Razel, 1985).

Five years later, Del was described as having mild paralysis of the left arm (Dennis, 1938). The exact role of the depriving conditions in this disability is unclear. Might this have been a physical disability intensified by the deprived conditions? Or would the end result have been the same no matter what the conditions? Though we will never know, it is clear that overall we cannot dismiss the effects of the deprived conditions as insignificant, and such a study should never be repeated.

Institutionalized infants, cradle-bound infants, and the twins Del and Rey all have in common long periods spent lying on their backs. Recall that muscle strength and balance appear to be two rate-controlling systems for walking; that is, they must develop to a certain point before infants can walk. If so, we might attribute the delayed onset of walking in deprived infants to their limited opportunity to develop trunk and leg strength and to practice balance in an upright position.

## Training and Enrichment

The lasting beneficial effects of training or enriching the environment may also demonstrate the existence of sensitive periods for motor development.

### The Gesell and Thompson Twin Study— "T" and "C"

Gesell and Thompson (1929, 1934, p. 315, 1941, 1943) used a co-twin method, realizing that training one twin could give twins of identical genetic background different environments. They worked with a pair of identical twins living in an institution, starting at approximately 11 months of age. The twin called "T" for treatment was trained 20 minutes a day, 6 days a week, for 6 weeks. Training consisted of climbing, crawling, pulling up to a standing position, assisted walking, and fine-motor play with cubes. The twin called "C" for control received only 2 weeks of training on stair climbing, starting 1 week after T finished her program. T was able to climb stairs 5 weeks sooner than C, but C learned to climb quickly once her training began. T stood alone 6 weeks earlier than C and took her first step alone 4.5 weeks earlier. T also performed better than C on tests of fine-motor coordination. T maintained an edge over C on various motor tasks throughout childhood and into adolescence (Gesell & Thompson, 1941). The experimenters emphasized that C, learning skills at an older age, learned at a faster rate than T. They concluded that training had not transcended maturation (Gesell & Thompson, 1941, p. 216). An alternative interpretation is that early motor training yielded a lasting advantage (Razel, 1985, p. 176).

### The McGraw Twin Study— Johnny and Jimmy

McGraw (1935) conducted a well-known motor development study that dealt with the issue of critical periods and enrichment activities. She worked with two twins, Johnny and Jimmy. Unfortunately, subsequent researchers later suspected that McGraw's set of twins were fraternal rather than identical and therefore that their heredity was not identical (Dennis, 1951). Several aspects of the study, however, are still noteworthy.

McGraw first observed the twins from age 21 days to 22 months. One twin, Johnny, was exercised in motor activities whereas the other, Jimmy, spent most of his time in a crib. McGraw brought the twins to her laboratory during the day and they went home every evening. Their ages at the onset of the important motor skills were recorded and compared during the 1st year. There was little difference between the two boys.

During their 2nd year, Johnny's training consisted of instruction on a variety of tasks, including

- swimming and diving,
- skating,
- climbing, and
- traveling 40-degree and 61-degree inclines.

Johnny came to perform these tasks with ease whereas Jimmy could not perform any of them. In fact, Jimmy typically cried or clung to the experimenter when challenged with these tasks. When Jimmy was 22 months old, McGraw gave him special training on similar tasks for 2.5 months. Despite his advanced age compared to Johnny's age at mastery of the skills, Jimmy took longer to learn all of the skills except bicycling. When observed at 6 and 10 years of age, Johnny was still superior to Jimmy in motor performance and demonstrated more confidence, agility, and smoothness in his movements (McGraw, 1939).

McGraw's interpretation of these findings was that infantile reflexes and acquisition of the motor milestones cannot be altered by training, but skills that individuals learn variably can be enhanced by training. Razel (1985, 1988) suggests that researchers often overlook an important consideration in the Johnny and Jimmy study. Johnny was the twin chosen for the spe-

cial treatment because his development lagged behind Jimmy's at birth. He was flaccid and demonstrated weak reflexive behavior as a newborn. Hence, an alternate explanation is that Johnny's training was advantageous in the 1st year since he performed similarly to his brother despite his beginning at a disadvantage (Razel, 1985).

## Child Rearing in Kenya

More recently, Super (1976) documented child-rearing practices in Kenya. Kenyan mothers deliberately facilitate motor skills, specifically the upright skills of sitting, standing, and walking. Kenyan infants achieve the upright skills approximately a month earlier in their development than American infants. Yet they acquire the prone skills (rolling over, crawling), which their mothers do not emphasize, later than Americans. We might link their advantage in some skills, then, to training, not to genetic differences between Kenyan and American infants.

Similar results were found in a study of infant walker use. Crouchman (1986) studied infants who spent varying amounts of time upright in infant walkers and recorded the age at which they acquired milestone skills. Those who spent a large portion of the day in infant walkers reached prone locomotor milestones later than the others, but not upright skills such as sitting. Taken together, these training and enrichment studies emphasize that the time an infant spends in a particular posture affects when he or she acquires milestone skills. Spending a lot of time in a particular posture facilitates those skills associated with the posture. When infants spend little time in a posture, they often acquire those skills associated with the posture at a later age than average.

## Motor Development Training Programs

Several programs for maximizing motor development exist, but they have undergone little objective assessment. Ridenour (1978) reviewed these programs and categorized them as *programming plan* or *no-programming plan* depending on whether or not a program of prepracticing skills is advocated. Advocates of the programming plan suggest that it is beneficial to have infants prepractice the motor skills they will soon acquire. For example, the Prudden Infant Fitness Program calls for 20 minutes a day of mother-infant activities during the infant's 1st year. The activities include manipulating the limbs and trunk, and the use of infant walkers and baby bouncers is encouraged.

In contrast, advocates of the no-programming plan discourage prepracticing skills, manipulating infants, and using special equipment. Instead, they allow infants to achieve new postural positions (upright sitting, standing) on their own. Toys are placed near the infant, for the infant to obtain on his or her own initiative. An adult never places them in the infant's hand. The Pikler Program at the National Methodological Institute for Infant Care in Budapest is an example of the no-programming plan (Pikler, 1968). Pikler reports that the age at onset of the motor milestones is not appreciably delayed in these infants and that their quality of movement is better than that of instructed children. However, Razel (1985) pointed out that Pikler's comparisons show that her infants reached 29 of 36 milestone skills later than the norms.

---

In the absence of research information, it seems sensible for parents to provide an environment that facilitates the infant's natural motor development but to avoid activities the infant is obviously not ready to perform. Parents should also avoid programs that promise unrealistic acceleration of their child's motor development.

---

Researchers have conducted very little independent research on the merits of such programs. No reported studies have assessed programs from both categories simultaneously. It is difficult, then, to judge the value of programs that claim to optimize motor development.

## Analyzing the Studies on Sensitive Periods

It is important that we be aware of the perspectives of those who interpret research data. Researchers exploring the existence of sensitive periods in motor development during the 1930s had a maturation perspective. They interpreted the onset of skills within a normal age range and a faster rate of learning, even at a later age, as consistent with that viewpoint. Hence, they concluded that neuromuscular maturation drives skill acquisition, whereas variations in the environment play only a minor role in motor development—in other words, basic motor skills develop regardless of the environment.

From a dynamic systems perspective, deprivation and training can be associated with developmental progress in various systems. Those working from this perspective acknowledge the important role of neural development as well as the roles of other systems, especially the muscular and postural systems. An individual needs a certain degree of muscular strength and postural balance to achieve most of the milestone skills. Conditions that provide infants little opportunity to develop strength and balance potentially delay motor development. In contrast, conditions that facilitate strength and balance development potentially accelerate motor development. Other systems not yet studied extensively might be equally influential. Therefore, the environment, practice, and experience take on increased importance.

A particular aspect of the aforementioned studies of sensitive periods deserves our attention. The majority of these studies used just one method of assessing motor development—the acquisition of new skills. It is possible that in the long term, deprivation or enrichment affects not so much skill acquisition as the movement process or the movement product. Recall that in 1939 McGraw reported differences between Jimmy and Johnny in agility and smoothness. Perhaps this was an early tip that more qualitative aspects of movement deserve attention in regard to the existence of sensitive periods. Unfortunately, researchers did not heed this tip, and little research exists on the effects of deprivation or training on qualitative aspects of movement. We likewise know little about the role of providing early but appropriately timed practice experiences on building a child's confidence to perform motor skills. We have long recognized the importance of integrating perceptions of our environment with our actions. A new line of research is currently exploring this integration, and we will examine this topic in chapter 6. We need more study of all these aspects of early motor development, especially the interrelationships among neurologic, postural, and musculoskeletal development and an individual's opportunities to undertake and practice motor skills.

## REVIEW 3.4

Deprivation is likely to slow the rate of motor development, particularly if it affects the development of one or more systems that are rate controllers for a particular skill. In contrast, appropriate and well-timed training might speed the rate of motor development. The onset of a skill, however, is related to development of particular systems. No amount of training will bring about the development of a skill before the individual systems have advanced to a certain point. Researchers rarely investigate aspects of skill performance other than age at acquisition in regard to the existence of sensitive periods. A lack of opportunity to attempt skills may affect the quality of movement, and children's level of confidence about their movement abilities may depend on the extent of their

early motor experiences. Future research must encompass a variety of measures of motor development and the development of individual systems.

## SUMMARY

In the months following birth, infants acquire an amazing number of new skills. At birth, infants make random movements and reflexive responses to specific stimuli. The purpose of the infantile reflexes is still debated among developmentalists, but these reflex responses and random movements demonstrate that the nervous system can control relatively coordinated movements. Shortly after birth, infants begin to learn purposeful skills in a relatively fixed sequence. Developmentalists are interested in the body systems that serve as rate controllers for the onset of these skills. Environmental conditions can also influence the onset of new skills. If infants are placed in restricted or deprived conditions, the opportunity to learn and master new skills may be lost. In contrast, an enriched environment allows infants to attempt new skills as soon as they are ready for them.

With adequate opportunity, infants enter early childhood well on their way to mastering basic locomotion and grasping. Their next challenge is to acquire more complex locomotor and manipulative skills, such as jumping, hopping, running, skipping, catching, throwing, and striking. The next chapter begins by discussing the acquisition and refinement of these basic motor skills.

## Key Terms

bimanual reaching
co-contraction
co-twin method
crawling
creeping
criterion-referenced scale

infantile reflexes
locomotor reflexes
mark-time pattern
motor milestones
motor scale
movement pattern generators
movement process
movement product
norm-referenced scale
postural reactions
prereaching
primitive reflexes
reflexes
reversion/regression
visually elicited reaching
visually guided reaching

## Discussion Questions

1. What are the various ways we can gauge motor development? Pick a skill, such as jumping, and give an example of improvement for each of the five ways progress can be gauged.
2. How are an infant's supine kicks similar to an adult's walking steps? How are they different?
3. What are the three categories of reflexes? Give an example of each.
4. Contrast the maturation and dynamic systems perspectives on the role of reflexes in motor development. Do the same for their views of the locomotor milestones and reaching and grasping milestones.
5. By what age do infants achieve control of the upper body? Of the entire trunk?
6. What might account for differences in the average age at onset of a skill across various studies or scales?
7. From a dynamic systems perspective, what systems are likely rate controllers for walking?

8. How does the size of an object affect the grip an infant uses? How might this influence where an infant falls on Halverson's prehension sequence?
9. What are the three types of reaching used by infants? Define each and indicate when it predominates.
10. How can the motor scales published decades ago be used today? Are there any drawbacks to their use?
11. How can a deprived environment affect an infant's motor development?
12. How does an enriched environment or an infant training program affect motor development? What might limit any acceleration of the age at onset of the milestone skills?

## Suggested Readings

Bard, C., Fleury, M., & Hay, L. (Eds.) (1990). *Development of eye-hand coordination across the life span*. Columbia, SC: University of South Carolina Press.

McGraw, M.B. (1939). Later development of children specially trained during infancy. *Child Development*, **10**, 1-19.

Peiper, A. (1963). *Cerebral function in infancy and childhood*. New York: Consultants Bureau.

Ridenour, M.V. (1978). Programs to optimize infant motor development. In M.V. Ridenour (Ed.), *Motor development: Issues and applications* (pp. 39-61). Princeton, NJ: Princeton Book Company.

Woollacott, M.H., & Shumway-Cook, A. (Eds.) (1989). *Development of posture and gait across the life span*. Columbia, SC: University of South Carolina Press.

## Chapter 4

# Motor Behavior During Childhood

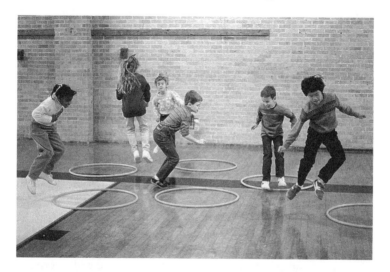

**4.1**
Our observations of developmental change in basic skill performance benefit from application of the laws of motion and stability.

**4.2**
Children's skill development includes qualitative changes that mark steps in a developmental sequence.

Infants begin to walk when they are about a year old, and soon thereafter they attempt other basic skills. They learn to run and jump during their 2nd year, and other forms of locomotion follow in early childhood. Children might try throwing and kicking as early as the 2nd year, depending on the opportunity and encouragement they receive from family members, but their initial attempts at these basic skills typically are crude and inconsistent. Compared to skilled adult performers, young children are mechanically inefficient although their movement patterns may be appropriate for their body size, strength, and level of coordination.

As children grow, gain more experience, receive instruction, and imitate others, they become more proficient in their basic skill performance. This improvement happens gradually, often in steps, with the child continually refining the skills to more closely approximate a form consistent with the mechanical principles of movement that optimize performance. Many of the improvements an individual achieves in childhood are due to increases in body size and strength, and therefore in ability to produce force. Yet size and strength alone do not account for how children progress from unskilled to skilled performance. Though their size and strength increase gradually over childhood, sudden, qualitative changes occur in skill performance.

A good example is the skill of overhand throwing. A 2-year-old usually performs this skill by pointing the elbow toward the target, extending the lower arm, and then releasing the ball; there is no leg or trunk action. Using such a movement pattern, even a fully grown adult could not throw a ball very far. To maximize performance, a person needs to use a movement pattern that capitalizes on mechanical principles as well as size and strength.

Because our observations of basic skill development benefit from a knowledge of the mechanical principles, we will consider motor development during childhood by first examining the pertinent mechanical laws, and then the process by which children progress, given the appropriate environment and opportunity to perform the skills.

## LAWS OF MOTION AND STABILITY

Movements occur in an environment that is governed by certain principles of motion and stability. Think about gravity as an example of an environmental factor. Gravity causes objects in flight to take a parabolic path. It dictates that an individual activate certain postural muscles to assume and maintain a position, even while executing a skilled movement. A person jumping must work against gravity to become airborne, and so on. So, aspects of the environment influence the movement patterns that performers use. Likewise, characteristics of the performer influence the movement pattern undertaken. A person throws using a movement pattern that is dictated by the shape and structure of the human body and limbs—that is, how the bones are shaped and connected to each other; how the muscles are shaped, placed, and connected to the bones; how strong the muscles are; how well the nervous system can coordinate muscle contractions; and so on. So the performer, with a task goal in mind, and the environment interact to shape or constrain a movement pattern.

Some movement patterns optimize the product of skill performance whereas others do not. To develop their skills, children must learn to use movement patterns that optimize performance. This process is complicated by the changes taking place in children's bodies. Growth changes an individual's overall size and proportions. As children grow and mature, their skeletal, muscular, and nervous systems allow them to produce greater force. As the body changes, the interaction between the body and the environment changes. Children discover qualitatively different movement patterns that improve the outcome of their skill performance by taking the best advantage of the laws of motion and stability. So young children, given their body size, shape, and strength, might execute what is for them the most efficient movement patterns possible. But as they grow, mature physiologically, and gain experience, other movement patterns become possible, and these allow children to execute skills with greater proficiency.

It is important for us, in observing motor performance, to know the laws of motion and stability so we can appreciate which movement patterns are likely to produce optimal results and which are not. Knowledge of the laws also helps us to focus on critical aspects of movement that often distinguish skilled movement patterns from unskilled ones. For these reasons, we will review the basic laws of motion and stability as they apply to basic skill performance. Biomechanics, the mechanics of muscular activity, is an area of study in itself and is beyond the scope of this text. You can find a more detailed explanation of these principles in any biomechanics text (cf. Hay & Reid, 1982; Kreighbaum & Barthels, 1990).

---

**CONCEPT 4.1**

Our observations of developmental change in basic skill performance benefit from application of the laws of motion and stability.

---

## Application of Force

*Newton's first law of motion* states that an external force must act on a resting object to cause it to move or to change an object already moving. Therefore, to throw a ball, one applies force to it. One can maximize performance by applying this force over the greatest distance possible. In executing motor skills, a person increases performance by taking a step forward when projecting an object; this motion increases the linear (straight-line) distance over which force is applied. Using a full range of body motion to increase the rotary distance over which force is applied also increases performance. Using a preparatory windup puts the performer in a position to maximize both the linear and rotary distance of force application. The preparatory positioning also stretches the muscles the performer will use, thus readying them for maximal contraction. These actions permit the person to project the object at a greater velocity than could be accomplished without a windup and a full range of motion. So, optimal skill performance is characterized in part by two phases: preparation, and the application of force through a full range of motion.

## Action and Reaction

*Newton's third law of motion* states that for every force one body exerts on another, the second body exerts an equal force on the first in the opposite direction. For example, when sprinters round the curve on a track, they push backward and to the right so they are projected forward and to the left. On the straightaway, they push directly backward. Any forces they exert in a plane other than that of the direction they wish to move detract from their performance. Athletes attempting maximal performance, such as long jumping for the greatest distance possible, want to exert as much force on the ground as they can to get the biggest possible return push. This maximal effort is characterized by full extension (straightening) of the push-off limbs—in this case, the legs.

We also see this *action-reaction law* applied among parts of the body. For example, in locomotor skills such as running, the lower body twists one way and the upper body twists the opposite way; so one leg swings forward, and the arm on that side of the body swings backward in reaction. The leg on one side of the body and the arm on the opposite side swing forward and back in unison. This familiar pattern is termed the *opposition* of arm and leg movement and is a characteristic of skilled locomotor movements.

## Extension of the Projecting Limb

When an athlete performs a ballistic task, projecting an object, the athlete's limb traces part of a circle—the arm travels in an arc in throwing, the leg in an arc in kicking. Releasing or striking an object causes it to fly away from this curved path in a straight line from the release or impact point. An object's velocity when it leaves this path is a product of its rotational velocity (speed along a curved path) and the radius of the circular path it is tracing. In other words, the object's straight-line velocity is determined by how fast an athlete's limb is moving

and the length of the limb. If the athlete's limb is already moving as fast as possible when he or she attempts a maximal performance, such as throwing or kicking a ball, the only other way to increase the projecting velocity of the object is to increase the length of the limb. The athlete achieves this increase by straightening or extending the limb just before release in a throw, or just before impact in a kick or strike.

So skilled performers begin a maximal effort with their limbs bent or cocked, and then extend them. Why not keep the limb straight throughout the throw, kick, or strike? It takes more effort to move the weight of an extended limb (and any held object) than of a bent or flexed limb. We see this conservation of effort when skilled sprinters bring the recovering (returning) leg forward in a bent position. To conserve energy in maximal efforts, athletes move their limbs bent, but they maximize the velocity of a projection by straightening their limbs just before release or impact.

## The Open Kinetic Chain

A person can toss or kick an object a short distance easily with a small movement of the arm or leg. But a maximal ballistic effort must involve more body parts moving in a sequence. The sequence must be timed so that the performer applies the force of each succeeding movement just after the previous movement to accelerate the object. As a brief example, recall that in a throw, the thrower steps forward and rotates the pelvis, then rotates the upper trunk as the throwing arm comes forward, extends, and rotates inward, all in a sequence of movements. We term a sequence such as this the *open kinetic chain* of movements.

---

One of the most significant changes we see in the skill development of children is how they make the transition from using a single action to executing skills via a pattern of efficient, properly timed sequential movements.

---

# Force Absorption

Earlier, we identified the benefit of applying maximal force over distance. The natural reverse of this principle is that one can minimize force by dissipating it over distance. In addition, one can dissipate force over area. The greater the distance and larger the area over which force is dissipated, the more gradually force is absorbed. To make a catch, then, a person should meet the ball well in front of the body and let the hands and arms "give" to absorb the force. When landing from a jump, a person flexes the legs after touchdown to increase the distance over which the force can be absorbed. To decrease the force of a fall, a person rolls to spread the impact of the fall over a larger area of the body.

# Base of Support

The stability of any object is related in part to the size of its *base of support*. A refrigerator lying on its side is more difficult to tip over than one standing upright. To become more stable, a person can increase the body's support base by spreading the feet apart if that person is standing, or by spreading the hands apart if that person is doing a handstand. The reverse is true if the aim is to lose stability. In locomotor skills, a person momentarily sacrifices stability (two-footed support base) in order to move by alternately losing and gaining balance (one-footed support base). The body's weight is pushed forward, ahead of the support base, and the person moves the leg forward to regain balance.

Young children first learning locomotor skills attempt to control their stability by keeping a wide base of support. For example, they walk with their toes out and feet planted out to the side. As they gain greater muscle control, experience, and confidence, they narrow their base of support.

Skilled performers use a base of support just wide enough to give them stability.

## REVIEW 4.1

The qualitative changes in motor performance that occur during childhood reflect changes in the interaction between the growing child and the environment. Children's progress is characterized by their selection of movement patterns that more and more often optimize the movement product, consistent with the principles of motion and stability. The major mechanical principles involved in efficient, skilled movement include the application and absorption of force, action and reaction, linear and rotational velocity, sequentially timed movements, and stability in the base of support. A knowledge of these principles will allow us to generalize across various basic skills. We need not approach developmental changes in each one of the basic skills as a completely new study because some aspects of change in other skills overlap, especially within the categories of locomotor, ballistic, reception, and weight-transfer skills.

# QUALITATIVE CHANGES IN MOTOR SKILLS

Basic skill development in children is a gradual process of refining skills. Often this process includes a qualitative change in the skill, such as beginning to take a step forward when throwing. Some authors have described development of a particular skill through successive steps. These developmental sequences are based on qualitative changes in critical features of the skill, which indicate how close the performance is to a mechanically optimal execution of the skill. Examples of critical factors that mark steps along a *developmental sequence* are swinging the nonsupport leg in hopping or using leg-and-arm opposition in running. In other words, the steps are based on qualitative change in the movement pattern rather than quantitative change in performance outcome such as hopping longer distances or running faster.

---

**CONCEPT 4.2**

Children's skill development includes qualitative changes that mark steps in a developmental sequence.

---

## Developmental Sequences

We can apply developmental steps to skill development in two different ways. In one method, we describe all the characteristic positions or movements of the various body components for the initial step, or Step 1, then we describe them for a more advanced level, Step 2, and so on, to the most advanced level (Seefeldt & Haubenstricker, 1982). A description of Step 1 performance would outline, perhaps, the leg action, the trunk action, and the arm action.

The alternative method, proposed by Roberton (1977, 1978b, 1978c), is a component model. In this method we follow each separate body component through whatever number of steps accounts for the qualitative changes observed in that component over time. The basic unit of description, then, is the body component, rather than the step. For example, we might describe the leg action in terms of four steps and the arm action in terms of five steps, and so on. This can result in a different number of steps for each component; we do not force the number of steps for each component to adapt to the number of steps necessary for the whole body, as in the previous method.

Further, the transition from one step to the next can occur at different times (ages) for the various body segments. We could classify an individual child's leg action in hopping as Step 2 and arm action as Step 3. This means that individual children can reach optimal performance levels in different ways: Sally's leg action might be more advanced than her arm action as she learns to throw, but Tommy's arm action in throwing might be ahead of his leg action.

Later in this chapter, when we consider jumping, we will look at developmental sequences for both the whole body and body components that illustrate the similarities and differences between the two methods. From now on in this text, we will use the component model.

---

Observing one body component at a time is well suited to students of motor development, and categorizing the behavior by body component follows more easily.

---

As a final point, remember that at times, children will be in transition between steps. If we were to observe their skill performance during a transition period, they might use less advanced movements when attempting a motor skill one time and more advanced movements when attempting the skill another time. In such a case, we would categorize the children into a step based on the developmental level they show most often—that is, their *modal level* (Roberton & Halverson, 1984). If neither level predominates in a certain child, we can note his or her level as "in transition" between Step 2 and Step 3, for example, or perhaps as Step 2-1/2.

## Locomotor Skills

The locomotor skills are those used to change the location of the body, to move it through space. We will consider seven locomotor skills here:

1. Walking
2. Running
3. Jumping
4. Hopping
5. Galloping
6. Sliding
7. Skipping

## Walking

Walking might seem too simple to interest us when compared to more complex sport skills. Most individuals acquire a near-adult walking pattern by the time they are 5 years of age. Yet walking involves most of the mechanical characteristics of locomotion in general. Once these characteristics become familiar to us we can apply them to the other forms of locomotion. As noted earlier, a child usually begins walking alone between 9 and 17 months of age. The developmental transitions we see in children from the time they learn to walk until they are about 5 years of age provide us a rich opportunity to study the influence of rate-controlling systems on the development of locomotion.

### Characteristics of Early Walking

The walking pattern an infant first uses is characterized by short steps with limited leg and hip extension. Figure 4.1a shows a child who has just learned to walk. The step is flat-footed and the knee is bent, thus accentuating vertical leg lift. The toes point out (out-toeing), and the feet are spread wide apart when planted, as the infant attempts to maintain lateral balance (see Figure 4.1b). There is little (if any) trunk rotation, which is consistent with the short stride. The hands and arms are carried high in a bent position, often termed the *high guard position*. They are fixed and do not swing with each stride. The high guard position is common in beginning walkers because it assists their unsteady balance and provides some protection in case of a fall. As the child continues to de-

velop, the arms will drop to about waist level (middle guard position) and later to an extended position at the sides (low guard position), but they still will not swing (see Figure 4.1c). When children begin to use the arm swing, it frequently is unequal and irregular; both hands might swing forward together (Roberton, 1984).

### Proficient Walking

An infant's initial attempts to walk are qualitatively different than an adult's walking pattern.

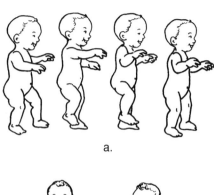

a.

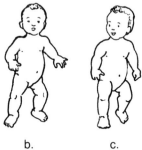

b.                    c.

**Figure 4.1** (a) A beginning walker. Note the short stride and high guard arm position. (b) To maintain balance beginning walkers often plant the feet wide apart with the toes out. (c) Rather than swinging the arms in time with the legs, beginning walkers often hold their arms in a middle or low guard position.
(a and c are drawn from film tracings from the Motor Development and Child Study Laboratory, University of Wisconsin–Madison; b is redrawn from Wickstrom, 1983.)

An adult's walking pattern, as shown in Figure 4.2, reflects certain developmental changes:

- Absolute stride length must increase, reflecting greater application of force and greater leg extension at push-off. Also, as children grow, increased leg length contributes to a longer stride.
- Planting the foot on the ground must change to the heel-then-forefoot pattern, which results from an increased range of leg motion.
- The individual must reduce out-toeing and narrow the base of support laterally to keep the forces exerted in the forward-backward plane.
- The skilled walker must adopt the double knee-lock pattern to assist the full range of leg motion. In this pattern the knee extends at heel strike, flexes slightly as the body weight moves forward over this supporting leg, then extends once more at foot push-off. Because the knee extends twice in one step cycle, we call this pattern the double knee-lock.
- The pelvis must rotate to allow the full range of leg motion and oppositional movement of the upper and lower body segments.
- Balance must improve and forward trunk inclination be reduced.
- The skilled walker must coordinate oppositional arm swing, with the arms extended at the sides, with the legs. This is consistent with the principle of action and reaction; that is, the opposite arm and leg move forward and back in unison. The arm swing must become relaxed and move from the shoulders with a slight accompanying movement at the elbow.

## Developmental Changes in Walking

Children usually achieve the developmental changes in walking early; by age 2 most of them have the essential ingredients of an advanced walk. For example, children exhibit pelvic rotation on the average at 13.8 months, knee flexion at midsupport at 16.3 months, foot contact within a trunk-width base of support at 17.0 months, synchronous arm swing at 18.0 months, and heel-then-forefoot strike at 18.5 months (Burnett & Johnson, 1971). The length of time that one foot supports body weight while the other swings forward increases, especially from 1.0 year to 2.5 years (Sutherland et al., 1980).

Stride length increases through midadolescence, partly because of the fuller range of motion at the hips, knees, and ankles and partly because of the increase in leg length resulting from growth. The velocity of the walk increases, especially between 1.0 and 3.5 years of age (Sutherland et al., 1980). The rhythm and coordination of a child's walk improve observably until age 5 or so, but beyond this age, pattern improvements are subtle and probably not detectable to the novice observer.

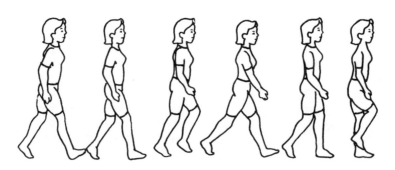

**Figure 4.2** An advanced walker. Note the double knee-lock pattern, trunk rotation, and oppositional arm swing.

## Observing Walking Patterns

It is easier to understand the characteristics of walking if you spend time watching infants and young children walk. Critical observation of movement is a skill you must practice. You need to focus on specific body components to assess the quality of the movement pattern. You must focus attention on one body segment at a time, such as the legs; it is also important that you position yourself where you can see these body segments clearly. For example, when watching walking from the side, you can check first for the heel-strike pattern, then for full extension at push-off, knee flexion at mid-support, and the range of leg motion. It is difficult to see the several aspects of leg action all at once. Focusing on one body part (such as the knee) through several steps in the movement pattern is the best observation strategy. Experienced observers can see several aspects of the pattern at once, but most focus on only a limited number of critical features at any one time.

---

*Novice observers best focus on one critical feature at a time.*

---

Next, you can direct attention toward arm position and opposition to leg action, which are also easy to observe from the side. From the front or rear, you can observe foot angle (to check for out-toeing or in-toeing), the width

## Observing Motor Skill Patterns

An instructor of motor skills must be able to critically observe children's skill patterns. The instructor needs to give students feedback, provide further practice experiences, and formally assess their skills. The observation process requires a disciplined, systematic focus on the critical features of a skill pattern rather than on the outcome or product of a skill. The observer must learn observation techniques and practice them like any other skill before they become automatic.

Barrett (1979) has provided a guide for improving the observation skills of instructors and coaches based on three principles:

1. Analysis
2. Planning
3. Positioning

To analyze developmental movement, the observer first must know the developmental sequences of the skill, including the critical features that characterize a given developmental step, and the mechanical principles involved in proficient performance.

Observers must organize and plan their observations to prevent their attention from wandering once activity begins. They may find it helpful to have written observation guidelines, many of which can be based on the developmental sequences suggested by researchers. However, one can design suitable observation guidelines by simply listing the critical features of the skill to be watched. It might also be a good idea for observers to watch a given feature of a skill many times (two tries, three, etc.).

The third principle is positioning. Many new observers rivet themselves to one location and attempt to watch everything from there. Some critical features of motor skills can be seen only from the side; others are best seen from the front or back. It is important, then, for the observer to move about to be able to watch the performer from several angles.

The process of motor skill observation demands focused attention: New observers must plan ahead, know the critical features of the skill to be watched, position themselves properly, and practice.

of the support base, and the degree of trunk rotation.

Videotaping an individual performing a skill quickly is particularly helpful in your initial attempts to analyze the skill. You can view movements several times at normal speed, in slow motion, and in stop action.

## Running

Running is a more advanced motor skill than walking, but many of the critical features of the two movement patterns are similar. By definition, running has a period of "flight" when neither foot is touching the ground; in walking, one foot is always in contact with the ground. Children typically achieve this flight phase around 6 to 7 months after they begin to walk. Their earliest running attempts are probably very fast walking.

Sometimes, a child who attempts more complex skills exhibits less mature movement patterns than he or she does attempting other, less complex skills. For example, even though the child previously "outgrew" less efficient movement patterns in walking, observers often note examples of regression to those less efficient patterns in very early running attempts (Burnett & Johnson, 1971). When first learning to run, the child may adopt a wide base of support, a flat-footed landing, leg extension at

midsupport, and the high guard arm position. This regression probably reflects that the child is attempting to simplify some parts of the task, such as the arm swing, until he or she acquires more experience. As the child practices the running stride and gets used to its balance demands, he or she will put the arm swing back into the movement pattern.

### Characteristics of Early Running

Some of the characteristics of early running are pictured in Figure 4.3. Focus first on the leg action in Figure 4.3a. You will see a period of flight, but the legs still have a limited range of motion. The rear leg does not extend fully at push-off. The recovering thigh comes forward with enough acceleration that the knee bends, but not with enough acceleration to carry the thigh to a level parallel with the ground at the end of the leg swing. Therefore, the range of motion is limited, and the stride length is short.

Look next at the arm swing, and note the opposition of the arms to the legs. The arms swing to accompany the trunk's rotation, though, rather than driving forward and back as they would in a skilled sprinter. The elbows extend when they swing back, which is unnecessary movement; the arms even swing out slightly to the side, wasting energy. Beginning runners sometimes swing their arms horizon-

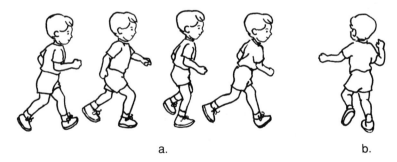

a.                                                                              b.

**Figure 4.3** (a) A beginning runner. The legs have a limited range of motion. The arms extend at the elbow and swing slightly to the side rather than driving forward and back. (b) The thigh and arms swing out rather than forward and back.
(a is drawn from film tracings from the Motor Development and Child Study Laboratory, University of Wisconsin–Madison; b is redrawn from Wickstrom, 1983.)

tally, across the body rather than forward and back; this is probably to aid their unsteady balance.

Figure 4.3b portrays some characteristics of early running that one can observe from the rear. As the child swings the recovering thigh forward, it inefficiently rotates to the side rather than moving straight forward. The arm swings to the side, away from the body, probably to assist with balance, but again, this movement pattern wastes energy that could be directed toward running forward.

## Proficient Running

As with early walking, the movement patterns a child uses in early running are qualitatively different than an adult's running pattern. Applying the mechanical principles discussed earlier, we can identify the developmental changes needed for beginning runners to optimize their performance, as pictured in Figure 4.4, as follows:

- Stride length must increase, indicating that the runner is applying greater force. As greater force is used, several characteristics of mature running emerge: The rear leg is fully extended at push-off; the heel is tucked close to the buttocks as the thigh swings forward with greater acceleration; and before foot strike, the thigh has come parallel to the ground. When the recovery

leg is swung forward in a tucked position, the runner's effort is conserved.
- The runner must eliminate lateral leg movements so that forces are kept in the forward-backward plane.
- For extended running, each foot must strike the ground heel first, then forefoot, or strike the ground in an approximately flat pattern.
- The runner must eliminate out-toeing and narrow the base of support.
- The runner's support leg must be allowed to flex at the knee as the body's weight comes over the leg.
- Trunk rotation must increase to allow for a longer stride and better arm-leg opposition. The trunk should lean slightly forward.
- The arms must swing forward and back, with the elbows approaching right angles, and move in opposition to the legs.

## Developmental Changes in Running

As children grow, then, these qualitative changes in running pattern, together with increased body size and strength and improved coordination, typically result in improved quantitative measures of running speed and time in flight. Such changes have been well documented in several University of Wisconsin studies of children between ages 1.5 and 10.0

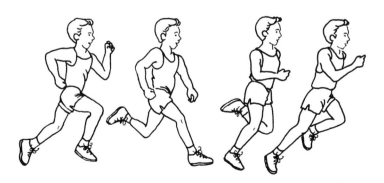

Figure 4.4   An advanced runner. Note the fuller range of leg motion.

years (Beck, 1966; Clouse, 1959; Dittmer, 1962). Therefore, we can expect improvement in both the process and the product of running performance as children grow. Improvements in the product of running performance—increased speed, for example—certainly may continue through adolescence. However, not every individual achieves all of the improvements in running pattern during childhood. Most teenagers continue to refine their running form, and it is not uncommon to observe inefficient characteristics in adults' running, especially out-toeing, lateral leg movements, and limited stride. Perhaps these reflect skeletal and muscular imbalances in individual runners. So age alone does not guarantee perfect running form; adolescents and adults alike may have inefficient running patterns.

Both walking and running are symmetrical patterns. Each leg makes a cycle: toe-off, swing, heel strike, support, and return to toe-off. At any point in one leg's cycle, the other leg is halfway to that point. This is termed *50% phasing*. The legs perform the same movement but at opposite times in the step cycle. We will discuss other locomotor skills later in this chapter, and it will be interesting to compare their timing to the 50% phasing of walking and running.

### Observing Running Patterns

As with walking, observing running patterns in people of all ages will help you better understand the critical features of running. You can observe running from the side, the front, or the back, focusing on one particular aspect of the running pattern at one time, as outlined for walking.

## Jumping

Typically, children attempt jumping tasks at a young age, often achieving the simplest forms before age 2. In jumping, the child propels the body from a surface with either one or both

feet and lands on both feet (see Table 4.1). Children also acquire specialized forms of jumping during childhood, such as hopping and leaping. Hopping requires taking off and landing on the same leg, often repeatedly. Leaping is a run with a projection forward from one foot to a landing on the other. Table 4.1 outlines several examples of hopping and leaping. Let us first look at jumping.

### Characteristics of Early Jumping

We can gauge developmental changes in jumping in various ways:

- The age at which a child can perform certain kinds of jumps (age norms)
- The distance or height of a jump (the product)
- The maturity of the jumping pattern (the process)

Early developmentalists determined age norms for preschool children's jumping achievements (Wickstrom, 1983). These norms appear in Table 4.2. The table indicates that children learn to step down off a higher surface from one foot to the other before jumping off the floor with both feet. Children then learn to jump down from progressively greater heights onto both feet. Later, they master forward jumps,

**Table 4.1  Types of Jumps Arranged by Progressive Difficulty**

---

Jump down from one foot to the other foot.
Jump up from two feet to two feet.
Jump down from one foot to two feet.
Jump down from two feet to two feet.
Run and jump forward from one foot to the other.
Jump forward from two feet to two feet.
Run and jump forward from one foot to two feet.
Jump over object from two feet to two feet.
Jump from one foot to same foot rhythmically.

---

Reprinted by permission from Wickstrom, 1983.

jumps over objects, and hopping a few times on one foot. By the time children reach school age, they usually can perform all of these jumps.

Due to a secular trend, the exact ages at which children today can perform the various jumps might be younger than those in Table 4.2, but the order in which they acquire those jumping skills still applies. Developmentalists frequently use product assessments—that is, they measure the horizontal or vertical distance jumped—to assess jumping skill after the children have refined the movement process. We will focus here on the movement process, because the measurement of distance jumped is rather self-explanatory and straightforward.

Several published developmental sequences aid us in examining the developmental changes that occur in jumping movement patterns. Such sequences identify the steps children achieve in making the transition from inefficient to proficient movement patterns. The advancements reflect the children's adoption of movements that are more and more mechanically efficient. We can see improvements in both the vertical and the horizontal (standing long) jump, but those developmental sequences researchers have suggested thus far are based on the standing long jump (Clark & Phillips, 1985; Roberton, 1984).

It is helpful to first identify some of the characteristics of beginning jumpers in both the vertical jump and the standing long jump. Most young jumpers begin by executing a vertical jump, even if they intend to jump horizontally. Look at the beginning jumpers in Figures 4.5, 4.6, and 4.7. A vertical jump is shown in Figure 4.5 and a horizontal or standing long jump in Figures 4.6 and 4.7. Note that in all three jumps, the preparatory crouch is slight, and the legs are not fully extended at lift-off. In fact, the vertical jumper in Figure 4.5 tucks the legs to leave the ground rather than extending them at takeoff to project the body up. In this example, the head is no higher at the peak of the jump than at takeoff.

**Table 4.2  Jumping Achievements of Young Children**

| Achievement | Motor age (mo) | Source |
|---|---|---|
| Jump from 12 in. height; one foot | 24 | M&W |
| Jump off floor; both feet | 28 | B |
| Jump from 18 in. height; one foot | 31 | M&W |
| Jump from chair 26 cm high; both feet | 32 | B |
| Jump from 8 in. height; both feet | 33 | M&W |
| Jump from 12 in. height; both feet | 34 | M&W |
| Jump from 18 in. height; both feet | 37 | M&W |
| Jump from 30 cm height; both feet | 37.1 | B |
| Jump forward 10 to 35 cm from 30 cm height; both feet | 37.3 | B |
| Hop on two feet 1 to 3 times | 38 | M&W |
| Jump over rope 20 cm high; both feet | 41.5 | B |
| Hop on one foot 1 to 3 times | 43 | B |

Reprinted by permission from Wickstrom, 1983. Adapted from information in studies by Bayley (1935) (B) and McCaskill & Wellman (1983) (M&W).

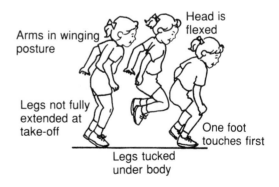

**Figure 4.5**  Sequential views of a vertical jump. The form here is inefficient. The legs are tucked up under the body rather than fully extending to project the body off the ground. Notice that one foot touches down first. The arms do not assist the jump. The jumper simply holds them in the winging posture.
(Redrawn from Wickstrom, 1983.)

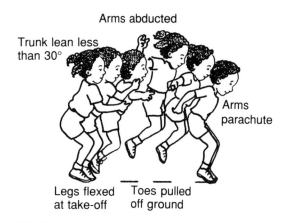

Arms abducted

Trunk lean less
than 30°

Arms
parachute

Legs flexed        Toes pulled
at take-off        off ground

**Figure 4.6** A beginning long jumper. As the
jumper's weight shifts forward, the toes are pulled
off the floor to "catch" the body at landing. The
trunk lean at takeoff is less than 30 degrees from
vertical. The arms are used at takeoff but are in
an abducted position, laterally rotate in flight, and
"parachute" for the landing.
(Drawn from film tracings from the Motor Development
and Child Study Laboratory, University of Wisconsin–
Madison.)

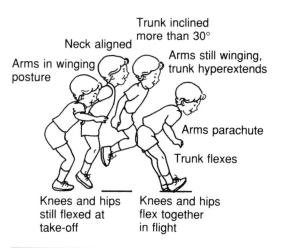

Trunk inclined
more than 30°

Neck aligned

Arms in winging
posture

Arms still winging,
trunk hyperextends

Arms parachute

Trunk flexes

Knees and hips        Knees and hips
still flexed at        flex together
take-off              in flight

**Figure 4.7** A beginning jumper. The leg action
is in Step 3 at takeoff because the knees extend
at the same time the heels leave the ground. The
knees and hips flex together during flight, and
knees then extend before landing. The trunk is
somewhat erect at takeoff. The trunk hyperextends in flight, then flexes for landing. The arms
wing at takeoff, Step 1, before parachuting for
the landing.

Another characteristic of beginning jumpers
is that they do not use a two-footed (symmetrical) takeoff or landing, as shown in Figure 4.5,
even when they intend to do so. A one-footed
takeoff, or step-out, is the lowest level of leg
action in the developmental sequence for the
standing long jump takeoff (see Table 4.4). The
legs may also be asymmetrical during flight. To
improve this leg action, the jumper needs to
first, make a symmetrical, two-footed takeoff,
flight, and landing; and second, fully extend the
ankles, knees, and hips at takeoff, following a
deep preparatory crouch. The knees and hips
flex together in the flight phase of the standing
long jump, following a full and forceful extension of the legs at takeoff.

To jump a long distance (standing long jump),
the skilled performer leans the trunk forward
at least 30 degrees from the vertical. By age
3, children can change their trunk angle at takeoff to make either a vertical or a horizontal

jump (Clark, Phillips, & Petersen, 1989). Yet
beginning jumpers often keep the trunk too
erect during a horizontal jump. When a skilled
jumper leans the trunk forward to facilitate
jumping for distance, the heels usually come
off the ground before the knees start to extend
(Clark & Phillips, 1985). Skilled jumpers appear to tip forward at the start of the takeoff.
The leg action wherein "heels up" begins the
takeoff is the most advanced step in the developmental sequence for the leg action of the
horizontal jump.

Lack of coordinated arm action also char-
acterizes beginning vertical and horizontal
jumpers. Rather than to assist the jumping action, they may use their arms asymmetrically,
hold them stationary at the sides, or keep them
in a high guard position as a precaution against
falling. Arms may *wing* (extend backward) in-
effectively during flight (see Figure 4.5) or *para-*

*chute* (extend down and out to the side) during landing (see Figure 4.6). To achieve a proficient jump, the jumper must use the arms symmetrically to lead the jump from a preparatory extended position to an overhead swing. The developmental sequence for the arm action of the standing long jump progresses from no arm action to limited arm swing; to extension, then partial flexion; and to extension, then complete arm swing overhead.

### Proficient Jumping

Through these developmental changes, performers can develop a proficient jumping pattern, as shown in Figures 4.8 and 4.9. To execute proficient jumps, they do the following:

- Get into a preparatory crouch that will stretch the muscles and allow the legs to apply maximal force as they fully extend at the moment of lift-off.
- Take off for a horizontal jump with the heels coming off the ground and both feet leaving the ground at the same time.
- Extend the arms backward, then initiate the takeoff with a vigorous arm swing forward to a position overhead.

In a jump for height, they do the following:

- Direct force down and extend the body throughout flight. If they are to strike an object or touch something overhead, the dominant arm reaches up and the opposite arm swings down. The person jumping gains height through a lateral tilt of the shoulders.
- Keep the trunk relatively upright throughout the jump.
- Flex the ankles, knees, and hips upon touchdown to allow the force of landing to be absorbed.

In a jump for distance, they do the following:

- Direct force down and back by beginning the takeoff with the heels leaving the

ground before the knees extend. The trunk appears to tip forward.
- Flex the knees during flight, then bring the thighs forward to a position parallel with the ground.
- Swing the lower legs forward for a two-footed landing.
- Let the trunk come forward in reaction to the thighs flexing, putting the body in a jackknife position.
- Flex the ankles and knees when the heels touch the ground to absorb the momentum of the body over distance as the body continues to move forward.

### Developmental Changes in Jumping

With practice, children can eventually make the refinements in jumping pattern just described. Continuous growth in body size and strength also contributes to quantitative improvements in how far children can jump. During the elementary school years, children average increases of 3 to 5 inches a year in the horizontal distance they can jump and approximately 2 inches a year in vertical height jumped (DeOreo & Keogh, 1980). Qualitative improvements in jumping vary among children. For example, Clark and Phillips (1985) observed that fewer than 30% of the 3- to 7-year-olds they filmed had the same level of leg and arm action. Most had more advanced leg action than arm action, but some had more advanced arm action than leg action. If one component was more advanced than the other, it was usually by only one step, but some children were two steps more advanced in one component than another. So we see many different movement patterns among developing children.

Developmental changes for all body components at one time are shown in Table 4.3, whereas Table 4.4 shows the developmental sequence using the component approach. Note that the developmental sequence for the whole body is first organized by step number, and all the characteristics of performance at

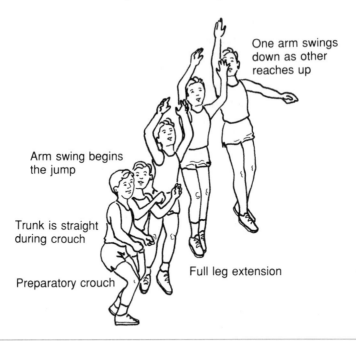

One arm swings
down as other
reaches up

Arm swing begins
the jump

Trunk is straight
during crouch

Preparatory crouch

Full leg extension

**Figure 4.8** An advanced vertical jump for the purpose of reaching high. From a preparatory crouch, this basketball player swings his arms forward and up to lead the jump. The hips, knees, and ankles extend completely at takeoff. Near the peak of the jump, one hand continues up while the other comes down, tilting the shoulder girdle to assist the high reach. Note that the trunk tends to remain upright throughout. (Redrawn from Wickstrom, 1983.)

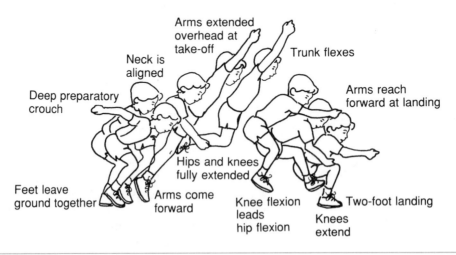

Arms extended
overhead at
take-off

Trunk flexes

Neck is
aligned

Deep preparatory
crouch

Arms reach
forward at landing

Hips and knees
fully extended

Feet leave
ground together

Arms come
forward

Knee flexion
leads
hip flexion

Two-foot landing

Knees
extend

**Figure 4.9** An advanced long jump. The feet leave the ground together and touch down together. The legs fully extend at takeoff beginning with ''heels up.'' The knees then flex in flight, followed by hip flexion and finally knee extension to reach forward for landing. The trunk is inclined more than 30 degrees at take-off, and the jumper maintains this lean in flight until the trunk flexes for landing. The arms lead the jump and reach overhead at takeoff. They then lower to reach forward at landing.

**Table 4.3  Developmental Sequence of the Standing Long Jump for the Whole Body by Step**

**Step 1**  Vertical component of force may be greater than horizontal, resulting jump is then upward rather than forward. Arms move backward, acting as brakes to stop the momentum of the trunk as the legs extend in front of the center of mass.

**Step 2**  The arms move in an anterior-posterior direction during the preparatory phase, but move sideward (winging action) during the "in-flight" phase. The knees and hips flex and extend more fully than in Step 1. The angle of takeoff is still markedly above 45 degrees. The landing is made with the center of gravity above the base of support, with the thighs perpendicular to the surface rather than parallel as in the reaching position of Step 4.

**Step 3**  The arms swing backward and then forward during the preparatory phase. The knees and hips flex fully prior to takeoff. Upon takeoff the arms extend and move forward but do not exceed the height of the head. The knee extension may be complete, but the takeoff angle is still greater than 45 degrees. Upon landing, the thigh is still less than parallel to the surface, and the center of gravity is near the base of support when viewed from the frontal plane.

**Step 4**  The arms extend vigorously forward and upward upon takeoff, reaching full extension above the head at "lift-off." The hips and knees are extended fully with the takeoff angle at 45 degrees or less. In preparation for landing the arms are brought downward and the legs are thrust forward until the thigh is parallel to the surface. The center of gravity is far behind the base of support upon foot contact, but at the moment of contact the knees are flexed and the arms are thrust forward in order to maintain the momentum to carry the center of gravity beyond the feet.

*Note.* Degrees are measured from horizontal.
Adapted by permission from Seefeldt, Reuschlein, & Vogel, 1972.

that level are described. The body component sequence is first organized by body area, and then the developmental steps for only that body component are described.

The developmental steps in Table 4.4 describe body positions and movement magnitudes. For example, we distinguish Steps 3 and 4 of arm action at takeoff by how far the arms swing. Skilled jumpers also extend their knees faster than young children, perhaps due in part to greater leg strength (Clark et al., 1989). So developmental differences involve differences in limb and joint position and movement speeds.

The difference between a vertical jump and a standing long jump also involves a difference in position and movement speed. For example, in the standing long jump, the hips are more flexed than in the vertical jump as the jumper makes the transition from the preparatory crouch to the takeoff. The hips extend faster

in the standing long jump whereas the knees and ankles extend faster in the vertical jump. Other characteristics of jumping remain stable across developmental steps and type of jump. Clark et al. (1989) found that 3-, 5-, 7-, and 9-year-olds and adults all used the same pattern of leg coordination. In addition, all used that same pattern for both standing long jump and vertical jump. Specifically, the timing of hip, knee, and ankle joint extension at takeoff was similar in all groups. Perhaps this reflects the mechanics involved in propelling the body's mass off the ground. The neuromuscular system must use a leg coordination pattern that gets the body off the ground, but limb positions and movement speeds change as the jumper is better able to optimize jumping distance or adapt the jump to a specific task, like shooting the basketball jump shot.

It is clear that all persons do not master jumping in childhood or even in adolescence.

**Table 4.4   Developmental Sequence for the Standing Long Jump Takeoff**

*Leg action component*

**Step 1**   One-foot takeoff. From the beginning position the jumper steps out with one foot. There usually is little preparatory leg flexion.

**Step 2**   Knee extension first. The jumper begins to extend the knee joints before the heels come off the ground, resulting in a jump that is too vertical to achieve maximum horizontal distance.

**Step 3**   Simultaneous extension. The jumper extends the knees at the same time the heels come off the ground.

**Step 4**   Heels up first. The jump begins with the heels coming off the ground, then the knees extend; the jumper appears to start the takeoff by tipping forward.

*Arm action component*

**Step 1**   No action. The arms are stationary. After takeoff they may "wing" (shoulder girdle retracts).

**Step 2**   Arms swing forward. The arms swing forward at the shoulder from a starting position at the sides. The arms also might swing out to the side (abduct at the shoulder).

**Step 3**   Arms extend, then partially flex. The arms extend back together during leg flexion, then swing forward together at takeoff. Arm swing never reaches a position overhead.

**Step 4**   Arms extend, then fully flex. The arms extend back together during leg flexion, then swing forward to a position overhead.

Adapted by permission from Clark & Phillips, 1985.

Zimmerman (1956) found many inefficient jumping characteristics in college women, including limited arm swing and incomplete leg extension at takeoff. In order for children and teens to receive assistance from their instructors in perfecting an advanced jumping pattern, instructors must be able to critically observe and analyze jumping performance.

### Observing Jumping Patterns

As with the skills we discussed previously, it is necessary that you practice the observation of jumping. You can easily observe most aspects of jumping from the side: arm swing, leg extension at takeoff, body angle, leg action in flight, and leg action in landing. Lateral movements of the arms, though, are best seen from the front or back. It can be difficult to see whether "heels up" or knee extension occurs first in the standing long jump unless you videotape the jumpers and view the tape in slow motion.

Jumpers who begin with their heels up, though, appear to tip forward, whereas jumpers who begin with knee extension appear too upright.

### Hopping

Adults rarely use hopping to move around, yet to become a skillful mover, an individual should develop hopping skills during childhood. To hop, especially repeatedly, one must project and absorb body weight with just one limb and maintain balance on the small base of support that one foot provides. Complex sport and dance skills often incorporate these movement abilities.

### Characteristics of Early Hopping

Remember that children might move through the levels of arm action and leg action at different rates. Look at the two early hoppers shown in Figures 4.10 and 4.11. The leg action of

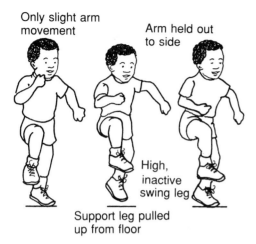

Only slight arm movement

Arm held out to side

High, inactive swing leg

Support leg pulled up from floor

**Figure 4.10** An early hopping attempt exhibiting Step 1 leg action and Step 1 arm action. The support leg is pulled off the floor to produce only momentary flight. The swing leg is held high and remains inactive in the hop. The arms are high, and one is held out to the side. They are not working in opposition.
(Drawn from film tracings from the Motor Development and Child Study Laboratory, University of Wisconsin–Madison.)

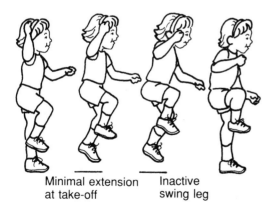

Minimal extension at take-off

Inactive swing leg

**Figure 4.11** This girl uses some leg extension to leave the ground, but her swing leg is still inactive. She is in Step 2 of the developmental levels of leg action.
(Drawn from film tracings from the Motor Development and Child Study Laboratory, University of Wisconsin–Madison.)

the hopper in Figure 4.10 is ineffective. The child momentarily lifts the support leg from the floor by flexing it rather than projecting the body up by leg extension, and the swing leg is inactive. The arms are also inactive; this child's leg and arm action fall into the first developmental step. The hopper in Figure 4.11 has achieved some leg extension; this child is in the second step of leg action but still the first step of arm action.

### Proficient Hopping

To become proficient hoppers, children need to make the following improvements:

- The swing leg must lead the hop.
- The support leg must extend fully.
- The hopper must use the arms, which should move in opposition to the legs.
- The hopper must flex the support leg at landing to absorb the force of the landing and to prepare for extension at the next takeoff.

The hopper in Figure 4.12 has made one of these improvements by moving the arm opposite the swing leg in opposition, but the other arm does not move in a consistent way. The advanced hopper in Figure 4.13 assists the hop with both arms moving in opposition to the legs, in accordance with the mechanical law of action and reaction. The hopper in Figure 4.12 extends the support leg at takeoff, reflecting good force application, and uses the swing leg, but not vigorously. The hopper in Figure 4.13 has made this improvement—the swing leg leads the takeoff, allowing the momentum of several body parts to be chained together, then swings back behind the support leg to lead the next takeoff.

### Developmental Changes in Hopping

Many of the mechanical principles that apply to jumping are involved in hopping as well. Roberton and Halverson (1984) suggested the developmental levels for hopping in Table 4.5.

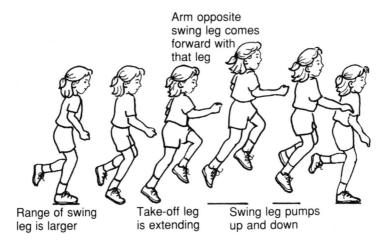

Arm opposite
swing leg comes
forward with
that leg

Range of swing
leg is larger

Take-off leg
is extending

Swing leg pumps
up and down

**Figure 4.12**  A more advanced hop, Step 3 in the developmental sequence of leg action, Step 4 in arm action. The swing leg leads the hop. Although the range of the swing leg is larger, it could still be larger. The arm opposite the swing leg comes forward with that leg, but the other arm is not working in opposition.
(Drawn from film tracings from the Motor Development and Child Study Laboratory, Univeristy of Wisconsin–Madison.)

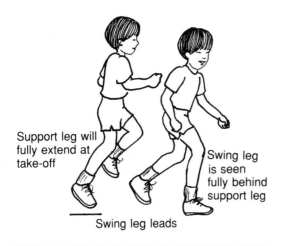

Support leg will
fully extend at
take-off

Swing leg
is seen
fully behind
support leg

Swing leg leads

**Figure 4.13**  This boy demonstrates Step 4 leg action because the range of the swing leg is sufficient to carry it completely behind the support leg. Both arms move in opposition to the legs.
(Drawn from film tracings from the Motor Development and Child Study Laboratory, University of Wisconsin–Madison.)

This sequence has been modified and validated by Halverson and Williams (1985). The authors used a component approach, so they have identified levels for leg action and for arm action separately. They suggested four levels of leg action and five levels of arm action. Notice that the lower steps describe the characteristics of early hopping, and the higher steps describe proficient hopping.

Few children under age 3 can hop repeatedly (Bayley, 1969; McCaskill & Wellman, 1938). Developmentalists often cite the preschool years as the time children become proficient hoppers (Gutteridge, 1939; Sinclair, 1973; Williams, 1983). Yet Halverson and Williams (1985) found that over half a group of 63 children (3-, 4-, and 5-year-olds) were in Step 2 of both arm and leg action. They observed few attempts that they could classify at the advanced levels, and hopping on the non-preferred leg was developmentally behind hop-

**Table 4.5  Developmental Sequence for Hopping**

*Leg action*

**Step 1**  Momentary flight. The support knee and hip quickly flex, pulling (instead of projecting) the foot from the floor. The flight is momentary. Only one or two hops can be achieved. The swing leg is lifted high and held in an inactive position to the side or in front of the body.

**Step 2**  Fall and catch; swing leg inactive. Body lean forward allows the minimal knee and ankle extension to help the body "fall" forward of the support foot and, then, quickly catch itself again. The swing leg is inactive. Repeat hops are now possible.

**Step 3**  Projected takeoff; swing leg assists. Perceptible pretakeoff extension occurs in the hip, knee, and ankle in the support leg. There is little or no delay in changing from knee and ankle flexion on landing to extension prior to takeoff. The swing leg now pumps up and down to assist in projection. The range of the swing is insufficient to carry it behind the support leg when viewed from the side.

**Step 4**  Projection delay; swing leg leads. The weight of the child on landing is now smoothly transferred along the foot to the ball before the knee and ankle extend to takeoff. The support leg nearly reaches full extension on the takeoff. The swing leg now leads the upward-forward movement of the takeoff phase, while the support leg is still rotating over the ball of the foot. The range of the pumping action in the swing leg increases so that it passes behind the support leg when viewed from the side.

*Arm action*

**Step 1**  Bilateral inactive. The arms are held bilaterally, usually high and out to the side, although other positions behind or in front of the body may occur. Any arm action is usually slight and not consistent.

**Step 2**  Bilateral reactive. Arms swing upward briefly, then are medially rotated at the shoulder in a winging movement prior to takeoff. It appears that this movement is in reaction to loss of balance.

**Step 3**  Bilateral assist. The arms pump up and down together, usually in front of the line of the trunk. Any downward and backward motion of the arms occurs after takeoff. The arms may move parallel to each other or be held at different levels as they move up and down.

**Step 4**  Semi-opposition. The arm on the side opposite the swing leg swings forward with that leg and back as the leg moves down. The position of the other arm is variable, often staying in front of the body or to the side.

**Step 5**  Opposing-assist. The arm opposite the swing leg moves forward and upward in synchrony with the forward and upward movement of that leg. The other arm moves in the direction opposite to the action of the swing leg. The range of movement in the arm action may be minimal unless the task requires speed or distance.

*Note.* This sequence has been partially validated by Halverson & Williams (1985).
Reprinted by permission from Roberton & Halverson, 1984.

ping on the preferred leg. Figure 4.14 shows that many more children were at Step 1 when hopping on their nonpreferred leg than when hopping on their preferred leg. Few children were beyond Step 2 when hopping on either leg. If the children in this study are representative of this age group, hopping continues to develop well past the age of 5.

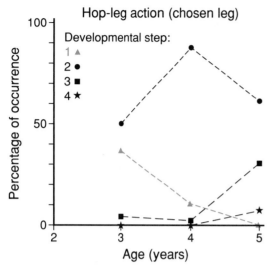

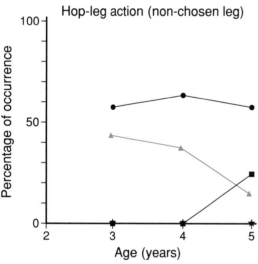

Figure 4.14 The developmental level of leg action in 3-, 4-, and 5-year-old hoppers on their preferred leg (top) and nonpreferred leg (bottom). Note that more children were at Step 1 when hopping on their nonpreferred leg than when hopping on their preferred leg. Only at age 5 were any notable portion of the children at Step 3. (Reprinted by permission from Halverson & Williams, 1985.)

Why do children advance from one developmental level of hopping to another? Several researchers attempted to answer this question by examining the force of landing in hopping (Getchell & Roberton, 1989; Roberton & Halverson, 1988). Note that in Step 2 the hopper lands flat-footed and holds the swing leg still. By Step 3 the hopper uses a softer landing (more leg flexion to cushion the landing, followed by extension to the next takeoff) and swings the nonhopping leg. The researchers confirmed that the force of landing in a Step 2 hop rises sharply upon landing, whereas in a Step 3 hop it rises gradually. To achieve the soft landing, the neuromuscular system probably prepares ahead of time (ahead of the landing) to moderate the force of landing by allowing the leg to "give" (flex). Perhaps, then, once children achieve a Step 2 hop, their ability to project the body higher and to travel faster, and perhaps their increasing body weight, increases the force of the landing. Once that force reaches a critical value that could cause a damaging, jarring landing, the neuromuscular system changes children's hopping movements to allow a safer, more cushioned landing. Hence, children advance to the next developmental level.

*Observing Hopping Patterns*

As with the other locomotor skills, a novice observer must practice hopping assessment. Halverson (1983; see also Roberton & Halverson, 1984) suggests a systematic pattern of observation that focuses on the body parts one at a time. As novice observers, you should observe leg action from the side. Initially, pay attention to the swing leg. Is it active? If so, does it move up and down or swing past the support leg? Next, observe the support leg. Does it extend at takeoff? Does it flex upon landing and extend during the next hop? Look at arm action from both the side and the front. Watch first to see whether the arm movement is bilateral or opposing. If it is bilateral, you can then categorize arm movements as inactive, reactive, or backward in direction. If arm movement is opposing, note whether one or both arms move synchronously with the legs.

## Galloping, Sliding, and Skipping

Galloping, sliding, and skipping all involve the fundamental movements of stepping, hopping, or leaping. Galloping and sliding consist of a step on one foot, then a leap-step of the other foot. The same leg always leads with the step. The difference between galloping and sliding is the direction of movement. In galloping, the individual moves forward; in sliding, the movement is sideways. Skipping is a step and a hop

on the same foot, with alternating feet: step-hop (on right foot), step-hop (on left foot), step-hop (on right foot), and so on. The movement is usually forward (see Figure 4.15a and b).

### Characteristics of Early Skill Patterns

Children's early attempts at these skills are usually arrhythmical and stiff, as shown in Figure 4.16. The arms are rarely involved in projecting the body off the floor. Children might hold their arms stiffly in the high guard position or out to the side to aid their balance. Their stride or step length is short, and they land flat-footed. Little trunk rotation is used, and they exaggerate vertical lift. In early galloping attempts, a child's trailing leg may land ahead of the lead leg.

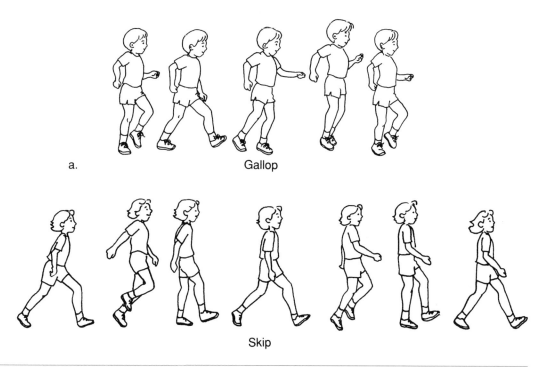

a.                          Gallop

b.                          Skip

**Figure 4.15** (a) Galloping is a step on a lead leg and a leap-step on the trailing leg. (b) Skipping is a step then a hop on one foot and a step then a hop on the other foot, alternately continuing. (Redrawn from Clark & Whitall, 1989.)

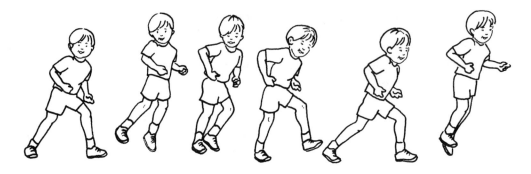

**Figure 4.16** A beginning galloper. The arms are held stiffly, the stride length is short, and vertical movement is exaggerated.

### Proficient Skill Patterns

In contrast, children proficient at galloping, sliding, and skipping are rhythmical and relaxed, as seen in Figure 4.17. Proficiency in these skills includes the following characteristics:

- The arms are no longer needed for balance.
- In skipping, arms swing rhythmically in opposition to the legs and provide momentum.
- The child can use the arms for another purpose during galloping and sliding, such as clapping.
- Heel-forefoot or forefoot landings prevail.
- The knees "give" on landing, remaining flexed while they support the body's weight, and then extend at takeoff, especially when the child is traveling quickly.

### Developmental Changes

Galloping is the first of these three patterns to emerge. It develops sometime after the child has firmly established the running pattern (around age 2) and usually before hopping (at age 3 or 4). Galloping is the first asymmetrical locomotor pattern a child learns. You'll recall that walking and running have 50% phasing—the legs make the same movement, but the cycle of one leg is halfway behind the cycle of

the other. Galloping is uneven. The step takes longer than the leap-step. Gallopers, regardless of age, tend to use one of two timing patterns: The step takes either approximately twice as long as the leap-step (a 66%/33% phasing) or three times as long (a 75%/25% phasing) (Clark & Whitall, 1989b; Whitall, 1988b). Children master sliding next, but in both galloping and sliding, they develop the ability to lead with the nondominant leg much later than with the dominant leg.

Skipping is usually the last of the locomotor patterns to emerge, usually between 4 and 7 years of age. A little more than half of 5-year-olds demonstrate early skipping (Branta, Haubenstricker, & Seefeldt, 1984). At first, a child might perform a unilateral step-hop—that is, a skip with the dominant leg and just a running step with the other leg. When the child begins to skip with both legs, occasional breaks with a step or gallop interjected are common (Gutteridge, 1939; Wickstrom, 1987).

Though no one has validated developmental steps for skipping, several changes are obvious. A beginning skipper uses a high hop and knee lift. The skip appears jerky. Perhaps this reflects the need for much effort to project the body off the ground for the hop. Eventually, the child partially extends the leg on the hop and uses a lower but smoother knee lift, making the skip smoother and more rhythmic. Perhaps

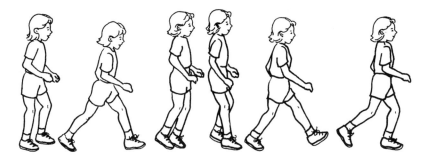

**Figure 4.17**   An advanced galloper. The arms move in opposition to the legs. Movements are rhythmical and landings are not flat-footed.

greater leg strength allows the child to get the body off the ground with only partial leg extension.

Several changes in arm action occur. Beginners use the arms inconsistently, often swinging one or both arms up to the side. Then, skippers begin to use the arms bilaterally, swinging them sometimes forward and back in circles, sometimes forward and down. Skilled skippers can use their arms in opposition to their legs (Wickstrom, 1987).

It is easy to speculate as to why skipping is the last fundamental locomotor skill that children develop. The coordination between the legs is symmetrical, but within each leg the pattern of movement is asymmetrical. Girls typically perform these locomotor skills at an earlier age than boys, perhaps reflecting their slight edge in biological maturity for chronological age, imitation of other girls, or possibly encouragement from family and friends.

*Observing Galloping,*
*Sliding, and Skipping Patterns*

While observing galloping, you should first take a side view and note where the trailing foot lands in relation to the lead foot. You can also see the extent of vertical lift from the side. You can watch the arms from any angle. In proficient galloping, the trailing foot lands alongside or behind the lead foot; the flight pattern is low; and the arms are free to swing rhythmically, to clap, or to engage in another activity. You should note whether a child can lead with just the dominant leg or with either leg.

Sliding is best observed from the front. Focus on the knees to see if they are stiff, as in early sliding, or relaxed so that the child's steps have the spring characteristic of proficient sliding. Note whether the arms are in an inefficient guard position or are relaxed and free to be used for another task. As with galloping, you should see if a child can slide to just the dominant side or to both sides.

When watching skipping, observe whether the child skips with one leg and runs with the other, or skips with both. If the child skips with both legs, look at the height of the hop and the knee lift from the side. Lower height and knee lift characterize a more proficient, smoother skip. Finally, watch the arm pattern to see if it is bilateral or, in a more proficient skipper, in opposition to the leg movement.

## Developmental Transitions in Locomotor Skills

In chapter 3 we examined the factors that might be responsible for the initiation of early skills such as creeping and walking. Now let's consider what might initiate the locomotor skills of running, galloping, hopping, and skipping. To do so, it is useful to adopt the dynamic systems perspective. According to this perspective, new movement patterns may emerge as a result of an increase (also called a scaling up) of some factor, such as speed. Thus far, few researchers have attempted to identify these factors for the later developing locomotor skills, but Clark and Whitall (1989b) have speculated upon what they might be:

- In running there is a period of flight, so to run, an individual must be able to exert sufficient force at toe-off to produce a reaction force that propels the body into flight. The rate-controlling factor for running might be the ability to generate sufficient force, which in turn might be related to increases in muscle mass or improved nervous system control of the muscles to generate a forceful thrust. Recall that running follows walking by 6 to 7 months. The postural system also must be capable of keeping the body upright to generate greater force at toe-off.

- The transition from running to galloping might be possible when the neuromuscular system can generate different levels of force in each limb. Recall that in galloping one leg takes a step while the other takes a leap-step, so the legs require different levels of ground reaction force. In addition, the postural system must be able to handle the new balance requirements of galloping. In either case, it takes at least 6 months after the individual has established running for the rate-controlling systems to develop to allow galloping.

- Hopping likely depends on the postural system's ability to balance the body on one limb for a succession of hops. Also, the individual must be able to generate enough force to lift the body with one limb, recover, and quickly generate the force again to hop repeatedly. Too long a recovery rate for muscle contraction might be a limiting factor for repeated hopping.

- The emergence of skipping does not appear to be limited by generation of force for the hop, because children hop before they skip; or by balance, because it is more difficult to balance while hopping than while skipping. As mentioned earlier, however, skipping is the most complex locomotor pattern. Skipping might not appear until the individual's neuromuscular system can coordinate the two limbs that are each performing a complex pattern.

It is hoped that developmentalists will soon test Clark and Whitall's hypotheses. Understanding the rate controllers for the fundamental locomotor skills will help us understand how performers acquire even more complex skills.

## Ballistic Skills

*Ballistic skills* are those in which a person applies force to an object in order to project it. The ballistic skills of throwing, kicking, and striking have similar developmental patterns because the mechanical principles involved in projecting objects are basically the same. The ballistic skill researchers have studied most is the forceful overhand throw for distance. Much of the discussion on throwing also applies to kicking and striking, which we will examine next.

### Overarm Throwing

Throwing takes many forms. The two-handed underhand throw (windup between the legs) and one-handed underhand throw are common in young children. There is also a sidearm throw and a two-handed overarm throw. The type of throw people use, especially children, often depends on the size of the ball. Our focus, though, is on the one-handed overarm throw. It is the most common type of throw people use in sport games and has been studied more widely than other types. Many of the mechanical principles involved in the overarm throw also apply to other types of throws.

Researchers often make product assessments using accuracy, distance, and ball velocity as criteria to gauge throwing skill development. However, product measures have several drawbacks. Researchers often must change an accuracy assessment task when working with children of different ages. Young children need a short distance over which to throw in order to reach the target. A short distance, though, makes the task too easy for older children who might all achieve perfect scores. So researchers must increase the distance or decrease the target size for older groups. Also, scores on throws for distance often reflect factors such as body size and strength in addition to throwing skill. Two children may have equal throwing skills but quite different distance scores, because one child is bigger and stronger. Finally, measuring ball velocity at release requires specialized equipment that may not be readily available. Thus, we could argue that product scores are not as useful to teachers as knowing how a child throws. Let's now turn our attention to the quality of the throwing pattern.

### Characteristics of Early Overarm Throwing

It is helpful to contrast children's early attempts to throw with an advanced overarm throw. Young children's throwing patterns tend to be restricted to arm action alone. The child depicted in Figure 4.18 does not step into the throw or use much trunk action. This child merely positions the upper arm, often with the elbow up or forward, and executes the throw by elbow extension alone. Figure 4.19 shows more movement but little gain in mechanical efficiency. Obviously, these children demonstrate minimal throwing skill.

### Proficient Overarm Throwing

By studying the characteristics of a proficient throw, we can identify the limitations in early

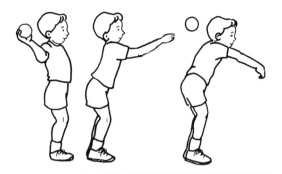

**Figure 4.18** A beginning thrower who simply brings the hand back with the elbow up and throws by extending the elbow without taking a step.
(Drawn from film tracings from the Motor Development and Child Study Laboratory, University of Wisconsin–Madison.)

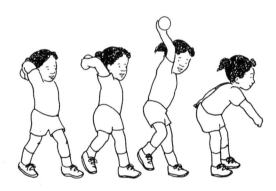

**Figure 4.19** A beginning thrower. Note the trunk flexion, rather than rotation, with the throw.
(Drawn from film tracings from the Motor Development and Child Study Laboratory, University of Wisconsin–Madison.)

throwing attempts. Thus, an advanced, forceful throw for distance has the following movement patterns:

- The weight shifts to the back foot, the trunk rotates back, and the arm makes a circular, downward backswing for a windup.

- The leg opposite the throwing arm steps forward to increase the distance over which the thrower applies force to the ball and to allow full trunk rotation.
- The trunk rotates forward to add force to the throw. To produce maximal force, trunk rotation is *differentiated*—that is, the lower trunk (pelvis) actually begins its rotation forward while the upper trunk (spine) is still "winding up" or moving backward. We also call this type of action *opening up*; this describes any action in which body parts move in opposite directions to exert force ultimately in one direction.
- The trunk bends laterally, away from the side of the throwing arm.
- The upper arm forms a right angle with the trunk and comes forward just as (or slightly after) the shoulders rotate to a front-facing position. This means that from the side, you can see the upper arm within the outline of the trunk.
- The thrower holds the elbow at a right angle during the forward swing, extending the arm when the shoulders reach the front-facing position. Extending the arm just before release lengthens the radius of the throwing arc.
- The forearm lags behind the trunk and upper arm during the forward swing. While the upper trunk is rotating forward, the forearm and hand appear to be stationary or to move down or back. The forearm lags until the upper trunk and shoulders actually rotate to the direction of the throw (the front-facing position).
- The follow-through dissipates the force of the throw over distance. The greater portion of wrist flexion comes during follow-through, after the thrower releases the ball. Dissipating force after release allows maximal speed of movement while the ball is in the hand.

- The thrower carries out the movements of the body segments sequentially, progressively adding the contributions of each part to the force of the throw. Generally, the sequence is as follows:

1. Step forward and pelvic rotation
2. Upper spine rotation and upper arm swing
3. Upper arm inward rotation and elbow extension
4. Release
5. Follow-through

### Developmental Changes in Overarm Throwing

Now that we have discussed the characteristics of an advanced, forceful throw, we can examine how an individual progresses through the developmental steps from initial throwing attempts toward advanced throwing skill. Several developmental sequences of overarm throwing have been proposed, beginning with a sequence outlined by Wild in 1938 and including that of Seefeldt, Reuschlein, and Vogel in 1972. More recently, Roberton proposed a developmental sequence for the overarm throw using the body component approach. Two of the component sequences, arm action and trunk action, have been validated as developmental sequences (Roberton, 1977, 1978a; Roberton & DiRocco, 1981; Roberton & Langendorfer, 1980). Carefully studying the developmental overarm throw sequence outlined in Table 4.6 will help you to compare these steps with the different characteristics of early throwers depicted in Figures 4.18 and 4.19 and the more advanced throwers in Figures 4.20 to 4.23.

Begin the comparison by focusing on the trunk action component. In the first step of the developmental sequence, you do not see trunk action or forward-backward movements before the thrower releases the ball (see Figures 4.18

**Table 4.6  Developmental Sequence for Throwing**

*Trunk action in throwing and striking for force*

**Step 1**   No trunk action or forward-backward movements. Only the arm is active in force production. Sometimes, the forward thrust of the arm pulls the trunk into a passive left rotation (assuming a right-handed throw), but no twist-up precedes that action. If trunk action occurs, it accompanies the forward thrust of the arm by flexing forward at the hips. Preparatory extension sometimes precedes forward hip flexion.

**Step 2**   Upper trunk rotation or total trunk "block" rotation. The spine and pelvis both rotate away from the intended line of flight and then simultaneously begin forward rotation, acting as a unit or "block." Occasionally, only the upper spine twists away, then toward the direction of force. The pelvis, then, remains fixed, facing the line of flight, or joins the rotary movement after forward spinal rotation has begun.

**Step 3**   Differentiated rotation. The pelvis precedes the upper spine in initiating forward rotation. The child twists away from the intended line of ball flight and, then, begins forward rotation with the pelvis while the upper spine is still twisting away.

*Backswing, humerus, and forearm action in the overarm throw for force*
*Preparatory arm backswing component*

**Step 1**   No backswing. The ball-in-the-hand moves directly forward to release from the arm's original position when the hand first grasped the ball.

**Step 2**   Elbow and humeral flexion. The ball moves away from the intended line of flight to a position behind or alongside the head by upward flexion of the humerus and concomitant elbow flexion.

**Step 3**   Circular, upward backswing. The ball moves away from the intended line of flight to a position behind the head via a circular overhead movement with elbow extended, or an oblique swing back, or a vertical lift from the hip.

**Step 4**   Circular, downward backswing. The ball moves away from the intended line of flight to a position behind the head via a circular, down and back motion, which carries the hand below the waist.

*Humerus (upper arm) action component during forward swing*

**Step 1**   Humerus oblique. The humerus moves forward to ball release in a plane that intersects the trunk obliquely above or below the horizontal line of the shoulders. Occasionally, during the backswing, the humerus is placed at a right angle to the trunk, with the elbow pointing toward the target. It maintains this fixed position during the throw.

**Step 2**   Humerus aligned but independent. The humerus moves forward to ball release in a plane horizontally aligned with the shoulder, forming a right angle between humerus and trunk. By the time the shoulders (upper spine) reach front-facing, the humerus (elbow) has moved independently ahead of the outline of the body (as seen from the side) via horizontal adduction at the shoulder.

**Step 3**   Humerus lags. The humerus moves forward to ball release horizontally aligned, but at the moment the shoulders (upper spine) reach front-facing, the humerus remains with the outline of the body (as seen from the side). No horizontal adduction of the humerus occurs before front-facing.

*Forearm action component during forward swing*

**Step 1**   No forearm lag. The forearm and ball move steadily forward to ball release throughout the throwing action.

*(continued)*

**Table 4.6** *(continued)*

**Step 2** Forearm lag. The forearm and ball appear to "lag," that is, to remain stationary behind the child or to move downward or backward in relation to him/her. The lagging forearm reaches its furthest point back, deepest point down, or last stationary point before the shoulders (upper spine) reach front-facing.

**Step 3** Delayed forearm lag. The lagging forearm delays reaching its final point of lag until the moment of front-facing.

*Action of the feet in forceful throwing and striking*

**Step 1** No step. The child throws from the initial foot position.

**Step 2** Homolateral step. The child steps with the foot on the same side as the throwing hand.

**Step 3** Contralateral, short step. The child steps with the foot on the opposite side from the throwing hand.

**Step 4** Contralateral, long step. The child steps with the opposite foot a distance of over half the child's standing height.

*Note.* Validation studies support the trunk sequence (Roberton, 1977; Roberton, 1978a; Roberton & Langendorfer, 1980; Langendorfer, 1982; Roberton & DiRocco, 1981). Validation studies support the arm sequences for the overarm throw (Halverson, Roberton, & Langendorfer, 1982; Roberton, 1977; Roberton, 1978a; Roberton & Langendorfer, 1980; Roberton & DiRocco, 1981) with the exception of the preparatory arm backswing sequence, which was hypothesized by Roberton (1983) from the work of Langendorfer (1980). Langendorfer (1982) feels the humerus and forearm components are appropriate for overarm striking. The foot action sequence was hypothesized by Roberton (1983) from the work of Leme and Shambes (1978), Seefeldt, Reuschlein, and Vogel (1972), and Wild (1937). Reprinted by permission from Roberton & Halverson, 1984.

and 4.19). In the second step, the thrower proceeds to a *block rotation* of the trunk; that is, the upper and lower trunk rotate together, or the upper trunk simply rotates alone. Block rotation occurs between the third and fourth positions in Figure 4.21. Often, you can see the most advanced trunk action, differentiated rotation, in pictures of baseball pitchers. In Figure 4.23, the pitcher has started to rotate the lower trunk toward the direction of the throw while the upper trunk is still twisting back in preparation to throw. We term this *differentiated rotation* because the different parts of the trunk rotate one at a time.

To analyze the complexity of arm movements in throwing, first study the preparatory backswing, then the upper arm (humerus) motions, and finally the forearm motions. An un-

skilled thrower often does not use a backswing (Figure 4.18). At the next step in the developmental sequence, a thrower will flex the shoulder and elbow in preparation for elbow extension, as in Figure 4.19. A more advanced preparation is to use an upward backswing, but the most desirable backswing is circular and downward. The thrower pictured in Figure 4.21 is using this pattern.

As an unskilled thrower begins to swing the upper arm forward to throw, he or she often swings it at an angle oblique to the line of the shoulders—that is, with the elbow pointed up or down. A desirable advancement is to align the upper arm horizontally with the shoulders, forming a right angle with the trunk, as seen in Figure 4.20. Even so, the upper arm may move ahead of the trunk's outline. This movement results in a loss of some of the momentum the thrower gains from moving the body parts sequentially for a forceful throw. In the most advanced pattern, the upper arm lags behind so that when the thrower reaches a front-facing position, you can see the elbow from the side

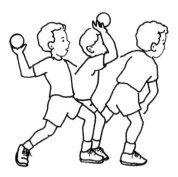

**Figure 4.20** A thrower with Stage 2 arm action. The forearm reaches its farthest point back before the shoulders rotate to front-facing, but the humerus then swings forward before the shoulders, and the elbow is consequently visible outside the body outline. Note the right angle between the humerus and trunk.
(Drawn from film tracings from the Motor Development and Child Study Laboratory, University of Wisconsin–Madison.)

within the outline of the trunk, as in Figure 4.21.

It is also desirable for the forearm to lag behind. The thrower in Figure 4.20 has some forearm lag, but the deepest lag comes before rather than at the front-facing position. The thrower in Figure 4.21 demonstrates the advanced pattern of delayed forearm lag.

Most unskilled throwers throw without taking a step, like the child in Figure 4.18. When a child learns to take the step, he or she often does so with the homolateral leg, the leg on the same side of the body as the throwing arm. This reduces the extent of trunk rotation and the range of motion needed for a forceful throw. When the child acquires the advanced pattern of a contralateral step, he or she may initially take a short step, as in Figure 4.19. A long step (more than half the thrower's height) is desirable.

The body component analysis of overarm throwing demonstrates that individuals do not achieve the same developmental step for all body components at the same time. For example, the thrower in Figure 4.19 is in Step 1 of trunk, humerus, and forearm action but in Step 3 of foot action. The thrower in Figure 4.21 is in Step 3 of humerus, forearm, and

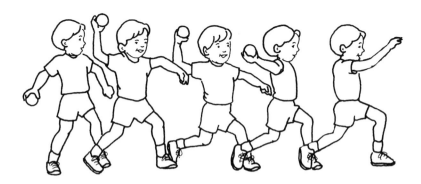

**Figure 4.21** A relatively advanced thrower. Arm, leg, and preparatory action are characteristic of the most advanced step, but the trunk action is characteristic of Stage 2, or block rotation, rather than differentiated rotation.
(Drawn from film tracings from the Motor Development and Child Study Laboratory, University of Wisconsin–Madison.)

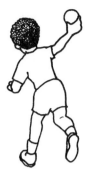

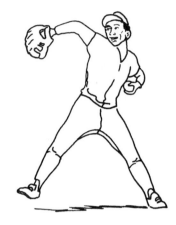

**Figure 4.22**  From the rear you can see that this advanced thrower flexes the trunk laterally away from the ball at release.
(Drawn from film tracings from the Motor Development and Child Study Laboratory, University of Wisconsin–Madison.)

**Figure 4.23**  This still drawing of a baseball pitcher captures the forward movement of the hips while the upper trunk is still back. This is called differentiated rotation because the hips and upper trunk rotate at different times.
(Drawn from film tracings from the Motor Development and Child Study Laboratory, University of Wisconsin–Madison.)

foot action but in Step 2 of trunk action. Children the same age may be at various levels of the body component sequences, so they look different from one another as they advance through the developmental sequence.

It is desirable for all individuals to move through the various developmental steps during childhood to achieve an advanced throwing pattern. They can then use throwing in a number of different physical activities, such as softball, football, and team handball. In fact, several authors noted that children have developed a skillful throwing pattern by age 6 (DeOreo & Keogh, 1980; McClenaghan & Gallahue, 1978; Zaichkowsky, Zaichkowsky, & Martinek, 1980). At least two studies present contradictory results. Halverson, Roberton, and Langendorfer (1982) filmed a group of 39 children in kindergarten and 1st, 2nd, and 7th grades and classified them according to Roberton's developmental sequence. Their analysis of upper arm action demonstrated that most of the younger boys were already at Step 2 of humerus action, and by Grade 7, more than 80% had achieved the most advanced level (Step 3). In contrast, approximately 70% of the girls were still in Step 1 of humerus action when initially filmed. By Grade 7, only 29% of the girls had reached Step 3.

This trend was also apparent for forearm action. Almost 70% of the boys demonstrated Step 2 forearm action when initially filmed. Some were still in this level by Grade 7, but considerably more, 41%, had reached Step 3. More than 70% of the girls began in Step 1, and the majority, 71%, were only at the second level in Grade 7. Gender differences in developmental throwing progress were even more apparent for trunk action. Almost all the boys started in Step 2, and 46% advanced to Step 3 by Grade 7. Similarly, almost 90% of the girls were in Step 2 in kindergarten, but by Grade 7, all the girls remained in Step 2, none having advanced to Step 3.

Another study (Leme & Shambes, 1978) focused on throwing patterns in adult women. The 18 women were selected because they had very low throwing velocities. All demonstrated inefficient throwing patterns, including block rotation, lack of a step forward with the throw, and lack of upper arm lag. Although these women were unique because of their low throwing velocities, the study certainly demonstrates that not all adults achieve an advanced throwing pattern. Perhaps these women lacked practice opportunities or good instruction in childhood. Together, these two studies suggest that progress through the developmental levels is not automatic and may not be completed during childhood or even adolescence.

### Observing Overarm Throwing Patterns

Overarm throwing is complex and difficult to observe in detail. The best procedure is to focus on a small number of components, or even a single component, at any one time. Some characteristics are best observed from the front or back:

- The trunk to upper arm angle
- The elbow angle
- Lateral trunk bend

You can see others from the throwing side:

- The step
- Trunk rotation
- Upper arm and forearm lag

Videotaping is particularly valuable in helping you learn to observe the overarm throw.

## Kicking

Like throwing, kicking projects an object; but unlike in throwing, the individual strikes the object. Children obviously must have the perceptual abilities and eye-foot coordination necessary to consistently make contact with the ball. Teachers can simplify the task for young children by challenging them to kick a stationary ball.

### Characteristics of Early Kicking

As with throwing, unskilled kickers tend to use a single action rather than a sequence of actions. As you can see in Figure 4.24, there is no step forward with the nonkicking leg, and the kicking leg merely pushes forward at the ball. The knee of the kicking leg is bent at contact, and an unskilled kicker may even re-

tract the leg immediately after contacting the ball. The trunk does not rotate, and the child holds the arms stationary at the sides. The child in Figure 4.25 demonstrates more advanced kicking skill by stepping forward with the non-kicking foot, thus putting the kicking leg in a cocked position.

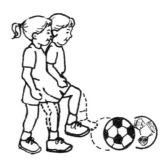

**Figure 4.24** A beginning kicker simply pushes the leg forward.
(Drawn from film tracings from the Motor Development and Child Study Laboratory, University of Wisconsin–Madison.)

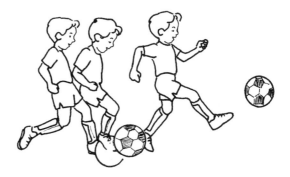

**Figure 4.25** This kicker has made some improvements compared to the beginning kicker. He steps forward, putting the leg in a cocked position, but the leg swing is still minimal. The knee is bent at contact, and some of the momentum of the kick is lost.
(Drawn from film tracings from the Motor Development and Child Study Laboratory, University of Wisconsin–Madison.)

## Proficient Kicking

Compare the characteristics of early kicking to the critical features of advanced kicking shown in Figure 4.26. The advanced kicker does the following:

- Starts with a preparatory windup. The kicker achieves this position, with the trunk rotated back and the kicking leg cocked, by leaping or running up to the ball. As a natural consequence of the running stride, the trunk is rotated back, and the knee of the kicking leg is flexed just after the push-off of the rear leg. Hence, the kicker is able to apply maximal force over the greatest distance. Running up to the ball also contributes momentum to the kick.
- Uses sequential movements of the kicking leg. The thigh rotates forward, then the lower leg extends (knee straightens) just before contact with the ball to increase the radius of the arc through which the kicking leg travels. The straightened leg continues forward after contact to dissipate the force of the kick in the follow-through.
- Swings the kicking leg through a full range of motion at the hip.
- Uses trunk rotation to maximize the range of motion. As a result of the complete leg swing, the kicker compensates by leaning back at contact.
- Uses the arms in opposition to the legs, as a reaction to trunk and leg motion.

## Developmental Changes in Kicking

The study of kicking development in children has not been as extensive as educators would like. Although we know the overall changes children must undergo to perform an advanced kick, the qualitative changes that each body part makes are not well documented. Recently, Haubenstricker, Seefeldt, and Branta (1983) found that only 10% of the 8.5- to 9.0-year-old children they studied exhibited advanced

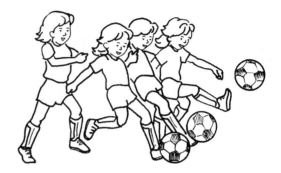

**Figure 4.26**   An advanced kicker. Note the full range of leg motion, trunk rotation, and arm opposition.
(Drawn from film tracings from the Motor Development and Child Study Laboratory, University of Wisconsin–Madison.)

kicking form. So we have reason to speculate that, as with throwing, children do not automatically achieve proficient kicking.

## Observation of Kicking Patterns

To give children adequate instruction in kicking, it is especially important to observe individual children. From the side, a teacher can look for

- placement of the support foot,
- range of motion and precontact extension in the kicking leg,
- range of trunk motion, and
- arm opposition.

Let us now turn to the development of punting—a special form of kicking for which researchers have hypothesized a developmental sequence.

## Punting

Punting is a ballistic skill that is mechanically similar to kicking. Yet punting tends to be more difficult for children to learn. To punt, a child drops the ball from the hands and must time the leg swing to the dropping ball.

## Characteristics of Early Punting

A beginning punter tends to toss the ball up rather than drop it and will often release the ball after the support leg contacts the ground, if the child even takes a step at all. The arms drop to the sides. The child might rigidly extend the kicking-leg knee or bend it at a right angle, as in Figure 4.27. The child typically holds the foot at a right angle to the leg so that the ball contacts the toes rather than the instep, resulting in an errant punt.

## Proficient Punting

To execute a sound punt, as shown in Figure 4.28, a child must do the following:

- Extend the arms forward with the ball in hand before dropping it as the final leg stride is taken.
- Move the arms to the side after releasing the ball, then move into an arm opposition pattern.
- Leap onto the supporting leg and swing the punting leg vigorously up to contact

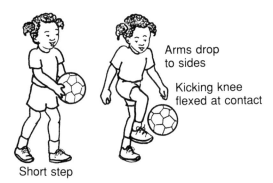

Short step

Arms drop to sides

Kicking knee flexed at contact

**Figure 4.27** A beginning punter takes only a short step and flexes the kicking leg knee 90 degrees at contact (Step 1). The ball is dropped from waist height (Step 3), but the arms drop to the sides at contact (Step 1).
(Drawn from film tracings from the Motor Development and Child Study Laboratory, University of Wisconsin–Madison.)

the ball such that the body leaves the ground with a hop of the supporting leg.
- Keep the kicking-leg knee nearly straight and the toes pointed at time of contact.

## Developmental Changes in Punting

Roberton (1984) hypothesized a developmental sequence for punting (see Table 4.7). Arm action is divided into two sequences, one for the ball-release phase and one for the ball-contact phase. The ball-release sequence outlines progress from tossing the ball up to begin the punt, to dropping the ball late, to timing the drop appropriately. The ball-contact sequence shows that the arms make a transition from nonuse to bilateral movement to the arm opposition pattern that characteristically accompanies forceful lower trunk rotation.

The leg action sequence reflects a developmental transition from a short step of the nonkicking leg to a long step, and finally to a leap. At contact, the ankle of the kicking leg changes from a flexed to an extended position.

## Observing Punting Patterns

Observing a punter from the side offers you a view of the ball drop, the arm position, and the foot position. You can clearly see the degree of foot extension at ball contact from this position.

# Sidearm Striking

Although many sports and physical activities incorporate striking, research data on the development of striking is sparse. Striking encompasses numerous skills. It can be done with various body parts, such as the hands or feet. People can also use a variety of implements in various orientations, such as swinging a bat sidearm, a racket overhand, or a golf club underhand. In our discussion, we will focus on one-handed sidearm striking with an implement and one-handed overarm striking with an implement.

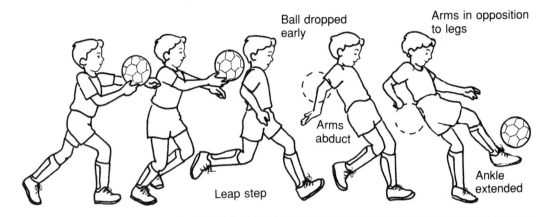

**Figure 4.28**　An advanced punter. The last step is a leap, the ankle is extended (plantar flexed) at ball contact, and the punt is completed with a hop on the support leg (Step 3). The ball is dropped early from chest height (Step 4), the arms abduct and move in opposition to the legs (Step 3).
(Drawn from film tracings from the Motor Development and Child Study Laboratory, University of Wisconsin–Madison.)

Of the basic skills we've discussed so far, striking involves the most difficult perceptual judgment. Success in meeting a moving object is limited in early childhood; therefore, it is difficult to assess striking of a moving object in young children. For this reason, teachers often adapt striking tasks for young children by making the ball stationary. Researchers often base developmental sequences for striking on striking a stationary ball so that they can describe the changes in young children's movement patterns.

We can apply the mechanical principles and developmental aspects of one-handed striking of a stationary object to other types of striking tasks. Keep this in mind as we examine the development of the striking pattern.

### Characteristics of Early Sidearm Striking

A child's first attempts to strike sidearm often look like unskilled attempts to throw overhand. The child chops at the oncoming ball by extending at the elbow, using little leg and trunk action. As in Figure 4.29, the child often faces the oncoming ball.

### Proficient Sidearm Striking

An advanced sidearm strike incorporates many of the characteristics of an advanced overarm throw. Such characteristics include the following:

- Stepping into the hit, thus applying linear force to the strike. The step should be a distance more than half the individual's standing height (Roberton, 1984). The preparatory stance should be sideways to allow for this step and the sidearm swing.
- Using differentiated trunk rotation to permit a larger swing and to contribute more force through rotary movement.
- Swinging through a full range of motion to apply the greatest force possible.
- Swinging in a roughly horizontal plane and extending the arms just before contact.
- Linking or chaining the movements together to produce the greatest force possible. The sequence is backswing and step forward, pelvic rotation, spinal rotation and swing, arm extension, contact, and follow-through.

**Table 4.7   Developmental Sequence for Punting**

*Ball-release phase: Arm component*

**Step 1**   Upward toss. Hands are on the sides of the ball. The ball is tossed upward from both hands after the support foot has landed (if a step was taken).

**Step 2**   Late drop from chest height. Hands are on the sides of the ball. The ball is dropped from chest height after the support foot has landed (if a step was taken).

**Step 3**   Late drop from waist height. Hands are on the sides of the ball. The ball is lifted upward and forward from waist level. It is released at the same time as or just prior to the landing of the support foot.

**Step 4**   Early drop from chest height. One hand is rotated to the side and under the ball. The other hand is rotated to the side and top of the ball. The hands carry the ball on a forward and upward path during the approach. It is released at chest level as the final approach stride begins.

*Ball-contact phase: Arm component*

**Step 1**   Arms drop. Arms drop bilaterally from ball release to a position on each side of the hips at ball contact.

**Step 2**   Arms abduct. Arms bilaterally abduct after ball release. The arm on the side of the kicking leg may pull back as that leg swings forward.

**Step 3**   Arm opposition. After ball release, the arms bilaterally abduct during flight. At contact the arm opposite the kicking leg has swung forward with that leg. The arm on the side of the kicking leg remains abducted and to the rear.

*Ball-contact phase: Leg action component*

**Step 1**   No/short step; ankle flexed. No step or one short step is taken. The kicking leg swings forward from a position parallel or slightly behind the support foot. The knee may be totally extended by contact or, more frequently, still flexed 90 degrees with contact above or below the knee joint. The thigh is still moving upward at contact. The ankle tends to be (dorsi-) flexed.

**Step 2**   Long step; ankle extension. Several steps may be taken. The last step onto the support leg is a long stride. The thigh of the kicking leg has slowed or stopped forward motion at contact. The ankle is extended (plantarflexed). The knee has 20 to 30 degrees of extension still possible by contact.

**Step 3**   Leap and hop. The child may take several steps, but the last is actually a leap onto the support foot. After contact, the momentum of the kicking leg pulls the child off the ground in a hop.

*Note.* This sequence was hypothesized by Roberton (1984) and has not been validated.
Reprinted by permission from Roberton & Halverson, 1984.

### Developmental Changes in Sidearm Striking

Researchers have not validated a complete developmental sequence for sidearm striking, but we can apply the sequences for foot and trunk action in the overarm throw to striking (see Table 4.6). Additionally, we know some of the qualitative changes individuals make in the arm action for sidearm striking. The arm action for sidearm striking is distinct from that for overarm and underarm (as in the golf swing) striking, but all three forms share many of the same mechanical principles. We will discuss sidearm striking first, but keep in mind that many of

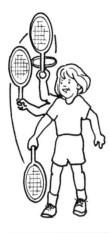

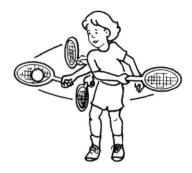

**Figure 4.30** This girl has made improvements compared to the beginning striker. She stands sideways and executes a sidearm strike, but does not involve the lower body.
(Drawn from film tracings from the Motor Development and Child Study Laboratory, University of Wisconsin–Madison.)

**Figure 4.29** This young girl executes a striking task with arm action only. She faces the ball and swings down rather than sideways.
(Drawn from film tracings from the Motor Development and Child Study Laboratory, University of Wisconsin–Madison.)

the qualitative changes in the arm action for sidearm striking and the mechanical principles involved will apply to overarm striking as well.

The first obvious change in sidearm striking from that shown in Figure 4.29 occurs when a striker stands sideways to the ball. By transferring the weight to the rear foot, taking a step forward, and transferring the weight forward at contact, a striker is able to improve his or her striking skills. The child in Figure 4.30 turns sideways but has not yet learned to step into the strike.

A second beneficial change is the use of trunk rotation. Individuals first use block rotation before advancing to differentiated (pelvic, then spinal) rotation, a developmental sequence similar to that in throwing. A skilled striker who uses differentiated trunk rotation appears in Figure 4.31.

Strikers also progressively change the plane of their swing from the vertical chop seen in Figure 4.29 to an oblique plane, and finally to a horizontal plane, as seen in Figure 4.30. They eventually obtain a longer swing by holding

their elbows away from their sides and extending their arms just before contact. A beginning striker frequently holds a racket or paddle with a *power grip*, where the handle is held in the palm like a club (see Figure 4.32a and b; Napier, 1956). With this grip the striker tends to keep the elbow flexed during the swing and to supinate the forearm, thus undercutting the ball. Although children often use the power grip with any striking implement, they commonly adopt it when given implements that are too big and heavy for them. Educators can promote use of the proper *shake-hands grip* by giving children striking implements that are an appropriate size and weight (Roberton & Halverson, 1984).

### Observing Sidearm Striking Patterns

As with many of the skills we've looked at thus far, studying a child's swing from more than one location yields the most information. From the "pitching" position you can observe the direction of the step, the plane of the swing, and arm extension. From the side, you can check the step, the trunk rotation, and the extent of the swing.

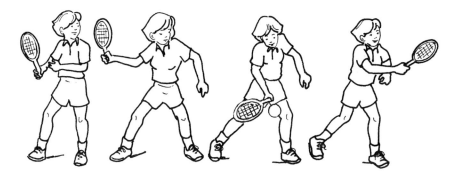

**Figure 4.31** An advanced striker. The swing arm moves through a full range of motion. The striker steps into the swing and uses differentiated trunk rotation.
(Drawn from film tracings from the Motor Development and Child Study Laboratory, University of Wisconsin–Madison.)

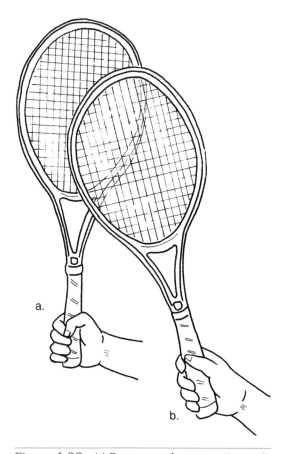

**Figure 4.32** (a) Beginners often use a "power" grip, causing them to undercut a ball. (b) A "shake hands" grip is desirable for sidearm striking.

## Overarm Striking

One can execute overarm striking without an implement, such as in the overarm volleyball serve, or with an implement, such as in the tennis serve. We will focus on overarm striking with an implement.

### Characteristics of Early Overarm Striking

A beginning striker demonstrates limited pelvic and spinal movement, swings with a collapsed elbow, and swings the arm and racket forward in unison, as in Figure 4.33. The collapsed elbow leads to a low point of contact between the racket and the ball. The movement pattern of early overarm striking, then, is similar to that of early overarm throwing and early sidearm striking.

### Proficient Overarm Striking

A person who is skilled at overarm striking, as depicted in Figure 4.34, will do the following:

- Rotate both the pelvis and the spine more than 90 degrees.
- Hold the elbow at an angle between 90 and 119 degrees at the start of forward movement.
- Let the racket lag behind the arm during the forward swing.

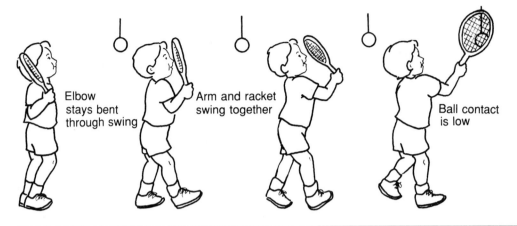

**Figure 4.33** Beginning overarm striking. Trunk movement is minimal. The elbow is collapsed, the arm and racket move together, and contact point is low.

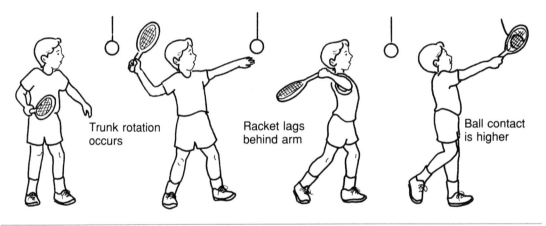

**Figure 4.34** Proficient overarm striking. Trunk rotation is obvious. The racket lags behind the arm during the swing.

Racket lag is consistent with the open kinetic chain principle described in concept 4.1 of this chapter and with the humerus and forearm lag: The humerus lags behind trunk rotation, the forearm lags behind the humerus, and the racket lags behind the forearm to create the chain of sequential movements.

### Developmental Changes in Overarm Striking

Langendorfer (1987) and Messick (1991) proposed developmental sequences for overarm

striking. Both based these sequences on cross-sectional studies and have not validated them with longitudinal research.

Overarm striking is similar to overarm throwing and sidearm striking, but it has unique features, too. Langendorfer identified eight component sequences from a study of children 1 to 10 years old. The trunk, humerus, forearm, and leg sequences are similar to those for overarm throwing (see Table 4.6). Sequences unique to overarm striking included pelvic range of motion, spinal range of motion, elbow angle, and racket action (see Table 4.8).

Messick observed 9- to 19-year-olds executing tennis serves. She identified elbow angle and racket sequences similar to those Langendorfer identified except that extending the forearm and racket up to contact the ball was char-

acteristic of the tennis serves. She also noted a developmental sequence of preparatory trunk action in tennis overarm striking, and this appears in Table 4.8.

Neither Langendorfer nor Messick found the developmental sequences for foot action in throwing to apply to overarm striking, although they observed age differences in weight shifting—older performers shifted their weight more than younger ones. Perhaps overarm striking requires a different sequence that has not yet been identified. This may be especially true in the context of tennis, where the rules specify that the server must not step on the baseline.

### Table 4.8  Developmental Sequence for Overarm Striking

*Preparatory phase: Trunk action component*

**Step 1**   No trunk action or flexion/extension of the trunk

**Step 2**   Minimal trunk rotation (< 180 degrees)

**Step 3**   Total trunk rotation (> 180 degrees)

*Ball-contact phase: Elbow action component*

**Step 1**   Angle is 20 degrees or less, or greater than 120 degrees

**Step 2**   Angle is 21 to 89 degrees

**Step 3**   Angle is 90 to 119 degrees

*Ball-contact phase:*
*Spinal range of motion component*

**Step 1**   Spine (at shoulders) rotates through less than 45 degrees

**Step 2**   Spine rotates between 45 and 89 degrees

**Step 3**   Spine rotates more than 90 degrees

*Ball-contact phase:*
*Pelvic range of motion component*

**Step 1**   Pelvis (below the waist) rotates through less than 45 degrees

**Step 2**   Pelvis rotates between 45 and 89 degrees

**Step 3**   Pelvis rotates more than 90 degrees

*Ball-contact phase: Racket action component*

**Step 1**   No racket lag

**Step 2**   Racket lag

**Step 3**   Delayed racket lag (and upward extension)

The preparatory trunk action and the parenthetical information in Step 3 of Racket Action are reprinted by permission from Messick, 1991. The remaining components are reprinted by permission from Langendorfer, 1987.

### Observing Overarm Striking Patterns

Observation of overarm striking is similar to that of sidearm striking. You might prefer, though, to watch from behind rather than from the "pitching" position, in addition to from the side.

## Reception Skills

Several *reception skills* are basic to sport performance. In these skills, a performer must gain possession or control of an object. The most common reception skill is catching. "Trapping" a soccer ball is a reception skill where the body or foot absorbs the ball's momentum such that the ball remains in a player's control and doesn't bounce away. Fielding in hockey also allows the player to control the ball (or the puck in ice hockey). Little research data are available for reception skills other than catching. However, many of the mechanical principles involved in catching apply to these other skills. The following discussion of the development of catching provides an overview of reception skills in general.

### Catching

The goal of catching is to retain possession of the object you catch. It is better to catch an object in the hands than to trap it against your body or opposite arm so that you can quickly manipulate the object—usually by throwing it.

### Characteristics of Early Catching

A child's initial catching attempts involve little force absorption. The young child pictured in Figure 4.35 has positioned the hands and arms rigidly. This catcher traps the ball against the chest rather than catching it with the hands. It is common to see children turn away and close their eyes in anticipation of the ball's arrival.

### Proficient Catching

In moving from novice to proficient catching skills, as shown in Figure 4.36, a child must do the following:

- Learn to catch with the hands and "give" with the ball, thus gradually absorbing the ball's force.
- Master the ability to move to the left or the right, forward or back, in order to catch the ball.
- Point the fingers up when catching a high ball and down when catching a low one.

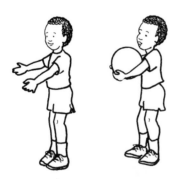

**Figure 4.35**  This young boy holds his arms and hands rigidly rather than "giving" with the ball to gradually absorb its force. Instead of catching the ball in his hands, he traps it against his chest.
(Drawn from film tracings from the Motor Development and Child Study Laboratory, University of Wisconsin–Madison.)

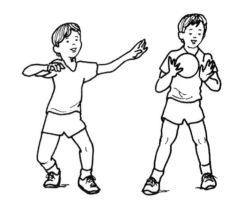

**Figure 4.36**  Proficient catching. The ball is caught with the hands and the hands and arms "give" with the ball.

### Developmental Changes in Catching

It is more difficult to identify developmental sequences for the reception skills than for the locomotor or ballistic skills because the sequence is specific to the conditions under which the individual performs the skill. Many factors are variable in catching: the ball's size, shape (e.g., a round basketball vs. a football), speed, trajectory, arrival point, and so on. Haubenstricker, Branta, and Seefeldt (1983) conducted a preliminary validation of a developmental sequence for arm action in two-handed catching. They used progressively smaller balls as children demonstrated better skill. The sequence, originally outlined by Seefeldt et al. (1972), is summarized in Table 4.9. At 8 years of age most of the boys and almost half the girls these investigators tested were at the highest level of arm action. Virtually all of the children had passed through Steps 1 and 2 by this time. Slightly higher percentages of boys than girls performed at higher levels at any given age, but overall this group demonstrated well-developed arm action by age 8.

Strohmeyer, Williams, and Schaub-George (1991) proposed developmental sequences for the hands and body in catching a small ball (see Table 4.9). A unique feature of this work is that it is based on catching balls thrown directly to

**Table 4.9  Developmental Sequence for Two-Handed Catching**

*Arm action component*

**Step 1**  Little response. Arms extend forward, but there is little movement to adapt to ball flight; ball usually trapped against chest.

**Step 2**  Hugging. Arms are extended sideways to encircle the ball (hugging); ball is trapped against chest.

**Step 3**  Scooping. Arms are extended forward again but move under object (scoop); ball is trapped against chest.

**Step 4**  Arms "give." Arms extend to meet object with the hands; arms and body "give"; ball is caught in hands.

*Hand action component*

**Step 1**  Palms up. The palms of the hands face up. (Rolling balls elicit a palms-down, trapping action.)

**Step 2**  Palms in. The palms of the hands face each other.

**Step 3**  Palms adjusted. The palms of the hands are adjusted to the flight and size of the oncoming object. Thumbs or little fingers are placed close together, depending on the height of the flight path.

*Body action component*

**Step 1**  No adjustment. No adjustment of the body occurs in response to the ball's flight path.

**Step 2**  Awkward adjustment. The arms and trunk begin to move in relation to the ball's flight path but the head remains erect, creating an awkward movement to the ball. The catcher seems to be fighting to remain balanced.

**Step 3**  Proper adjustment. The feet, trunk, and arms all move to adjust to the path of the oncoming ball.

The arm action component is adapted by permission from Haubenstricker, Branta, & Seefeldt, 1983. The hand and body action components are reprinted by permission from Strohmeyer, Williams, & Schaub-George, 1991.

the catcher as well as balls thrown high or to the side of the catcher. These sequences suggest that, as catchers improve, they

- are better able to move their bodies in response to the oncoming ball,
- catch the ball in their hands, and
- adjust their hands to the anticipated location of the catch.

The investigators tested their sequences on a cross section of children between 5 and 12 years old. All of the children over 8 made some adjustment in body position to the oncoming ball, and 11- to 12-year-olds successfully adjusted their body positions about 80% of the time. In contrast, this oldest group could properly adjust their hand positions to the ball only 40% of the time if the ball was thrown directly to them, and less than 10% of the time if it was thrown to various positions around them.

### Observing Catching Patterns

Catching can be observed from the front, allowing you to also toss the ball, or from the side.

### Factors Influencing Interception Skills

It is clear that catching is not a simple task for children. Let us consider some of the reasons that catching and striking an oncoming object are so difficult.

The characteristics of *interception skills* such as catching and striking oncoming objects can vary in many ways. For example, ball velocity, ball size, ball shape, ball trajectory, ball direction, and arrival point can all change. To be successful, performers must make accurate perceptual judgments about where and when they can intercept the object. In addition, they must anticipate this interception to initiate the proper movement beforehand. The goal is to complete the movement by the time of interception. We often term such tasks *coincidence-anticipation tasks*, because a performer anticipates the completion of a movement to coincide with the arrival of a moving object (Belisle, 1963).

Variations in task characteristics influence not only the product of performance—a hit or catch versus a miss—but also the process or movement pattern. For example, children who are capable of catching small balls in their hands may choose to scoop very large balls with their arms, perhaps as a surer means of retaining them (Victors, 1961). It is important that educators be aware of task characteristics for all skills, but this is especially relevant to the interception skills. Various levels and combinations of the task characteristics influence the difficulty of the task and the success of performers. A teacher who uses a developmental sequence periodically to assess progress must keep the task characteristics constant or acknowledge any variations. Let us consider how task characteristics influence performance of the interception, or coincidence-anticipation, skills.

A number of researchers have found that coincidence-anticipation performance improves throughout childhood and adolescence (Bard, Fleury, Carriere, & Bellec, 1981; Dorfman, 1977; Dunham, 1977; Haywood, 1977, 1980; Stadulis, 1971; Thomas, Gallagher, & Purvis, 1981). But the exact pattern of improvement with advancing age depends on task characteristics:

• Young children are less accurate as the movement required of them gets more complex (Bard et al., 1981; Haywood, 1977). So response complexity is one task characteristic that influences how well children perform on interception tasks.

• Children's accuracy decreases if the interception point is further away. For example, McConnell and Wade (1990) found that both the number of successful catches and the efficiency of the movement pattern used decreased if children 6 to 11 years old had to move 2 feet instead of 1 foot, left or right, to catch.

• Young children are more successful at intercepting large balls than small ones (Isaacs, 1980; McCaskill & Wellman, 1938; Payne, 1982; Payne & Koslow, 1981).

• A high trajectory also makes interception more difficult for young children because the ball changes location in both horizontal and vertical directions (DuRandt, 1985).

• Some ball color and background combinations influence young children's performance. Morris (1976) determined that 7-year-olds could better catch blue balls moving against a white background than white balls against a white background. The effect of color diminished with advancing age.

• The speed of the moving object affects coincidence-anticipation accuracy, but not in a clear pattern. A faster speed makes interception more difficult, especially when the object's flight is short. But researchers often note that children are inaccurate with slow velocities because they respond too early (Bard et al., 1981; Haywood, 1977; Haywood, Greenwald, & Lewis, 1981; Isaacs, 1983; Wade, 1980). Perhaps children prepare for the fastest speed an object might travel and then have difficulty delaying their responses if the speed is slower (Bard, Fleury, & Gagnon, 1990). Also, the preceding speeds might influence young children more than they do older performers. If the previous moving object came fast, young children judge the next object to be moving faster than it really is (Haywood et al., 1981). Educators should be aware, then, that when they vary the speed of an object in an interception task greatly from one repetition to the next, children can have difficulty adjusting their responses. This is particularly true if the object's flight is short or the response required is complex.

Clearly, educators must be aware of how the task characteristics may affect the performers they observe. Some conditions make interception tasks more difficult than others, affecting both the product and the process of performance.

---

Young children are just refining their perceptual judgments and are learning to coordinate complex movements. Difficult task conditions might affect their performance more than that of older children.

---

# Weight-Transfer Skills

Most motor skills require people to transfer or shift body weight—to support themselves on various limbs or parts of the trunk successively. A gymnast transfers weight to move across the balance beam or to attain and hold a new balance. A baseball batter or tennis player transfers weight from the rear foot to the front foot when striking a ball. Walking and running require continuous weight shifts from one foot to the other. Although most skills could be classified *weight-transfer skills*, some *rely* on appropriate and well-timed weight transfers for execution. We will focus on two of the latter.

The first is rising to stand from a supine (on your back) position. Compared to some sport skills, this skill might appear very simple. People can execute it throughout most of their lives, providing us the opportunity to study how the skill changes over many decades. Rising is also important to independence (VanSant, 1990). For example, someone who has suffered damage to the central nervous system might need someone's help just to stand. The other weight-transfer skill is the forward roll, a basic gymnastic skill that people also use when falling to better absorb the momentum of landing. Let us begin with rising to stand.

## Rising

In rising, an individual begins lying supine on the floor and ends in a standing position.

### Characteristics of Early Rising

Young children often rotate the trunk so that they rise from a kneeling or half-kneeling position by pushing on the floor with one or both hands. Most children between 4 and 7 years push and reach with the arms, rotate the trunk as they raise it, and come to an asymmetrical squat before standing (see Figure 4.37). Asymmetry, then, is characteristic of early rising patterns.

### Proficient Rising

An efficient pattern of rising from a supine position on the floor is shown in Figure 4.38 and is characterized by the following:

- Both hands push symmetrically against the floor; the person then raises the arms and uses them for balance.
- The head and trunk come forward past a vertical position, and the back extends to achieve an upright position.
- The legs flex to bring the heels near the buttocks to allow a squat, and then extend to stand; the individual might take a step.

### Developmental Changes in Rising

VanSant and her colleagues studied the motor task of rising from the floor to stand in individuals as young as 4 years and as old as 83. The developmental sequence resulting from this work appears in Table 4.10. The sequence is divided into three components:

1. The arms
2. The trunk (including the head)
3. The legs

As noted earlier, children's rising patterns typically consist of asymmetrical movement.

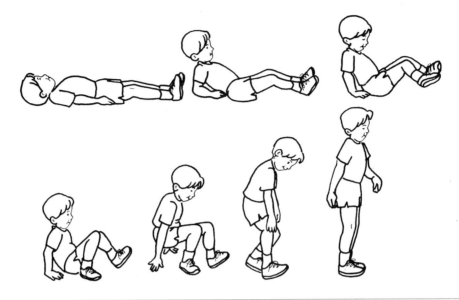

**Figure 4.37** Early rising. Asymmetry is characteristic of this stage. The right limbs push more than the left limbs (Arm Step 2, Leg Step 4). The head and trunk flex forward, then rotate left as the right limbs push (Step 4).

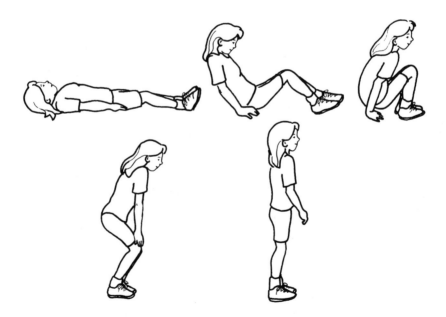

**Figure 4.38** Proficient rising. Movement is symmetrical. The arms push together, then swing forward together (Step 3). The knees flex together (Step 5). The trunk maintains alignment throughout the forward flexion and back extension to rise (Step 5).

**Table 4.10   Developmental Sequence for Rising to Stand**

*Arm action component*

**Step 1**    Push and reach to bilateral push. One hand is placed on the support surface beside the pelvis. The other arm reaches across the body and the hand is placed on the surface. Both hands push against the surface to an extended elbow position. The arms are then lifted and used for balance.

**Step 2**    Push and reach. One or both arms are used to push against the support surface. If both arms are used, there is asymmetry or asynchrony in the pushing action, or a symmetrical push gives way to a single arm push pattern.

**Step 3**    Symmetrical push. Both hands are placed on the surface. Both hands push symmetrically against the surface prior to the point when the arms are lifted synchronously and used to assist with balance.

**Step 4**    Bilateral reach. The arms reach forward, leading the trunk, and are used as balance assisting, throughout the movement. A front- or slightly diagonal-facing is achieved before the back extends to the vertical.

**Step 5**    Push and reach with thigh push. One or both arms are used to push against the support surface. If both arms are used, there is asymmetry or asynchrony in the pushing action, or a symmetrical push gives way to a single arm push pattern. The other arm is then placed on one knee and pushes, assisting in extension of the trunk or legs to the vertical.

**Step 6**    Push and reach to bilateral push with thigh push. One hand is placed on the support surface beside the pelvis. The other arm reaches across the body and the hand is placed on the surface. Both hands push against the surface to an extended elbow position. One or both arms are then lifted and placed on the thighs and push, assisting in extension of the trunk or legs to the vertical.

*Trunk action component*

**Step 1**    Full rotation, abdomen down. The head and trunk flex and rotate until the ventral surface of the trunk contacts the support surface. The pelvis is then elevated to or above the level of the shoulder girdle. The back extends up to the vertical, with or without accompanying rotation of the trunk.

**Step 2**    Full rotation, abdomen up. The head and trunk flex and/or rotate until the ventral surface of the trunk faces but does not contact the support surface. The pelvis is then elevated to or above the level of the shoulder girdle. The back extends from this position up to the vertical, with or without accompanying trunk rotation.

**Step 3**    Partial rotation. Flexion and rotation bring the body to a side-facing position with the shoulders remaining above the level of the pelvis. The back extends up to the vertical, with or without accompanying rotation.

**Step 4**    Forward with rotation. The head and trunk flex forward with or without a slight degree of rotation. Symmetrical flexion is interrupted by rotation or extension with rotation. Flexion with slight rotation is corrected by counterrotation in the opposite direction. One or more changes in the direction of rotation occur.

**Step 5**    Symmetrical. The head and trunk move symmetrically forward past the vertical; the back then extends symmetrically to the upright position.

*Leg action component*

**Step 1**    Kneel. Both legs are flexed toward the trunk and rotated to one side. A kneeling pattern is assumed. One leg is then flexed forward to assume half kneeling. The forward leg pushes into extension as the opposite leg moves forward and extends.

*(continued)*

**Table 4.10    (continued)**

**Step 2**    Jump to squat. The legs are flexed and rotated to one side. Both legs are then lifted simultaneously off the support surface and de-rotated. The feet land back on the surface with hips and knees flexing to a squat or semisquat position. The legs then extend to the vertical.

**Step 3**    Half kneel. Both legs are flexed toward the trunk as one or both legs are rotated to one side. A half kneeling pattern is assumed. The forward leg pushes into extension as the opposite leg moves forward and extends.

**Step 4**    Asymmetrical wide-based squat. One or both legs are flexed toward the trunk assuming an asymmetrical, crossed-leg, or wide-based squat. Internal rotation of the hips may cause the feet to be placed on either side of the pelvis. Asymmetry of hip rotation is common. The legs push up to an extended position. Crossing or asymmetries may be corrected during extension by stepping action.

**Step 5**    Symmetrical squat. The legs are brought into flexion with the heels approximating the buttocks in a narrow-based squat. Stepping action may be seen during assumption of the squat, or balance steps (or hops) may follow the symmetrical rise.

Reprinted by permission from VanSant, in press.

VanSant and her colleagues found that most adolescents use a symmetrical hand push and symmetrical trunk flexion with an asymmetrical squat. About one third of adolescents could use the symmetrical squat. Therefore, symmetry is characteristic of the movement patterns individuals attain by adolescence. Young children might rotate and use asymmetrical positions because they cannot control the direction and amount of force they need to keep their balance throughout the rising task.

Note that the most efficient upper extremity pattern in Table 4.10 is Step 3 of the sequence. Because this sequence is a life span sequence, Steps 4, 5, and 6, which are enclosed by dotted lines, may represent movement patterns that middle and older adults use and that are not as mechanically efficient as the movements in Step 3. The next chapter will give you information about adult movement patterns to help you develop a life span view of performance of this motor task.

### Observing Rising Patterns

To best observe rising, view it from the side, with the individual's head and feet extending to your right and left. From this position you can see any trunk rotation as well as hand pushes. When the individual makes symmetrical movements, you will not be able to see the far limb or side of the body outside the outline of the near limb or side.

### Forward Rolling

To complete a forward roll, an individual moves along the ground, beginning and ending on the feet, with the hands, the back of the head, the upper back, the lower back, and the hips successively supporting the body's weight in between. Young children often call this skill a somersault, but technically a somersault is an aerial skill.

### Characteristics of Early Forward Rolling

In their early attempts to roll, children might be ineffective in executing symmetrical movements, as seen in Figure 4.39. A child might push more with one support arm than with the other or push off with one leg rather than two. A child needs sufficient arm and shoulder strength to support the body's weight and suffi-

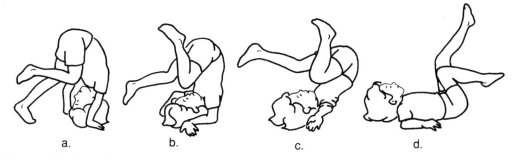

**Figure 4.39** A beginning roller places weight on the head (Step 1) and pushes off with one leg (Step 1). Arm action does not assist the roll (Step 1). The roll is continued by gravity (Step 1), and the knees and hips extend to a layout position (Step 1).
(Drawn from film tracings from the Motor Development and Child Study Laboratory, University of Wisconsin–Madison.)

cient abdominal strength to maintain the tuck position. Otherwise, the head and trunk lag behind and the child must extend the legs as a counterweight to bring the head and trunk up, resulting in a "sitting" finish (Roberton & Halverson, 1984).

### Proficient Forward Rolling

To become a proficient roller, as in Figure 4.40, a child must make the following changes:

- Instead of using the head to support the body's weight, the proficient roller supports the body's weight on the hands, tucking the chin to let the head slide through the arms.
- Instead of keeping the arms back as the lower back takes the weight, the proficient roller brings the arms forward to continue the roll's forward momentum.
- Instead of letting the head and trunk lose their tuck position after the hips start downward, the proficient roller maintains the tuck so that each body area leaves the surface as the next one takes weight.
- Instead of using a one-leg push-off that tends to make the roller go sideways, the proficient roller pushes off with two legs.
- Instead of extending the hips and knees when the lower back touches the ground,

the proficient roller keeps the hips and knees flexed throughout the roll so as to land on the feet and stand when the roll is complete.

### Developmental Changes in Forward Rolling

Roberton (1984) hypothesized developmental sequences for the forward roll from the work of Williams (1980) and Roberton and Halverson (1977) (see Table 4.11). She divided the sequence into two phases: an initial phase with head and arm action and leg action components; and a completion phase with arm action, head and trunk action, and leg action components. The sequential steps outline transitions toward supporting the body's weight with the arms and maintaining a tuck position throughout the roll. We can observe many of these developmental trends in the execution of other types of rolls (shoulder rolls, backward rolls, etc.).

### Observing Rolling Patterns

Observe the movement patterns in forward rolling from the side. A view along the direction of the roll can also help you note sideward rolls that indicate uneven leg and arm pushes. It is important to observe whether the child uses the arms to support the body's weight. Using the arms to pull the body forward to completion and maintaining a tucked position are additional keys to efficient rolling.

The transitions children make in these two weight-transfer skills reflect several improvements. They are increasingly able to use symmetrical movements. This might reflect both better control of bilateral movements and improved strength such that the dominant side of the body does not have to lead a movement. The transitions also reflect more refined control of balance so that the child can smoothly transfer momentum without pausing.

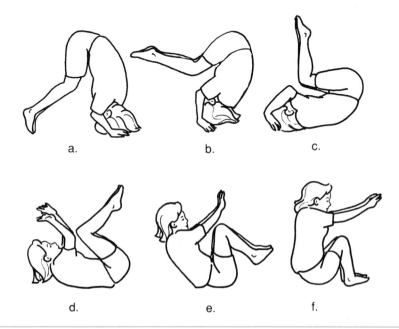

a.   b.   c.

d.   e.   f.

**Figure 4.40**　An advanced roller supports weight on the arms (Step 3), and both legs push equally to initiate the roll (Step 2). The arms are swung forward as weight is transferred to the shoulders (Step 3). The curl is maintained as the head and trunk come off the surface (Step 3), and the knees and hips remain flexed (Step 3).
(Drawn from film tracings from the Motor Development and Child Study Laboratory, University of Wisconsin–Madison.)

**Table 4.11　Developmental Sequences for the Forward Roll**

Initial phase

*Head and arm action component*

**Step 1**　Head support. Little weight is taken on the arms and hands. The hands are often placed on the surface even with the line of the head. The angle at the elbow is approximately 45 degrees. The child may be unable to hold the weight evenly, so the body collapses to one side.

**Step 2**　Head and arm support. The arms and hands partially accept the body weight. The base of support of the hands tends to be wide from side to side and behind the head toward the feet. The angle at the elbow is greater than 90 degrees.

**Step 3** Arm support. The arms and hands now accept the weight as the roll begins, permitting the head, with the chin tucked, to slide through the arms.

*Leg action component*

**Step 1** One-leg push. One leg leads in leaving the surface, then the knee and hip of the lead leg flex while the other leg extends on the push-off.

**Step 2** Two-leg push. Both legs push off equally. The knees flex to about 90 degrees as the balance is lost.

## Completion phase

*Arm action component*

**Step 1** Little assistance. The arms may remain back by the head until pulled off by the forward motion of the body.

**Step 2** Incomplete assist. The arms swing forward to assist in the completion of the roll when the shoulders and/or middle of the back have touched the surface. The elbows are extended during the assist. The hands may be used to push the body to the feet at the end of the roll.

**Step 3** Continual arm assist. The arms swing forward to assist in continuing the momentum of the roll, as soon as the weight has transferred to the shoulders. The arms continue to assist in a forward-upward direction until the weight is over the feet.

*Head and trunk component*

**Step 1** Head and trunk lag. As the hips begin the forward-downward movement, the child abandons the body to gravity. The upper trunk and hips land on the surface almost simultaneously. As the middle of the back and hips land, the head and upper back lag behind, often remaining close to or just off the surface, even when the lower back has made contact.

**Step 2** Partial head and trunk lag. The shoulders touch the surface before the middle of the back and hips, but the head and shoulders do not then leave the surface again until the middle of the back has touched. The body usually continues the roll in a semipiked position over the pelvis.

**Step 3** No head and trunk lag. The head leaves the support surface just after the shoulders touch. Both the head and trunk continue moving forward and upward throughout the roll. By the time the lower back contacts the surface, the head and shoulders are well off the mat.

*Leg action component*

**Step 1** Knees extend; hips extend. The legs tend to hold their push-off position until the lower back or pelvis touches the support surface. At this point, extension in the hip increases, contributing to the loss of curl in the roll. The knees either increase in extension or continue in an extended position. The angle at the hip may reach approximately 120 degrees and is then held if the body continues rotating over the pelvis.

**Step 2** Knees flex; hips extend. Leg action begins as in Step 1. When the middle of the back touches the support surface, extension at the hips increases, also as in Step 1, but the knees flex rather than continuing in an extended position. The roll may continue with the body in this position or the hips may flex.

**Step 3** Knees flex; hips flex. The knees begin flexion just after the hips begin the forward-downward movement in the roll and maintain that flexion throughout the roll. The hips continue flexion throughout the roll.

*Note.* These sequences have been hypothesized from Williams (1980) and Roberton and Halverson (1977). Reprinted by permission from Roberton & Halverson, 1984.

## Assessing the Movement Process

Assessment instruments that focus on qualitative change in basic skill development are not as well known as quantitative skill measures and are used less often. The person administering a qualitative assessment must be thoroughly familiar with the developmental sequence for the skill to be assessed and must have experience in observing the critical features of the movement pattern.

Observers can devise their own tools for assessing qualitative change using the developmental sequences described in this chapter. For example, an observer can list the steps for each component of the overhand throw on a page. After observing a child, the teacher places a check mark next to the appropriate step. By repeating this evaluation throughout the school year and for years to come, the teacher can chart each child's progress. Figure 4.41 presents an example of a checklist for an individual child's hopping performance. Teachers who work in preschools or elementary schools can design checklists that contain only those levels they will most likely observe in that group. For teachers who work with older children, the checklist can feature higher qualitative levels. Teachers who need to assess a large number of students in a short time can simplify the developmental sequences. For example, teachers assessing hopping could simply observe whether the child swings the nonsupport leg or holds it stationary. Figure 4.42 is an example of a simplified hopping checklist.

Ulrich (1985) developed a qualitative assessment of basic motor skills and reported its reliability and validity. The Test of Gross Motor Development (TGMD) is appropriate for children from 3 to 10 years of age. It has two subtests, one on locomotion that includes the run, gallop, hop, leap, horizontal jump,

Child: Jones, Randy   Classroom: S. Johnson
Motor Task: Hopping

| | Level Observed | | |
|---|---|---|---|
| Movement Component: *Leg Action* | Jan. 4 | | |
| Step 1.  Momentary flight | | | |
| Step 2.  Fall and catch; Swing leg inactive | | | |
| Step 3.  Projected takeoff; Swing leg assists | ✔ | | |
| Step 4.  Projection delay; Swing leg leads | | | |
| Movement Component: *Arm Action* | | | |
| Step 1.  Bilateral inactive | | | |
| Step 2.  Bilateral reactive | | | |
| Step 3.  Bilateral assist | | | |
| Step 4.  Semi-opposition | ✔ | | |
| Step 5.  Opposing assist | | | |
| Overall Movement Profile Legs | 3 | | |
| Arms | 4 | | |
| Movement Situation Teacher selected | | | |
| Child selected | ✔ | | |
| Observation Type Direct | ✔ | | |
| Video-tape | | | |
| Film | | | |
| Comments: | | | |

**Figure 4.41** A checklist for hopping based on the component sequences in Table 4.5 (p. 139). Such checklists can be designed from any of the component sequences available.
(Reprinted by permission from Roberton & Halverson, 1984.)

skip, and slide; and a second on object control that includes the two-handed strike, stationary bounce, catch, kick, and overhand throw. The test provides norms so that educators can identify children with deficient motor develop-

*(continued)*

**Assessing Fitness** *(continued)*

Motor task: hopping

Child's name _____ Teacher _____

| Movement component | Level observed | | |
|---|---|---|---|
| | Jan. 4 | | |
| Leg action | | | |
|     Step 1. Non-support leg inactive | | | |
|     Step 2. Non-support leg active | X | | |
| Arm action | | | |
|     Step 1. Arms inactive | | | |
|     Step 2. Bilateral arm movement | X | | |
|     Step 3. Arms opposing | | | |

**Figure 4.42** A simplified checklist for hopping.

ment or screen them out of a larger group for special instruction.

Educators can also use test results to plan their instruction in order to help children reach the next level and ultimately master the movement pattern. This is a criterion-referenced interpretation as opposed to a norm-referenced interpretation. The TGMD provides educators with a standardized assessment that emphasizes the quality of the movement pattern children use rather than the outcome or product of performance.

Several other qualitative assessments are available, but we know little about their validity and reliability (Herkowitz, 1978c). These assessment tools vary considerably in the number of developmental steps they use, even for the same skill. For example, the Fundamental Movement Pattern Assessment Instrument (McClenaghan & Gallahue, 1978) describes three steps for each of five motor patterns

(running, long jumping, kicking, throwing, and catching). The authors describe the motor patterns relative to body components. A second measure, the OSU Sigma Test (Loovis, 1976), describes four levels for each of 11 motor skills. The Developmental Sequences of Fundamental Motor Skills (Seefeldt, 1973, cited in Herkowitz, 1978c) categorizes each of 10 motor skills into four or five steps. Yet another measure, DeOreo's Fundamental Motor Skills Inventory (DeOreo, 1974), evaluates both the product and the process of 11 basic skills. These assessment tools are initial attempts to give educators a means for evaluating the process of children's performance. Educators must use them with caution, however, because little information is available on their standardization procedures. Further, we know little about their validity, and only a few have been examined for reliability (Herkowitz, 1978c).

## REVIEW 4.2

During childhood, basic skill performance improves. As children advance in age, they tend to progress to movement patterns that optimize their performance, consistent with the laws of motion and stability. This transition is marked by qualitative changes in their movement patterns. These qualitative changes can be the critical features in a developmental sequence. Researchers have proposed several such sequences, and a few have been validated. A useful feature of many developmental sequences is that they categorize qualitative change by body component. Individuals do not necessarily move to the next developmental step through simultaneous changes in all body components. Hence, sequencing by body component allows us to assess a child's developmental level while recognizing these variations. Children do not look the same as they advance through the developmental sequences; some may have more proficient leg action than arm action, some more proficient arm action than leg action, and so on.

Ideally, childhood is the time when individuals learn the movement patterns that optimize their performance. During adolescence individuals can continue to improve the product of their performance, learn to combine basic skills, and perform skills in a wide variety of situations. In chapter 5 we turn to motor development in adolescents and adults.

## SUMMARY

Children acquire the basic locomotor and manipulative skills as they grow, but there is a big difference between a child's first crude attempts at a skill and a mature athlete's smooth, powerful movements. Individuals acquire efficient movement patterns in stages. Step by step, a child can find movement patterns that are more and more mechanically efficient. These changes are qualitative—that is, they improve the quality of the movement. They probably reflect a complex interaction among the growing child, the task the child attempts, and the environment, including the space and equipment available. Opportunities for a child to attempt skills facilitate this interaction. Children do not automatically acquire efficient movement patterns just by growing older.

Professionals who guide children's motor development can manipulate practice opportunities. They can give children space and various types of equipment and can challenge them with various appropriate goals. Fundamental to this guidance, though, should be an understanding of what type of change will benefit children the most. It is often better to guide a child to the next step in a developmental sequence than to encourage adultlike performance when a child is at beginning levels.

Professionals who are familiar with the developmental sequences for basic skills can identify the next level or step to which children should move. Moreover, a knowledge of the physical laws of motion and stability facilitates an understanding of developmental sequences, because children change in the direction of more mechanically efficient movement. Professionals must sharpen their observation skills, too, so they know where children are within the sequence and can then help them progress through the next developmental steps.

---

### Key Terms

ballistic skills
base of support
block rotation
coincidence-anticipation tasks
developmental sequence
differentiated (trunk) rotation
50% phasing
interception skills
modal level
open kinetic chain

opening up
opposition
parachute
power grip
reception skills
weight-transfer skills
wing (winging)

## Discussion Questions

1. What distinguishes walking from running? Hopping from jumping? Galloping from skipping?
2. What distinguishes kicking from punting?
3. Which principles of motion and stability can we identify in proficient performance of all the locomotor skills? All the ballistic skills?
4. Growing older does not guarantee optimal skill performance. What factors might contribute to adolescents or adults having less than perfect movement patterns in performing basic skills?
5. What are the major qualitative changes in the development of hopping? Of throwing? Of catching? Of rolling forward?

6. What qualitative changes are common to throwing and striking?

## Suggested Readings

Espenschade, A.S., & Eckert, H.D. (1980). *Motor development* (2nd ed.). Columbus, OH: Charles E. Merrill.

Roberton, M.A. (1984). Changing motor patterns during childhood. In J.R. Thomas (Ed.), *Motor development during childhood and adolescence* (pp. 48-90). Minneapolis: Burgess.

Roberton, M.A., & Halverson, L.E. (1984). *Developing children—their changing movement*. Philadelphia: Lea & Febiger.

Wickstrom, R.L. (1983). *Fundamental motor patterns* (3rd ed.). Philadelphia: Lea & Febiger.

## Chapter 5

# Motor Behavior in Preadolescence Through Adulthood

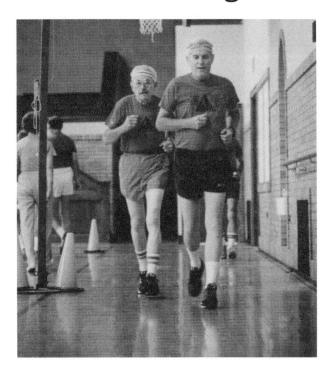

## CHAPTER CONCEPTS

**5.1**
During preadolescence and adolescence, the product (quantity) of skill performance improves.

**5.2**
Adults can refine and perfect their skills, but the aging process affects skill performance.

During the preadolescent and adolescent years, individuals typically improve the product of their skilled performance—running speed, throwing distance, jumping height, and so on. Part of this quantitative improvement is the result of continued growth, especially during the adolescent growth spurt, and accompanying increases in strength and endurance. Improved coordination undoubtedly contributes to skill improvement, too. This is not to say that all children automatically emerge from childhood having achieved the highest developmental step of qualitative change in their skill patterns. Although childhood is a period of great progress in basic skill performance and movement pattern, many adolescents (and adults) do not perform basic skills efficiently (Halverson et al., 1982; Haubenstricker, Branta, et al., 1983; Zimmerman, 1956). Thus, during the preadolescent and adolescent years, individuals ideally will overcome any remaining deficits in their motor pattern efficiency.

Preadolescents and adolescents who have acquired relatively advanced basic skills begin learning to combine and sequence the basic skills into more complex sport-related skills. For example, an infielder runs to catch a bouncing ball, pivots, and throws to first base, not as three individual skills but as one continuous movement. To perform sport-related skills, an individual also must be able to adapt the basic movements to a wide variety of situations. Adolescence, then, can be a period of great progress in skill performance. Individuals can develop to a level of proficient performance in a variety of activities they enjoy.

## MOTOR PERFORMANCE IN PREADOLESCENCE AND ADOLESCENCE

Researchers have studied a variety of motor skills that describe motor development in young people between 7 and 18 years old. Usually they assessed quantitative measures of these skills. Changes in basic skills, such as running, jumping, and throwing, when measured for performance, speed, distance, or accuracy, reflect quantitative improvement in motor per-

formance. The researchers also measured *functional strength* (e.g., the flexed-arm hang) and flexibility (e.g., the sit-and-reach test) to gauge changes in motor performance during adolescence (Branta et al., 1984).

---

**CONCEPT 5.1**

During preadolescence and adolescence, the product (quantity) of skill performance improves.

## Quantitative Improvement in Motor Performance

Although we will review specific performance scores in this section, we will emphasize the trends in improved performance that such scores outline rather than the actual scores in feet or seconds. Specific scores are easily influenced by test administration procedures, type of equipment used (size and weight), and even the clothing and shoes worn by participants. Thus, from a developmental perspective, our discussion focuses on relative changes in motor performance during this period.

### Running

The common quantitative measures of running ability are speed over a short distance (such as a 30-yd or 27.4-m dash) and speed in an agility run. After reviewing studies of dash performance in 1960, Espenschade concluded that running speed increased in boys and girls from an average rate of just under 4 yd/s at age 5 to just over 6 yd/s (3.7 m/s to 5.5 m/s) at age 13. Boys continued to improve to just over 7 yd/s (6.4 m/s) by age 17, but girls leveled off and actually regressed slightly during this age period. These trends are pictured in Figure 5.1a. Haubenstricker and Seefeldt (1986) compiled the results of 14 studies published since 1960, as shown in Figure 5.1b. These studies confirm the same trend, although children's scores are slightly faster, and the performance of adolescent girls plateaued rather than regressed. This "improvement" may reflect increased opportunities for girls to practice, improved instruction, and broadened social acceptance of girls giving an all-out effort in sport activities.

Running agility tests are quite variable in design. The agility run requires, in addition to speed, frequent changes in direction. The length of such tests typically ranges from 120 ft to 400 ft (36.6 m to 121.9 m), with

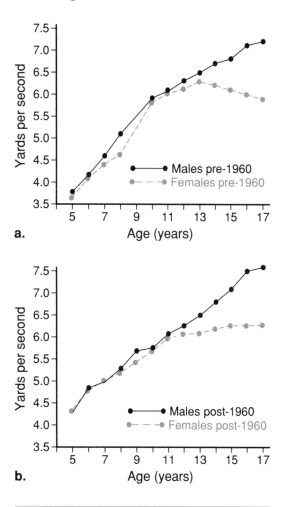

**a.**

**b.**

Figure 5.1   Running (dash) performance in boys and girls aged 5 to 17. (a) The compiled results of studies published before 1960. (b) The results of 14 studies published after 1960.
(Reprinted by permission from Haubenstricker & Seefeldt, 1986.)

variations in the number and type of directional changes. Such variations hinder our comparisons of the different studies reporting adolescents' performance. In a shuttle run, the performer runs back and forth between two points, changing direction at each point. Researchers using the 120-ft shuttle run reported a consistent improvement for boys between ages 5 and

18, with times of approximately 13 to 16 s at 5 years improving to approximately 10 s in the midadolescent years. The trend and scores for girls were similar, although the best average score in midadolescence was approximately 11 s (Branta et al., 1984). Two cross-sectional studies reported a regression in girls' scores in early adolescence (AAHPERD, 1976; Campbell & Pohndorf, 1961), but longitudinal studies have found improvement at all ages (Branta et al., 1984). Both boys and girls, then, improve their average running performance in dashes and agility runs during preadolescence and adolescence.

## Jumping

The most commonly used jumping tests are the horizontal and vertical jumps. Espenschade (1960) determined that boys and girls improved the distance they could jump horizontally from approximately 33 in. (0.84 m) at 5 years of age to 50 in. (1.27 m) at 9 years, as shown in Figure 5.2a. Thereafter, boys continued to improve to approximately 90 in. (2.28 m) at age 17, whereas girls improved gradually, then plateaued at slightly over 60 in. (1.52 m). More recent studies have confirmed this trend (Haubenstricker & Seefeldt, 1986), although the scores reported for girls have often been higher and not as far below the average performance of boys as the scores reported in earlier studies of young adolescents. Girls regressed slightly in midadolescence (see Figure 5.2b). Vertical jumping performance follows a similar trend, improving from approximately 7 in. (17.8 cm) at age 5 to almost 17 in. (43.2 cm) at age 14 in boys and approximately 12 in. (30.6 cm) in adolescent girls (Haubenstricker & Seefeldt, 1986).

## Throwing

Researchers most often use throwing distance to measure throwing performance, although

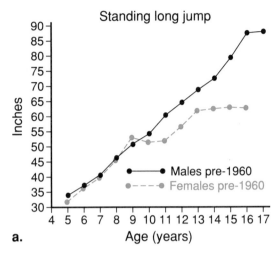

**a.**

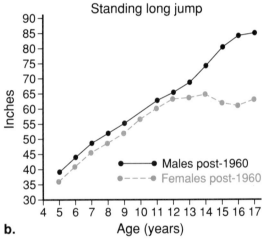

**b.**

**Figure 5.2** Standing long jump performance by boys and girls aged 5 to 17. (a) The compiled results of studies published before 1960. (b) The results of 14 studies published after 1960.
(Reprinted by permission from Haubenstricker & Seefeldt, 1986.)

they have also assessed speed and accuracy. Unlike in running and jumping performance, differences in the distance throw performance of boys and girls exist from even young ages. For example, Espenschade (1960) found that boys improved from approximately 24 ft (7.3 m) at 5 years of age to 153 ft (46.7 m) at

17 years, as shown in Figure 5.3a. In contrast, girls threw only 14.5 ft (4.4 m) at age 5, then improved to 75.7 ft (23.1 m) at 15, but declined slightly to 74.0 ft (22.6 m) at 16. As shown in Figure 5.3b, recent studies duplicated Espenschade's findings except that adolescent

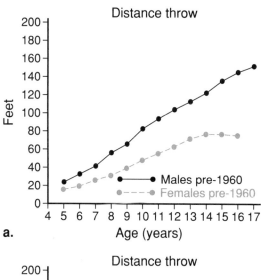

a.

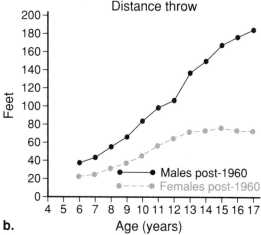

b.

Figure 5.3   Distance throw performance by boys and girls. (a) The compiled results of studies published before 1960. (b) The results of 14 studies published after 1960.
(Reprinted by permission from Haubenstricker & Seefeldt, 1986.)

boys demonstrated even better performance (Haubenstricker & Seefeldt, 1986).

Although both sexes' performances improve dramatically from childhood to adolescence, many researchers have reported large differences in performance level. Additionally, later studies have noted no trend of improved scores for girls. You'll recall from chapter 4 that Halverson et al. (1982) noted significant gender differences in throwing efficiency in 7th graders (children approximately 13 years old).

Few studies have measured changes in throwing speed over age, but Roberton, Halverson, Langendorfer, and Williams (1979) reported that boys improve their throwing speed 5.5 ft/s each year (1.7 m/s) from kindergarten to 7th grade. Girls improve at a rate of 3.9 ft/s each year (1.2 m/s) over the same span. Therefore, the trend of dramatic improvement but large gender differences in throwing speed parallels the results found in studies of throwing distances.

## A Meta-Analysis of Gender Differences

Thomas and French (1985) employed a statistical method to pool the results of 64 research studies that compared boy's and girls' motor performance. Though this statistical analysis technique, the *meta-analysis*, is beyond the scope of our discussion, you should know that this technique allows researchers to express differences between two groups on a scale that is independent of the specific measurement used in each of the research studies. This standardized difference is called an *effect size* and is expressed in units of standard deviation. For example, an effect size of 0.5 is one half of a standard deviation. Standardized academic tests such as the Scholastic Aptitude Test (SAT) and the Graduate Record Exam (GRE) are set up so that one half of a standard deviation is 50 points. An effect size of 0.20 represents a small difference between two groups, 0.50 a medium difference, and 0.80 or greater a large difference.

Thomas and French confirmed that the running dash, standing long jump, and agility run, along with sit-up performance and grip strength, followed the pattern of gender differences identified earlier. Boys perform slightly better in early childhood, widen the gap somewhat in middle childhood, then perform substantially better after puberty. Figure 5.4 is a plot of the effect size for the running dash, long jump, and agility (shuttle) run. Notice that the effect size is moderate, around 0.5, indicating that boys perform somewhat better until early adolescence. Then it increases throughout adolescence and is very large by late adolescence, indicating that boys perform much better than girls. The dotted lines in Figure 5.4 show a 95% *confidence interval*. This means that we can be 95% sure that the actual effect size falls within the dotted lines.

Thomas and French also confirmed through their meta-analysis that gender differences in throwing tend to be large and to favor the boys, even in childhood. Figure 5.5 is a plot of the effect size for both throwing distance and throwing velocity. The effect size is about 1.5 in early childhood and continues to increase, reaching values around 3.5.

Balance performance and two laboratory tasks that involve eye-hand coordination, but not strength or power, show a different pattern. One task is tapping: The performer is challenged to tap as many times as possible in a prescribed area within a time limit. The other task is pursuit rotor tracking, wherein the performer follows a moving target with a stylus as accurately as possible. The effect size for these three—balance, tapping, and tracking—is about zero until puberty, then it rises slightly, indicating that boys perform somewhat better (see Figure 5.6). Gender differences on other tasks such as coincidence-anticipation and reaction time tasks were not age-related. In fine eye-motor coordination and flexibility tasks, small gender differences favored girls. This vari-

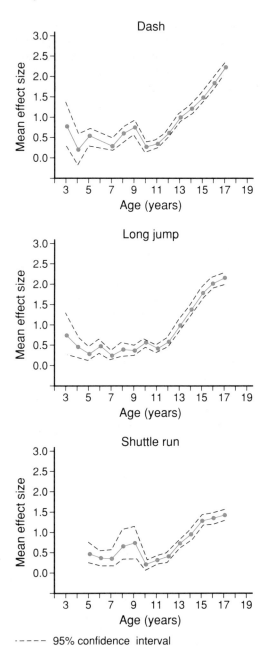

----- 95% confidence interval

**Figure 5.4** Effect size (solid line) indicating gender differences plotted over age for the running dash, standing long jump, and agility (shuttle) run. The dashed lines represent a 95% confidence interval, which means that it is 95% likely that the actual effect size falls within the dashed lines. (Reprinted by permission from Thomas & French, 1985.)

ation in gender differences implies that factors that are different for the two sexes influence quantitative performance. Let us examine some of those factors.

## Factors Influencing Quantitative Performance

Motor performance on the skills we've discussed clearly improves during preadolescence

and adolescence, but you must remember that quantitative performance reflects many factors, such as the developmental pattern used, body size and physique, body composition, strength, and coordination. The influence of these

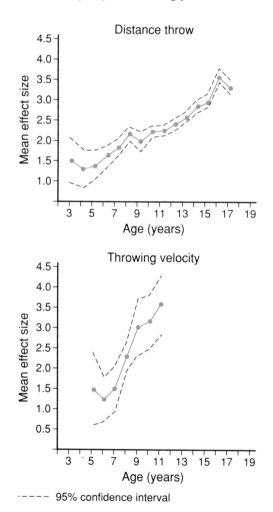

----- 95% confidence interval

**Figure 5.5**  Effect size indicating gender differences for throwing distance and velocity. Note that effect sizes are much larger than those plotted in Figure 5.4.
(Reprinted by permission from Thomas & French, 1985.)

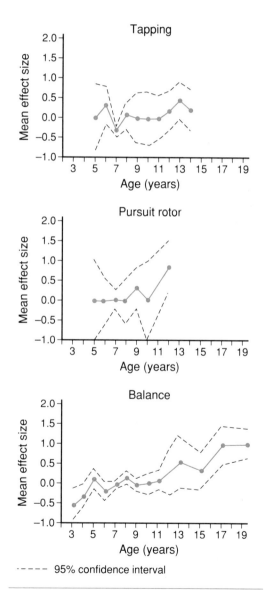

----- 95% confidence interval

**Figure 5.6**  Effect size indicating no gender differences for fine-motor skills and balance until puberty when moderate differences emerge.
(Reprinted by permission from Thomas & French, 1985.)

factors is particularly apparent at the extremes of the performance continuum (Malina, 1980). For example, an overweight or a very weak child will score poorly on quantitative tests. An early maturing, muscular child will score well. A single quantitative score also often confounds several factors. For example, a throw for distance confounds force and angle of projection. Some children score poorly because they have poor force production, whereas others score poorly because they throw at an ineffective projection angle. So one or a combination of body systems, environmental factors, or learning variables might be responsible for individual or group differences in quantitative scores. Even during adolescence one or more body systems can act as a rate controller for a given task.

One of the interesting group differences in the quantitative scores we have surveyed is the plateau or regression of girls' scores in mid-adolescence compared to the improvement in boys' scores (Espenschade & Eckert, 1974). Smoll and Schutz (1990) addressed the contribution of anthropometric variables to this gender difference. For over 2,000 Canadian students ages 9, 13, and 17 years, they measured height, percent body fat, lean body weight, and performance on six motor tasks:

1. Standing long jump
2. Catching (in a wall-pass test)
3. Running for 9 minutes
4. Sit-ups in 1 minute
5. Flexed-arm hang
6. Agility on a side-slide test

Recall that, typically, girls between 14 and 17 are past menarche, have achieved their adult stature, and as part of the maturation process have accumulated some additional fat weight. In contrast, boys gain substantial lean muscle tissue at puberty. Smoll and Schutz placed boys and girls by sex into relative groups of low, medium, and high levels of percent fat. The girls in the low percent fat group had higher fat percentages than the boys in their

low group. The researchers observed that excessive fatness was equally detrimental to the performance of boys and girls at any age and that fatness accounted for at least some of the gender differences, especially on weight-supporting tasks like the flexed-arm hang. At some point, extra adipose tissue likely hinders performance, particularly when it adds measurably to body weight. Height, body fat, and lean weight all accounted for gender differences on tasks such as the run and the wall pass. The effect of anthropometric differences on performance, then, can be task-specific.

Interestingly, less of the gender differences was accounted for by anthropometric factors at older ages (see Figure 5.7), which suggests that other factors still play a role in gender differences in late adolescence. For example, psychosocial factors could be related to the relatively poorer performance of girls. Some girls may lose interest in physical activities or come

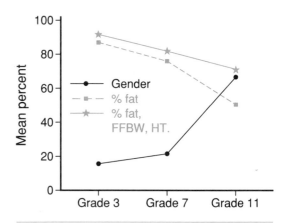

**Figure 5.7** The variance in performance averaged over the flexed-arm hang, standing long jump, and a timed run. Line (a) represents the variance due to gender alone, line (d) the gender differences due to percent fat, and line (e) the gender differences due to percent fat (% fat), fat-free body weight (FFBW), and height (HT). Note that the gender difference accounted for by the anthropometric measurements declines at older ages. (Reprinted by permission from Smoll & Schutz, 1990.)

to feel, through contact with significant friends and relatives, that a maximal effort in such activities is no longer appropriate to their gender role. This latter factor might have been particularly significant in groups tested before the 1970s, when the number of sport programs for girls increased. We will discuss the psychosocial factors that affect performance more fully in chapter 9, but for now keep in mind that such factors could account in part for the gender differences observed in performance.

Leisure pursuits could be another factor in gender differences. If teenage girls as a group tend to pursue more sedentary activities than teenage boys, they lose both the physical conditioning and practice opportunities that boys might gain in sport-type leisure activities. Remember, too, that these differences are stated in the average scores of groups of adolescent girls. Scores vary considerably within a group, and some girls probably continue to improve their performance. The more recent findings of improved running and higher jumping by adolescent girls might indicate a change in social attitudes toward girls' motor performance. Most newer studies have tested girls only to midadolescence. Continued measurement of girls into late adolescence in future studies will help place many of these contributing factors in perspective.

Smoll and Schutz (1990) measured just three anthropometric variables. Keep in mind that certain characteristics—greater height, leaner body composition, longer limb length, and more muscle tissue and strength—could give boys an advantage on specific tasks. But what about motor skills that require fine coordination and precision? Girls have outperformed boys on skills demanding speed and exactness of grasping (Yarmolenko, 1933) as well as hopping (Halverson & Williams, 1985; Jenkins, 1930). Recall that the Thomas and French (1985) meta-analysis documented an advantage for girls in fine eye-motor coordination tasks and flexibility.

Performance differences between the sexes depend in part upon the type of motor task involved. Individual variability is still the overriding rule, and the performance abilities of the boys and girls in a group overlap considerably. Some girls can outperform some boys.

## Quantitative Versus Qualitative Assessment

In studying the basic skills, you saw repeatedly that we can measure skill development by assessing the quality or process of the skill or the quantity or product of the skill. We can classify the performer into developmental steps relative to each body component or measure the distance of a jump or the speed of a throw.

When faced with assessing children, which method should teachers use, qualitative or quantitative? It depends both on who is being assessed and why. If the purpose is to plan instructional experiences for young children, qualitative assessment is the better method. Qualitative assessment is particularly useful as a formative evaluation, because it can help educators determine which educational experiences are appropriate for particular children or what instructions to give particular children. For example, using a qualitative assessment, the educator will see whether the child is taking a step with the throw, extending at the takeoff of a jump, and so on. Scores provided by quantitative assessment, such as the distance a child can throw a ball, give information about where an individual's motor development is compared to other individuals. However, the quantitative score alone does not indicate how an individual throws the ball. Particularly in the case of poor throwing ability, teachers need a qualitative assessment to determine instructional experiences and feedback to individuals on the skill patterns they are using. In contrast, once individuals have relatively proficient form, a teacher can use a quantitative assessment, especially one repeated at regular intervals, to chart a child's progress and compare it to norms for children of the same age and gender.

---

Most of the traditional assessment instruments available to educators yield quantitative scores (Herkowitz, 1978a), because quantitative measurement is straightforward. Professionals with little training in the movement sciences find quantitative measures of motor skill easier to administer. Educators should take care not to choose a quantitative assessment just because it is convenient or available.

---

## Stability in Motor Behavior

Some educators and coaches would like to identify the young boys and girls who have the potential to become elite athletes. These children could then receive special training and coaching to prepare them for Olympic or professional competition. Is this possible? Several investigators have examined this issue objectively by testing groups of children periodically and calculating a statistic called the *correlation coefficient* on the scores they obtained at different ages. This coefficient can range from −1.0 to 1.0 and is usually expressed as a two- or three-digit decimal number. When the coefficient is closer to 1.0, children tend to maintain

---

## Formal Quantitative Assessments

Several assessment instruments are available for evaluating quantitative skill performance. The most widely used is the Bruininks-Oseretsky Test of Motor Performance, a norm-referenced assessment (Bruininks, 1978). This is based on the Lincoln-Oseretsky Motor Development Scale, first published in 1923 in Russian and revised several times (Bailer, Doll, & Winsberg, 1973; DaCosta, 1946; Sloan, 1955). The Bruininks-Oseretsky Test consists of eight subtests, with a total of 46 gross- and fine-motor items. A shorter version of the test contains only 14 items, making it useful as a quicker screening tool. Some of the skills it tests are those discussed in this chapter, such as running agility (the shuttle run), catching a tossed ball, throwing a ball, and jumping horizontally. Some of the fine-motor skills tested are stringing beads, drawing and copying, cutting, and sorting cards. Two balance items and several strength measures are included. The test is appropriate for children between 4.5 and 14.5 years old.

Norms were derived from the testing of over 700 children varying in gender, race, community size, and geographic location. Reliability measures for the Bruininks-Oseretsky Test are high, and it has been used successfully to distinguish children with gross-motor dysfunctions from normal children (Haubenstricker, Seefeldt, Fountain, & Sapp, 1981).

A second example of a norm-referenced quantitative assessment is the Basic Motor Ability Test–Revised (Arnheim & Sinclair, 1979). This test also includes gross- and fine-motor items, including running, throwing, jumping horizontally, kicking, striking, balancing, and stringing beads, among others. The age range also is similar to that of the Bruininks-Oseretsky—from 4 to 12 years old. Norm-referenced assessments must be administered in a very specific way, according to the detailed instructions provided with the instrument, for comparisons to the norms to be meaningful.

their relative position in the group over the growth period. This means that children who perform better when they are young tend to perform better when the group is tested again years later. When the coefficient is closer to 0.0, children tend to trade relative positions within the group during the intervening period. A coefficient close to −1.0 indicates that children maintain their relative positions within the group, but in reverse order—the best performer at one time is the poorest the next time, and so on.

Rarick and Smoll (1967) repeated several motor tests—standing long (broad) jump, 30-yd dash, and throw for velocity—with a group tested each year from age 7 to age 12 and then again at age 17. They then calculated a correlation coefficient for the score of each test at each age with the age 12 score and the age 17 score (see Table 5.1). In general, the correlations were moderate. They were a bit higher over the years from 7 to 12, the lowest coefficient being .115 and the highest .924, than over the entire age span of 7 to 17, the lowest being .127 and the highest .596. Also, the coefficients were higher between two close ages, such as 11 and 12, than between two widespread ages, such as 7 and 17. Glassow and Kruse (1960) found that broad jump and 30-yd dash performance were moderately correlated, .74 and .70, respectively, between ages 6 and 7 and ages 12 and 13. Espenschade (1940) obtained correlations ranging from .29 to .66 and from .36 to .84, respectively, for boys and girls 13 to 16 years old on performance of a variety of tasks.

In summary, age-to-age correlations of motor performance in preteens and teens tend to be positive. Yet most of the correlations researchers have obtained are not high enough to justify their use for predicting adult performance from childhood scores. Too many skilled adult performers would have been dismissed as children with low potential for sport success.

---

Instructors are wise to avoid definitive judgments about children's long-term skill potential based on their status in late childhood.

---

## Skill Refinement

Improvement in the quantity of performance is only one aspect of skill progress that individuals must make in their teen years to achieve proficient skill. Children must also learn to combine the basic skills into integrated sequences and to respond to increasingly more *dynamic environments*. For example, a young ballplayer not only must improve in throwing velocity but also must learn to catch a bouncing ball, step on second base, turn, and throw quickly to first base over an oncoming runner. Unfortunately, educators do not presently have effective tools for systematically measuring these complex aspects of performance. Hence, we do not know much about how people acquire these aspects of skill; we just know that young athletes improve in their ability to combine skills as needed to meet the challenges of dynamic environments.

Another necessary improvement in skill performance is the ability to adapt a movement to a wide range of task demands and conditions. For example, basketball players making lay-up shots must adapt their movements to their starting positions in relation to the basket and the ever-changing positions of other players on the court. As with movement combinations, no system for comprehensively evaluating the development of this ability exists.

Educators can, however, specify the range of conditions that affect skill performance. For example, Herkowitz (1978b) suggested a developmental task analysis in which an educator creates a chart to list the factors involved in a specific task and the continuums along which the factors vary. Examples for throwing and striking appear in Figures 5.8 and 5.9. The

**Table 5.1  Age-to-Age Correlations of Motor Performance Measures**

| Measures | Age-to-age correlations (childhood) | | | | | Age-to-age correlations (childhood to adolescence) | | | | | |
|---|---|---|---|---|---|---|---|---|---|---|---|
| | 7 to 12 | 8 to 12 | 9 to 12 | 10 to 12 | 11 to 12 | 7 to 17 | 8 to 17 | 9 to 17 | 10 to 17 | 11 to 17 | 12 to 17 |
| Boys | | | | | | | | | | | |
| Broad jump | .484 | .534 | .663 | .849 | .780 | .596 | .563 | .694 | .788 | .665 | .728 |
| 30-yd dash | .386 | .424 | .460 | .694 | .780 | .181 | .138 | −.073 | .381 | .354 | .517 |
| Velocity throw | .501 | .308 | .479 | .580 | .501 | .278 | .136 | .378 | .455 | .330 | .404 |
| Girls | | | | | | | | | | | |
| Broad jump | .709 | .705 | .755 | .807 | .896 | .502 | .804 | .704 | .745 | .714 | .661 |
| 30-yd dash | .924 | .830 | .784 | .915 | .933 | .562 | .699 | .765 | .718 | .710 | .696 |
| Velocity throw | .115 | .534 | .462 | .361 | .552 | .127 | .252 | .204 | .225 | .290 | .295 |

Reprinted by permission from Rarick & Smoll, 1966.

| Factors | Size of the object being thrown | Distance object must be thrown | Weight of the object being thrown | Accuracy required of the throw | Speed at which target being thrown at is moving | Acceleration and deceleration characteristics of the target being thrown | Direction in which target being thrown at is moving |
|---|---|---|---|---|---|---|---|
| **Levels** — Simple | Small | Short | Moderately light | None | Stationary | No movement | No movement |
| | | | Moderately heavy | Little | Slow | Steady speed | Left to right of thrower |
| | | | | | | | Right to left of thrower |
| | Medium | Medium | | | | | |
| **Levels** — Complex | | | Light | Moderate | Moderate | Decelerating | Toward thrower |
| | Large | Long | Heavy | Much | Fast | Accelerating | Away from thrower |

Figure 5.8  General task analysis for throwing behavior.
(Reprinted by permission from Herkowitz, 1978.)

dotted lines in Figure 5.9 outline a relatively simple striking task, and the solid lines outline a complex task; note how the characteristics of the factors vary, such as the object struck and the implement used, between the levels of task difficulty.

Using such an analysis, an educator can generate many levels of difficulty. Research has not yet been conducted to show which factors developing children master first or what levels along the continuums most children easily achieve. It is clear that with sufficient guidance, experience, and practice, children can master such variations, and that such mastery is needed for sport and dance performance.

An educator can use a developmental task analysis to provide students with a variety of environmental situations. Children and adolescents will likely achieve advanced movement patterns in simple tasks before they achieve

them in complex tasks; also, skilled performers given simple tasks may use less efficient developmental patterns than they are capable of in challenging situations. That is, task complexity can drive the developmental level an individual demonstrates in a given performance. The environmental situation also affects the quantity of skill performance. One task can elicit a fast sprint, whereas another elicits an easy run. Educators can design educational experiences at the appropriate and desired level by manipulating task characteristics.

## REVIEW 5.1

Preadolescents and adolescents make steady, continued improvement in quantitative skill performance. Before adolescence, gender differences in performance are minimal in running and jumping but greater in throwing.

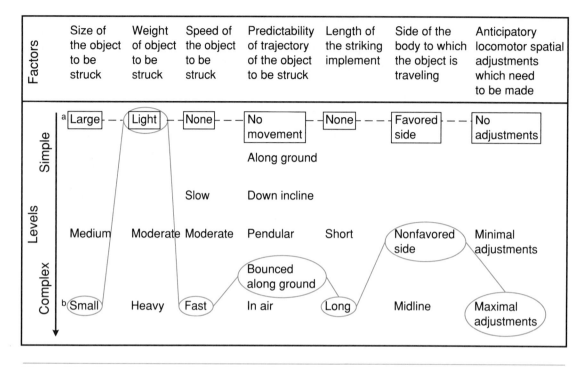

| Factors | Size of the object to be struck | Weight of object to be struck | Speed of the object to be struck | Predictability of trajectory of the object to be struck | Length of the striking implement | Side of the body to which the object is traveling | Anticipatory locomotor spatial adjustments which need to be made |
|---|---|---|---|---|---|---|---|
| Simple | [a]Large | Light | None | No movement | None | Favored side | No adjustments |
|  |  |  |  | Along ground |  |  |  |
|  |  |  | Slow | Down incline |  |  |  |
|  | Medium | Moderate | Moderate | Pendular | Short | Nonfavored side | Minimal adjustments |
|  |  |  |  | Bounced along ground |  |  |  |
| Complex | [b]Small | Heavy | Fast | In air | Long | Midline | Maximal adjustments |

**Figure 5.9**   General task analysis for striking behavior: (a) profile of a general task analysis for a relatively simple striking task (dotted line); (b) profile of a general task analysis for a relatively complex striking task (solid line).
(Reprinted by permission from Herkowitz, 1978.)

During adolescence the gap widens, in part because girls may plateau or even regress. Anthropometric differences account for some but not all of the performance differences between the genders. Environmental factors also might contribute to the differences.

Some environmental factors can be changed. For example, girls can eat properly and exercise to maintain their body fat in the optimal range. Parents and educators can encourage girls to succeed in physical activities and can provide opportunities for them to practice.

Additionally, the type of skill tested determines performance differences between the sexes. In skills involving body support or projection, boys perform better than girls, on average, yet in some other skills, girls outperform

boys. In all such cases, there is considerable overlapping of boys' and girls' scores. This reminds us of how important it is to consider each adolescent as an individual. Considering gender differences in performance as inevitable biological differences leads educators to lower their expectations for girls. As a result, gender differences persist when they actually could be narrowed by setting high but attainable goals for girls.

We know little about the specific way adolescents improve their ability to combine skills and respond to dynamic environments. Yet adolescence is a period of dramatic improvement in motor performance if children receive adequate instruction and experience. In fact, some adolescents achieve world-class status in their sports. When adolescents maximize their opportunities to learn skills well, they become adults who can use those skills in many enjoyable and beneficial physical activities.

Quantitative improvement in skill performance accompanies qualitative improvement and growth in size and strength. Educators can assess both the quantity and the quality of skills. Qualitative assessment helps educators plan practice experiences and provide formative feedback. Once an individual's movement pattern is relatively proficient, an educator can use quantitative assessment to compare it to that of other performers or to the individual's own previous performance.

## MOTOR PERFORMANCE IN ADULTHOOD

Once young adults attain a given level of performance for well-practiced skills, will they be able to maintain or improve that level in middle and older adulthood? This is a complex question, because the performance of skills is multifaceted. Some skills require accuracy, others speed, and others both accuracy and speed. Strength is a major factor in some skills, whereas others emphasize endurance or flexibility. Then, too, the gauge for maintenance and improvement may be either the movement process, the movement product, or both. It is likely that we can answer the question about performance in middle and older adults differently for various skills and methods of assessment because the aging process affects these factors differently. Middle or older adults may not retain at a young adult level skills whose major component is speed, but they may retain or improve skills emphasizing accuracy. Or they may maintain the quality of performance while the quantity declines.

Some types of skill performance by middle and older adults have received little attention.

For example, few researchers have examined the movement patterns of older adults; more have studied their cardiovascular and memory functions. As a result, we can form generalizations about some aspects of adult skill performance while questions about other aspects remain unresolved. Because we will discuss perception, fitness, and learning and memory later, the following discussion focuses on the qualitative and quantitative skill performance of adults. In many cases, we can make only tentative conclusions regarding adult skill performance.

> **CONCEPT 5.2**
> Adults can refine and perfect their skills, but the aging process affects skill performance.

## Rate Controllers in Adults

The prevailing stereotype of motor performance in middle and older adults is that of declining performance. To an extent this stereotype is understandable. You'll recall from chapter 2 that aging brings about physical changes, such as loss of bone and muscle mass, especially when adults become sedentary. We could speculate that such changes affect the mass of the various body parts, altering in turn the mechanical nature of skill performance. The central nervous system seems to be less adaptable in old age, and reaction and movement times tend to slow with increasing age. All of these factors might change the movement patterns an individual uses.

On the other hand, it is difficult to know if these changes are inevitable or if they result from declining activity levels or declining expectations of performance levels. Perhaps middle-aged adults who believe their performance is destined to decline actually fulfill their own beliefs. In fact, research has shown that the physical changes associated with aging are often minimal in older adults who remain fit and active and continue to participate in physical activities.

Whether small physical changes are significant enough to cause noticeable changes in movement patterns during skill execution is unclear at this time. We must take care in examining research on adult motor performance and recognize that results often reflect the sample of individuals studied. The range of abilities varies more among a sample of older adults than among other age groups. For example a researcher might study older adults confined to a nursing home or older adults of the same age living independently and participating in a community exercise program for seniors. Those studies showing significant declines in performance may reflect the effects of a sedentary lifestyle or of various disabilities rather than the potential for older adult performance.

The dynamic systems perspective is useful for examining adult motor performance. Recall that from this perspective, individual systems, such as the nervous sytem or muscular system, could be rate controllers—that is, the most slowly developing system or systems could prevent the onset of a new behavior until that system develops to a certain critical point. In the context of aging, a system that regresses also could change behavior. For example, if their muscle strength decreases or their nervous systems slow to a certain critical point, performers might need to change their movements by executing them less quickly, less forcefully, with a smaller range of motion, and so on. Let us keep this perspective in mind throughout our discussion of adult motor performance.

## Age at Peak Performance

One method to examine the course of skill performance in adults is to document the ages of athletes in elite competitive events or at the time of their peak performance. De Garay,

Levine, and Carter (1974) studied performance at the 1968 Olympics, and Malina, Bouchard, Shoup, and Lariviere (1982) looked at the 1976 Olympics. Partial results of these surveys are presented in Table 5.2. You can see that the ages of these elite performers vary considerably depending upon the type of skill they perform and their gender. For example, the men ranged in age from 14 to 49; swimmers and divers were typically the youngest, and weight lifters, fencers, and wrestlers were the oldest. Ages for women ranged from 12 to 38; gymnasts and swimmers were among the youngest, and divers and canoeists/rowers among the oldest.

If we consider the factors associated with this variability in ages, we can clarify the pattern of adult physical performance. First, the fitness component factors influence the pattern of age variability in elite performance. Some sports such as weight lifting require peak strength for peak performance. Because individuals achieve peak strength in their 20s (Burke, Tuttle, Thompson, Janney, & Weber, 1953), we can expect peak performance in weight lifting from those in their 20s or early 30s. In contrast, performance in activities such as rifle and pistol shooting requires less strength, but it benefits from years of practice and experience. An early survey of the ages at which championships were won confirmed this trend (see Table 5.3; Lehman, 1953). Although specific changes may have occurred in the years since Lehman completed this survey, it is still likely today that in the more physically demanding sports, especially those requiring speed, champions are younger than in the less physically demanding activities.

Social and cultural factors likely play a role in the age patterns in adult performance. Adults are expected to conform to societal norms, and these norms have often included "retirement" from sports and games by middle adulthood, especially for women. Recent emphasis on exercise and fitness throughout life may have

**Table 5.2   Ages of Performers in Various Olympic Events**

| Event | Year | Men | | | Women | | |
|---|---|---|---|---|---|---|---|
| | | Number | Mean | Age range | Number | Mean | Age range |
| Basketball | 1968 | 63 | 24.0 | 18-38 | | | |
| Boxing | 1968 | 142 | 22.9 | 17-35 | | | |
| | 1976 | 20 | 23.6 | 19-31 | | | |
| Canoeing | 1968 | 49 | 24.2 | 18-38 | 4 | 22.0 | 18-25 |
| Cycling | 1968 | 104 | 23.6 | 17-32 | | | |
| | 1976 | 22 | 22.8 | 17-32 | | | |
| Diving | 1968 | 16 | 21.3 | 16-30 | 7 | 21.1 | 16-38 |
| Gymnastics | 1968 | 28 | 23.6 | 18-31 | 28 | 23.6 | 18-31 |
| | 1976 | 11 | 24.8 | 20-33 | 15 | 17.0 | 13-20 |
| Rowing | 1968 | 86 | 24.3 | 18-40 | | | |
| | 1976 | 88 | 24.3 | 18-36 | 59 | 23.4 | 16-30 |
| Swimming | 1968 | 67 | 19.2 | 14-25 | 32 | 16.3 | 12-23 |
| | 1976 | 44 | 19.8 | 14-26 | 33 | 16.7 | 12-26 |
| Track | 1968 | 246 | 24.3 | 16-42 | 82 | 20.8 | 15-29 |
| Track and field | 1976 | 43 | 24.1 | 17-32 | 34 | 21.7 | 14-27 |
| Water polo | 1968 | 71 | 22.9 | 16-37 | | | |
| Weight lifting | 1968 | 59 | 26.7 | 17-49 | | | |
| | 1976 | 11 | 27.8 | 22-34 | | | |
| Wrestling | 1968 | 90 | 25.8 | 17-37 | | | |
| | 1976 | 16 | 21.9 | 17-27 | | | |

Data from deGaray, Levine, & Carter, 1974, and Malina, Bouchard, Shoup, & Lariviere, 1982.

begun to change such norms. It will be interesting to study changes in the participants' ages in elite competitions as attitudes change toward lifelong activity for men and women.

Studies of Olympic athletes or champions in various sports focus on elite performances. Yet many middle-aged athletes excel in competitive events below national and international levels, and many outperform the majority of younger adults. The decline in average performance levels of middle and older adults is often very slight, and individuals sometimes achieve their personal bests in their middle or late adult years. An examination of quantitative performance levels in middle and older adults illustrates how small the decline in performance really is.

## Quantitative Performance in Adults

The recent emphasis on lifelong exercise and fitness has made participation in Masters competitions and Senior Olympics popular. This in turn has given developmentalists more information on the quantitative levels of achievement adults can attain. Shea (1986a, 1986b) graphed results of the 1984 U.S. Masters National Swimming Championships in the 500-yd freestyle event (see Figure 5.10a). He averaged the top five times in each age group for both men and women. Note that the decline is very gradual in middle age; more noticeable after age 60, especially for women; and rather

**Table 5.3   Ages (yrs) at Which 1,175 Championships Were Won**

| Type of skill | N of cases | Median age | Mean age | Age range of maximum proficiency |
|---|---|---|---|---|
| U.S.A. outdoor tennis champions | 89 | 26.35 | 27.12 | 22-26 |
| Runs batted in: annual champions of the two major baseball leagues | 49 | 27.10 | 27.97 | 25-29 |
| U.S.A. indoor tennis champions | 64 | 28.00 | 27.45 | 25-29 |
| World champion heavyweight pugilists | 77 | 29.19 | 29.51 | 26-30 |
| Base stealers: annual champions of the two major baseball leagues | 31 | 29.21 | 28.85 | 26-30 |
| Indianapolis-Speedway racers and national auto-racing champions | 82 | 29.56 | 30.18 | 27-30 |
| Best hitters: annual champions of the two major baseball leagues | 53 | 29.70 | 29.56 | 27-31 |
| Best pitchers: annual champions of the two major baseball leagues | 51 | 30.10 | 30.03 | 28-32 |
| Open golf champions of England and of the U.S.A. | 127 | 30.72 | 31.29 | 28-32 |
| National individual rifle-shooting champions | 84 | 31.33 | 31.45 | 32-34 |
| State corn-husking champions of the U.S.A. | 103 | 31.50 | 30.66 | 28-31 |
| World, national, and state pistol-shooting champions | 47 | 31.90 | 30.63 | 31-34 |
| National amateur bowling champions | 58 | 32.33 | 32.78 | 30-34 |
| National amateur duck-pin bowling champions | 91 | 32.35 | 32.19 | 30-34 |
| Professional golf champions of England and of the U.S.A. | 53 | 32.44 | 32.14 | 29-33 |
| World record-breakers at billiards | 42 | 35.00 | 35.67 | 30-34 |
| World champion billiardists | 74 | 35.75 | 34.38 | 31-35 |

Reprinted by permission from Lehman, 1953.

dramatic after age 75. Shea also graphed world-record running times in the marathon for males 10 to 79 years old (Figure 5.10b). After increasing in adolescence and early adulthood, performance declines, following a trend similar to that for swimming.

Senior Olympic records established over the 10 years between 1980 and 1990 in the St. Louis region are graphed in Figure 5.11a-f. Although the records established in each 5-year age group decline with increasing age in almost every case, the decline over approximately 25 years is relatively small in most of the events. This is particularly true of changes between the 50- to 54-year-old group and the 70- to 74-year-old group. The declines are more dramatic after age 75.

The Masters and Senior Olympic events we have discussed so far are those with goals of maximal speed or distance. Consistent with our discussion of age at peak performance, we would expect the declines in these events to be more noticeable than in events that emphasize accuracy. Figure 5.12a-c shows performance

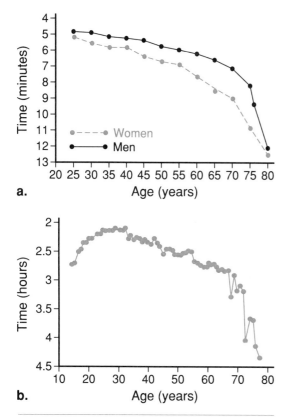

**a.**

**b.**

**Figure 5.10** (a) Results of the 1984 U.S. Masters National Swimming Championships in the 500-yd freestyle swim. (b) World-record marathon times for men.
(Reprinted by permission from Shea, 1986.)

results for several 1990 Senior Olympic events that emphasize accuracy—bowling (scratch scores), football throw for accuracy, and softball throw for accuracy. Notice that it is more difficult to find trends in these scores, except that scores for the 75- to 79-year-olds and the people over 80 are usually the lowest. For example, it is not uncommon for someone 60 to 64 years old to outscore the winner from a younger age group.

Speed and power are important even in these accuracy events. When ball velocity is slow, even small aiming errors can have a bigger impact on accuracy than when ball velocity is fast. Loss of strength and speed by those in

their late 70s and 80s could explain the large downturn in accuracy in these age groups.

A variety of factors surely contribute to the downward trend in quantitative performance with advancing age. Yet we should recognize that fewer adults are competing in the older age divisions. Fewer participants lower the chances of a truly record-setting performance. So a particular disadvantage of examining cross-sectional data in this case is the unequal number of participants in the groups being compared. It would benefit us to follow older adults longitudinally. For example, Helen Stephens won the 1936 Olympic gold medal in the 100-m dash with a time of 11.5 s at age 18. This Olympic record stood until 1960. As a Senior Olympian competing in the 65- to 69-year-old group, she ran the same event in 16.8 s. The difference between Helen Stephens's performance as an 18-year-old and her time in the same event over 45 years later was 5.3 s. This is a relatively small decline over the middle and older adult years. Unfortunately, large-scale longitudinal studies of data such as these are not available.

Our discussion of motor development in childhood and adolescence has emphasized the relationship between quantitative performance levels and qualitative change in movement patterns. It is possible that the slight declines in quantitative performance levels in older adults are related to qualitative changes in movement. Or the movement patterns might be stable, and the declines may relate to fitness factors such as loss of strength, or to societal norms that predict a decline and produce a self-fulfilling prophecy.

The following discussion examines the movement patterns of older adults. We will discuss fitness and social factors in later chapters.

## Qualitative Performance in Adults

Unfortunately, few research studies have looked at the movement patterns of middle and older adults. In part, this lack of research

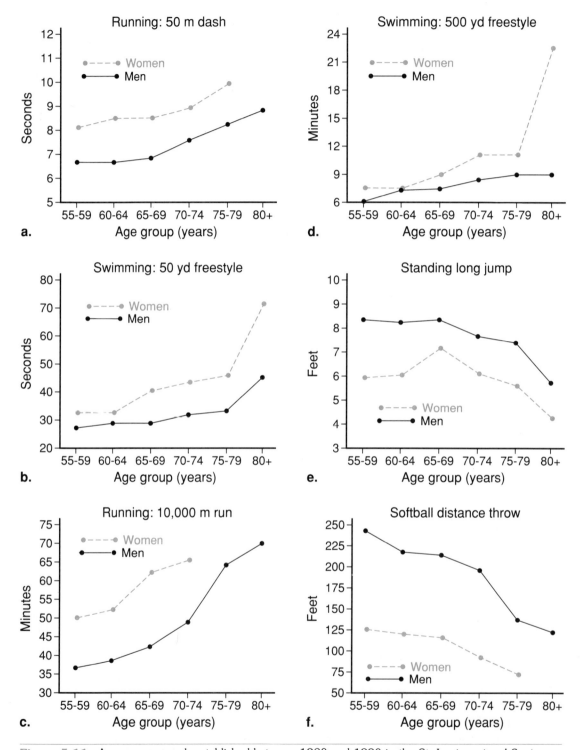

**Figure 5.11**　Age group records established between 1980 and 1990 in the St. Louis regional Senior Olympics for timed and distance events.

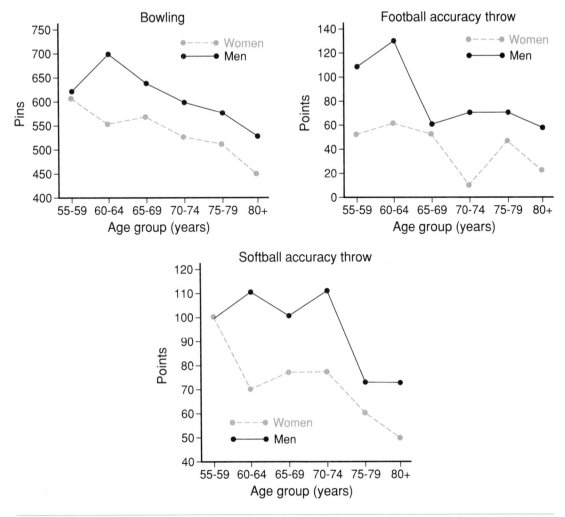

**Figure 5.12** Age group records established between 1980 and 1990 in the St. Louis regional Senior Olympics for accuracy events.

reflects the newness of technical advances that allow faster data analysis, but it also reflects the tendency of motor developmentalists to study children first. Researchers often feel the risk of injury is too great when they must ask older adults for maximal effort. In addition, older adults have been stereotyped as having sedentary lifestyles and little interest in activity.

## Walking

A large number of the existing studies on the movement patterns of older adults have fo-cused on walking. Murray and her co-workers (Murray, Drought, & Kory, 1964; Murray, Kory, Clarkson, & Sepic, 1966; Murray, Kory, & Sepic, 1970) conducted a series of studies on *gait patterns* in older men and women by measuring the linear and rotary dis-placements and the velocities of the limbs dur-ing walking. They found that the older men walked in a pattern similar to that of younger men but with these differences:

- The step length of the older men was ap-proximately 3 cm shorter.

- The older men toed out approximately 3 degrees more than younger men.
- The older men had a reduced degree of ankle extension.
- Pelvic rotation was diminished in older men.

Older women also showed greater out-toeing, shorter stride length, and less pelvic rotation than younger women.

Another common finding is that older adults walk more slowly than younger adults (Drillis, 1961; Gabel, Johnston, & Crowinshield, 1979; Molen, 1973). Schwanda (1978) confirmed the finding of a shorter stride length among older men and further demonstrated that most other aspects of the walking pattern (stride rate, time for recovering-leg swing, time on support leg, and vertical displacement of the center of gravity) remained similar to those of middle-aged men.

It is possible that shortened stride length and greater out-toeing reflect uncertainty in balance, but it is also true that some of these differences between older and younger adults are related to walking speed. When younger adults walk slowly, they, too, shorten their strides and decrease joint rotations (Craik, 1989; Winter, 1983). In an interesting study, Gabell and Nayak (1984) observed walking in a group of 32 older adults, 66 to 84 years old, who were selected from a group of 1,187. The researchers repeatedly screened members of the large group for various types of pathologies in order to arrive at the small healthy group. They found no significant differences between the walking of the 32 older adults and that of younger adults. So some of the changes in older adults' movement patterns might be related to diseases and injuries in the various body tissues, especially those that result in loss of muscle strength. Even so, these and other studies (Adrian, 1982) indicate that the changes in older adults' walking patterns are minor.

## Running

Researchers have studied a few other movement patterns in older adults. Nelson (1981) studied the walking and the running patterns of older women (ages 58 to 80). She asked the participants in her study to walk normally, walk as fast as possible, jog, and run as fast as possible. Average speed, stride length, and stride frequency all tended to increase over this sequence, but individuals varied greatly in how they changed from walking to jogging. The older women generally increased their walking speed by lengthening their stride, but they increased their running speed by increasing stride frequency, as do young women.

A major difference between younger and older women came in the pattern used for fast running:

- Older women did not tuck their recovering leg as completely.
- Older women had a shorter stride length.
- Older women took fewer strides than younger women.

The absolute speed of both jogging and running also differed among the age groups. Older women jogged more slowly (1.85 vs. 3.93 m/s) and ran more slowly (2.60 vs. 6.69 m/s) than a group of 20-year-old women (Nelson, 1981).

## Jumping

Klinger, Masataka, Adrian, and Smith (1980; cited in Adrian, 1982) included a vertical jump among several activities they studied in women over 60. As with the Nelson running study, the older women's jumping pattern appeared normal in the sequence of movements. Their maximal range of knee flexion, though, was smaller than that typically found in young adults, and the older women could not extend their legs as quickly. This is in agreement with measures of elbow extension speed in older women for throwing and striking. Older women's extension velocities were again much slower than those recorded from performances of young women.

## Throwing

A more extensive study of overarm throwing in older adults assessed both movement patterns and ball velocity. Williams, Haywood, and VanSant (1990, 1991) placed active older adult men and women between the ages of 63 and 78 into the developmental steps for overarm throwing (see Table 4.6 in chapter 4). These adults were active in a university-sponsored program but did not practice throwing or participate in activities with overarm movement pattterns. The developmental status of this group was only moderate. Most took a short, contralateral step (Step 3) and were categorized at Step 1 or 2 of humerus action and Step 1 or 2 of forearm action (see Figure 5.13). Almost all used block rotation of the trunk (Step 2). The researchers found gender differences similar to those in children; that is, men generally had better form. Yet qualitative throwing status also related to childhood and young adult experiences. Those who had participated in sports with overarm movement patterns had better form.

The ball velocities the older adults generated also were moderate; they were similar to velocities generated by 8- to 9-year-olds. The men averaged 54.4 ft/s (16.7 m/s), and the women averaged 39.1 ft/s (11.9 m/s). Hence, the older adults also confirmed the gender differences noted in youths.

Because the actions during the backswing in ballistic skills generally are related to ball velocity, Haywood, Williams, and VanSant (1991) closely examined the backswing used by older adults. The older adults who used a circular, downward backswing threw faster than those using an upward (therefore shorter)

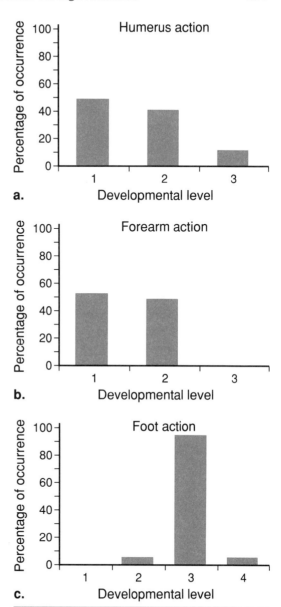

**Figure 5.13**   Qualitative performance of older adults throwing overarm for distance using the developmental categories in Table 4.6 (p. 147): (a) humerus action, (b) forearm action, (c) foot action. All older adult throwers demonstrated level 2 trunk action.

(Reprinted by permission from Williams, Haywood, & VanSant, 1991.)

backswing. Many older adults used backswing movement patterns that seemed different from those children use. For example, many started the circular, downward backswing (Step 4) but did not continue the circle. Instead, they bent the elbow to bring the ball up behind the head. A possible reason for this could be a change in the musculoskeletal system, such as decreased shoulder flexibility or a loss of fast-twitch muscle fibers. Because the throwers could not continue arm movement at the shoulder joint, or would experience pain in doing so, perhaps they reorganized the movement.

Though we need more research on this topic, we can see that the dynamic systems model can be applied to movement changes in older adults. One or more body systems might regress to a critical point at which a movement must change. The system or systems are therefore rate controllers for a movement behavior. Some of these new movement patterns might be unique to older adulthood, because declines in the various body systems that occur with aging might not be exactly the opposite of the advances that occur with physical growth.

The older adults in these studies were not observed as young adults, so we do not know if any or all of them reached the highest developmental level in all the body components when they were younger. We can only hypothesize that their moderate status as older adults reflects at least some change from the movement patterns of their youth. Some of the older adults were observed a year after the initial study (Williams et al., 1991), and the majority of throwers regressed a level in one or two body components. It appears that changes in the body's systems, lack of practice, or both contribute to less efficient movement. But the movement patterns, at least among these older adults in their late 60s and 70s, did not always regress to those used by young children. Rarely did any older adults use a homolateral step (Step 2) or an upper arm (humeral) flexion backswing (Step 2). They always used trunk rotation (Step 2), even though it was limited in extent.

Even if an 8-year-old and a 70-year-old produce identical ball velocities—a quantitative measurement—their throws might be qualitatively different. Older adults, especially those who had experience with a movement pattern in their youth, might maintain many aspects of an optimal movement pattern, but they might subtly change the extent of movement or fail to produce the force and speed they did as youths.

## Rising

VanSant's (1990) work on rising from a supine position also suggests that unique movement patterns emerge during the older adult years. In chapter 4 we described the developmental sequence for this task and discussed how children and adolescents perform it. One leg action category and two arm action categories in the developmental sequence reflect movement patterns observed in older adults, not children or adolescents (Leuhring, 1989; VanSant, in press; see Table 4.10). The unique leg action pattern includes pushing on the thighs in rising.

Cross-sectional observations of middle-aged and older adults showed a slow rate of regression to movement patterns common in childhood and to new but less efficient movement patterns (Leuhring, 1989; VanSant, 1990, in press). Young children and older adults, compared to adolescents and young adults, need more transitional positions in rising. They attain balance in these positions, in effect breaking the rising task down into segments, rather than transferring weight in a more fluid motion.

---

Changes in the muscular system that reduce force production and a decline in the posture and balance system might be the rate-controlling factors that cause older adults to change their movement patterns.

---

Although the number of studies providing information on older adults' patterns is limited, we can make several generalizations. Older adults generally maintain their movement patterns from younger adulthood. Although you might suspect that older adults revert to the patterns used by children, the extent of any such regression appears limited.

The movements of older adults are not as fast as those of younger adults. To what can we attribute this slower speed? Though physical factors such as strength could certainly be involved, Klinger et al. (1980) noted that half the older women in the aforementioned jumping study reported they had no sports background, and many indicated they had not attempted some of the activities tested since they had been in high school. Possibly, these women's lower limb velocities reflect a lack of practice and experience during the adult years or, perhaps, that these women never attained fast speeds when they were young adults. Adrian (1980) suggests that such lack of participation in sport activities might precede rather than follow bone, joint, and muscle changes with aging. If a person rarely moves rapidly through a large range of motion, the bones, joints, and muscles are never subjected to the beneficial levels of stress that contribute to improved strength and integrity of the tissues.

## REVIEW 5.2

Ideally, individuals should perfect the basic skills during childhood and adolescence so that by the time they are adults they can demonstrate mastery of the skills. Adulthood, then, should be a period of skill refinement and recombination wherein through additional practice and experience an individual improves his or her skill performance level. However, this is true of only some adults. Others may never master the basic skills. Nevertheless, the level of skill development a person achieves appears to be relatively stable in the middle and older adult years. Some declines are evident, though, in the quantity of performance, depending in part

on the physical or experiential demands of the specific skill.

It is difficult to determine how much of the decline in performance is related to an expectation that performance will decline or to a lack of practice and conditioning. Many of the adults studied may never have reached advanced movement patterns when they were younger. As more research is done on the movement patterns of older adults, including more research on a variety of individual lifestyles, developmentalists will gain a better understanding of the potential for performance in older adults.

## SUMMARY

Quantitative measurements are often used to gauge motor development in adolescents and adults. As individuals reach maturity, quantitative differences no longer reflect the rate of maturation, and greater emphasis is placed on optimizing performance of skills already learned and refined. Quantitative indicators reflect steady improvement of motor performance through adolescence. World-class athletes typically reach peak performance as young adults. Individuals can reach personal goals at older ages as they take up new activities or as they continue to practice and train. Movement patterns are well maintained in adulthood, but both quantitative performance levels and qualitative characteristics of movement can be affected as the body's systems contributing to performance undergo change. These changes can be brought about by lack of training and disuse, injury, disease, or natural aging. Individuals who actively train and are fortunate enough to avoid injury and disease can delay notable declines in performance until very old age.

Throughout our discussion of motor performance, we have mentioned factors related to the performance of skills, such as fitness and social norms. Our descriptions of growth, maturation, and motor development have often focused on the average or normal course of development, but factors related to skill performance introduce even more variations to the norm. Educators work with individuals. To achieve a more complete perspective on the range of factors that determine the performance levels of individuals as well as their skill potential, educators need to understand the correlates of motor development. We direct our attention to these factors in the next chapters.

## Key Terms

confidence interval
correlation coefficient
dynamic environments
effect size
gait patterns
meta-analysis

## Discussion Questions

1. How does skill performance change during preadolescence and adolescence in terms of quantitative measures of the movement product?
2. What factors might account for gender differences in quantitative motor performance scores?
3. To what extent can we predict skill ability in late adolescence from childhood scores?
4. What types of skills (strength, speed, accuracy) are most likely to show the earliest and sharpest quantitative declines as individuals move into older adulthood? Why?
5. Do movement patterns change as individuals reach older adulthood? Explain.

## Suggested Readings

Adrian, M.J. (1980). Biomechanics and aging. In J.M. Cooper & B. Haven (Eds.), *Proceedings of the Biomechanics Symposium*. Indianapolis, IN: Indiana State Board of Health.

Branta, C., Haubenstricker, J., & Seefeldt, V. (1984). Age changes in motor skill during childhood and adolescence. In R.L. Terjung (Ed.), *Exercise and sport science reviews* (Vol. 12, pp. 467-520). Lexington, MA: Collamore.

Craik, R. (1989). Changes in locomotion in the aging adult. In M.H. Woollacott & A. Shumway-Cook (Eds.), *Development of posture and gait across the life span* (pp. 176-201). Columbia, SC: University of South Carolina Press.

Eckert, H.M. (1987). *Motor development* (3rd ed.). Indianapolis: Benchmark.

Haubenstricker, J., & Seefeldt, V. (1986). Acquisition of motor skills during childhood. In V. Seefeldt (Ed.), *Physical activity and well-being* (pp. 41-102). Reston, VA: American Alliance for Health, Physical Education, Recreation and Dance.

Spirduso, W.W. (1986). Physical activity and the prevention of premature aging. In V. Seefeldt (Ed.), *Physical activity and well-being* (pp. 141-160). Reston, VA: American Alliance for Health, Physical Education, Recreation and Dance.

# Part III
# Correlates of
# Motor Development

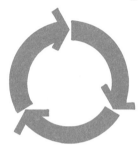

In Part III we survey factors that affect motor development, including perceptual change, physiological change in response to exercise, cognitive change, and psychosocial change.

In chapter 6 we trace the courses of visual, auditory, and kinesthetic development and explain the integration of these systems. Then we explore the development of balance in light of this integration. We conclude by discussing the importance of early experience in perceptual-motor activities.

You will learn about the age-related changes in physiological response to exercise in chapter 7. We review basic concepts of exercise physiology, including the physical fitness components of endurance, strength, flexibility, and body composition, emphasizing change in these components as a function of growth and training.

In chapter 8 we investigate the cognitive changes involved in information processing. We discuss age-related changes in such aspects as attention and response selection, along with the development of memory and knowledge structures.

In chapter 9, our final chapter, we examine sociocultural and psychosocial influences on motor development. Our initial focus is on how socialization affects participation in physical activities throughout life. Then we explore the development of one's self-esteem for skill performance in light of these social influences. The remainder of our discussion concentrates on how racial, socio-economic, and cultural factors alter children's environments and the resultant effects on physical growth and motor development.

## Chapter 6

# Perceptual-Motor Development

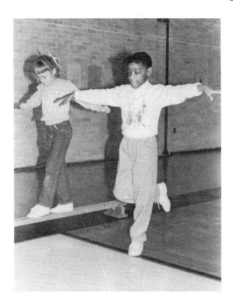

## CHAPTER CONCEPTS

**6.1**
Visual, kinesthetic, and auditory development contribute to skill development.

**6.2**
Intersensory integration improves during childhood.

**6.3**
Balance improves throughout childhood and adolescence; however, a loss of balance ability in older adulthood can lead to injury.

**6.4**
Early motor experience is important to perceptual-motor development.

Almost every motor act in one sense is a perceptual-motor skill; you base your movements on information about your environment and your position or location within it. For example, a softball infielder sees the location of the pitch, the batter striking the ball, and the ball bouncing on the ground; hears the hit and perhaps a runner on the base path; and feels the position of her body and arms. The player combines this sensory information with her memories of previous experiences and thus forms her perception of the surrounding world. Then, based on these perceptions, the infielder decides where and when she could intercept the ball, where to move, and how to position her body. After she catches the ball, she takes it from her glove and throws it to first base. The infielder then adds these perceptions of the environment and movements to her store of perceptions to help her in future performances.

You might think experienced platform divers could execute dives they've learned well without needing to hear and see the water below, because they know how far away it is. Yet a diver still must feel how gravity pulls his body and know where his trunk and limbs are relative to one another both before and during the dive.

Whether performance of a given skill relies predominantly on visual information, as in fielding a ball, or on kinesthetic information, as in diving, it is evident that perception is important to skilled performance.

## SENSORY AND PERCEPTUAL DEVELOPMENT

The term *perceptual-motor* used here describes movement that follows and depends on perceptual discriminations and judgments. We will focus on age-related changes in the sensory systems and the *perceptions* based on *sensations*.

We can attribute some improvements children make in their motor skills as they grow and mature to improvements in their sensory and perceptual functioning. As children learn to better select, process, organize, and integrate perceptual information and coordinate it with information from their increasing experiences, their motor skills improve. The result is refined motor skills and better performance. Much of the improvement in perception occurs in early childhood with subtle refinements coming in late childhood and early adolescence. Once perceptual-motor functioning is refined, developmentalists believe, it is maintained throughout adulthood.

We know very little about perceptual-motor changes in older adults, but researchers have identified many age-related changes in the sensory systems. Older adults probably adapt to many of the physical changes that take place in their sensory receptors and continue to perform well. Other changes may be detrimental to their performance; these changes warrant our attention. In the next section, we will review age-related changes in vision, kinesthesis, and audition over the life span. Later, we will discuss the integration of these systems as well as the importance of identifying perceptual-motor deficiencies in young performers.

---

**CONCEPT 6.1**

Visual, kinesthetic, and auditory development contribute to skill development.

---

## Visual Development

Vision plays a major role in most skill performance. To understand this role better, we need to examine age-related changes in both visual sensation and visual perception. Sensation is the neural activity triggered by some stimulus that activates a sensory receptor and results in sensory nerve impulses traveling the sensory nerve pathways to the brain. Perception is a multistage process that takes place in the brain and includes the selection, processing, organization, and integration of information received from the senses. It results in our knowing and understanding objects and events.

### Visual Sensation

During the 1st month of life, the visual system provides the infant with functionally useful but unrefined vision at a level approximately 5% of eventual adult *acuity* (sharpness of sight), or 20/800 on the Snellen scale of visual acuity (20/20 is desirable). The newborn's resolution of detail is such that she can differentiate facial features from a distance of 20 in.; beyond this, she probably cannot see objects clearly.

During the first 6 months after birth, the infant's vision shows rapid improvements in three areas:

- Accommodation
- Contrast sensitivity
- Acuity (Atkinson & Braddick, 1981)

*Accommodation* is the process by which the shape of the eye's lens (seen in Figure 6.1) adjusts to view objects at varying distances, which is important in performing motor skills. Newborns do not control accommodation very well, but by 5 to 6 months of age they show an accurate accommodation response. *Contrast sensitivity* describes our sensitivity to distributions of light and dark as they are spatially arranged in our field of view.

Improvements in acuity are related more to the increased number of neural connections in the visual cortex of the brain and to differentiation of the neurons in the part of the retina responsible for detailed vision (the fovea) than to changes in the size of the eye or its lens. Taken together, accommodation, contrast sensitivity, and acuity indicate how detailed visual information appears to the infant.

At about 6 months of age, then, as infants' motor systems are ready to begin self-propelled

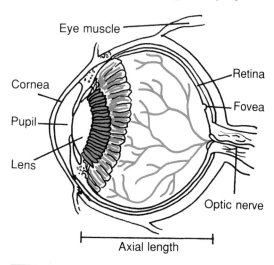

**Figure 6.1** The human eye.

locomotion, their visual systems perceive adequate detail to assist them in the task. From the dynamic systems perspective, vision is another system that must develop to an adequate level to facilitate locomotion. Many infants exhibit astigmatism, or blurred vision due to an imperfect curvature of the cornea. This phenomenon appears to be transient, however, and its incidence declines between 6 and 18 months (Braddick & Atkinson, 1979).

Visual sensation continues to improve during childhood, with slightly more rapid gains in acuity noted between ages 5 and 7 years and again between 9 and 10 years. On the average, 1-year-olds have visual acuity of about 20/100 to 20/50, 5-year-olds about 20/30, and by age 10, children without a visual anomaly score at the desired level of 20/20.

Refraction of light by the growing eye depends on the curvature of the cornea, the shape of the lens, and the axial length of the eye. These structures likely have a genetically determined growth target size, but they do not grow in synchrony. Some researchers have suggested that growth is controlled so that variations in one structure are balanced by another, minimizing refractive errors during growth. The role of visual experience in this process is unclear, but deprivation of vision during development is known to induce refractive errors in animals (Atkinson & Braddick, 1981).

If the axial length of the eye is such that the lens cannot focus light rays on the rear of the eye (retina), vision is blurred. Myopia or nearsightedness results from an axial length that is too long. Closer objects are seen clearly, but distant objects are blurred. Hyperopia or farsightedness results from an axial length that is too short. Near objects are blurred. Eyeglasses or contact lenses can help both these conditions. Individuals tend to become more nearsighted as they move through adolescence and into adulthood, and because of this, farsightedness in a young child will occasionally correct itself. Artificial lenses also can correct astigmatism.

Some children have an imbalance in the eye muscles and cannot direct their two eyes to move as a unit. This condition is termed strabismus, commonly known as lazy eye. If one or both eyes turn inward, it is called internal or convergent; if they turn outward, external or divergent. External strabismus especially can make reading difficult and result in headaches or even nausea. Children with strabismus usually see double images. Strabismus can range from mild to severe. For mild cases, an optometrist might prescribe eye muscle exercises or eyeglasses, but severe cases might require surgery. If strabismus remains untreated, vision in the nondominant eye eventually will be suppressed, and the child's *depth perception* will suffer. This would make play frustrating, especially games such as tag or catch in which the child must intercept moving objects or people.

## Visual Perception

The aspects of visual perception that are important to motor skills include perception of the following:

- Size constancy
- Figure-and-ground
- Whole objects versus parts
- Depth
- Spatial orientation
- Movement

Although you can find more detailed explanations of visual perception elsewhere (cf. Rosinski, 1977), we will confine our discussion to these topics and their development in children.

### Perception of Size Constancy

Consistent interpretation of the visual environment requires *perceptual size constancy*—that is, the ability to recognize that objects maintain a constant size even if their distance from the observer varies and their image takes up more or less space on the retina (Figure 6.2). Hence, you can recognize that two identi-

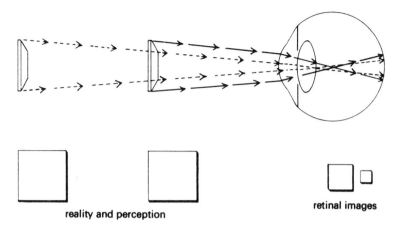

reality and perception                                  retinal images

**Figure 6.2**   Size constancy. The image of an object halves in size with each doubling of the distance of the object from the eye, but it does not *appear* to shrink so much; the brain compensates for the shrinking of the image with distance by a process called constancy scaling. (Reprinted by permission from Gregory, 1972.)

cal chairs are the same size, even if one is nearby and the other is across the room. Your brain recognizes that the smaller image is due to increasing distance from the eye, a process called *constancy scaling*. Similarly, you perceive the space or gap between two objects as constant whether the objects are near you or far away.

Another aspect of perceptual size constancy is the ability to judge accurately the sizes of different objects that are varying distances away. Young children tend to overestimate the space between two objects as they are placed farther and farther away from them. Such perceptual judgments gradually improve with age and are relatively mature in the average 11-year-old (Collins, 1976).

### Perception of Figure-and-Ground

A second aspect of visual perception, called *figure-and-ground*, allows an observer to locate and focus on an object (figure) embedded in a distracting background (ground) (Figure 6.3). This ability to extract figures seems to improve in spurts in growing children, particu-

larly between ages 4 and 6 years (Williams, 1983), and again between 6 and 8 years (Temple, Williams, & Bateman, 1979). Children can extract items from a background more successfully if the objects are familiar to them; they have considerable difficulty with abstract geometric forms. Children refine their figure-ground perception to a near-adult level after age 8 (Williams, 1983).

### Perception of Whole and Parts

The ability to discriminate the parts of an object, or a picture, from the whole is another important aspect of visual perception. This process allows adults to look at a stick man constructed from nuts and bolts and report seeing a man made from nuts and bolts. A young child with immature *whole-part perception* may report seeing only the man, only the nuts and bolts, or both but at different times. Later, by age 9, most children can integrate parts and the whole into the total picture (Elkind, 1975; Elkind, Koegler, & Go, 1964) (see Figure 6.4).

Adults often use whole-and-part perception. For example, if you are driving down the street

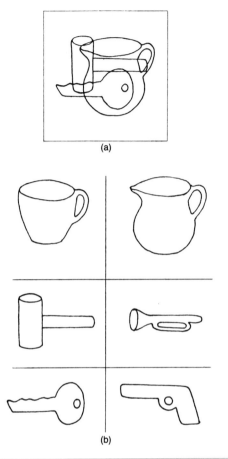

(a)

(b)

**Figure 6.3** A test plate from the Figure-Ground Perception Test of the Southern California Sensory Integration Test. A child must identify which of the six objects in (b) are present, or embedded, in picture (a).
(Reprinted by permission from Western Psychological Services, 1972.)

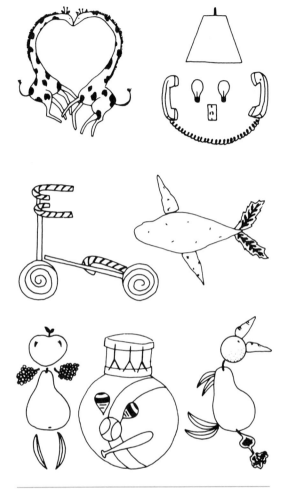

**Figure 6.4** The drawings used by Elkind, Koegler, and Go to study whole-part perception.
(Reprinted by permission from Elkind, Koegler, & Go, 1964.)

and see half a bicycle tire protruding from a row of parked cars and a child's head above it, you are not puzzled. You immediately perceive that a child on a bicycle is pulling into your path, and you slow down.

### Depth Perception

Depth perception is particularly important for performing motor skills. It enables a person to

judge the distance from his body to an object and to recognize that objects are three-dimensional. Because your two eyes are in different locations, each eye sees the visual field from a slightly different angle. This is termed *retinal disparity* (see Figure 6.5). The information you need to judge depth results from a comparison of the two slightly different pictures. Depth perception requires good visual acuity, too, because a sharper picture from

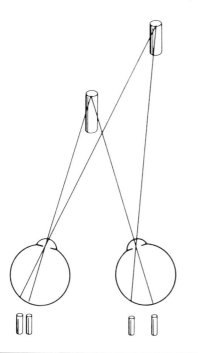

**Figure 6.5** Retinal disparity. Images on the left retina are closer together than the images on the right retina. The observer sees the two rods in depth.
(Reprinted by permission from Kaufman, 1979.)

each eye provides more information for the comparison.

Infants have at least some functional vision and, therefore, the mechanics for some degree of depth perception. In the well-known visual cliff experiments of Walk and Gibson (1961; Gibson & Walk, 1960; Walk, 1969), infants between 6 and 14 months of age, placed on one side of a drop-off (the visual cliff), stopped at the edge even though their mothers beckoned them from the other side. These studies demonstrated that even infants as young as 6 months had depth perception ability. On the other hand, 4-year-olds may err frequently in judging depth. Undoubtedly, as vision becomes more refined, so does depth perception. Individuals reach adult levels of visual acuity around age 10. Hence, Williams (1968) found that 12-

year-old boys judged depth as accurately as 16- and 20-year-olds.

## Spatial Orientation

*Spatial orientation* is the recognition of an object's orientation or arrangement in space. The importance of attending to or ignoring the orientation varies with the situation. In some cases, it is important to recognize that two objects are identical even if one is tipped to one side, upside down, or rotated. In other situations, an object's or symbol's orientation is critical to its meaning. Such is the case with letters such as *d* and *b*.

People also must perform many motor skills in defined spatial dimensions or with objects oriented in a particular way. As such, perception of spatial orientation is important in both everyday and sport tasks. Children are able to attend to spatial orientation before they are able to ignore it in situations where spatial orientation is irrelevant (Gibson, 1966; Pick, 1979). Three- and 4-year-olds can learn directional extremes such as high/low, over/under, and front/back, but they still consider intermediate orientations the same as the nearest extreme. Although children at this age can distinguish vertical from horizontal positions, they have difficulty with oblique lines and diagonals, often calling them vertical or horizontal. By age 8, most children have learned to differentiate obliques (various angles) and diagonals (45 degrees) but may still confuse left and right (Naus & Shillman, 1976; Williams, 1973).

## Perception of Spatial Relationships

One of the most basic perceptions involves the relationships among objects located in the environment and the relationships between the self and those objects. These perceptions permit us to move through our environment efficiently and safely, either on foot or when driving a vehicle. Researchers often study the development of spatial relationships by observing infants and placing barriers between them and a goal, usually a toy or the infant's mother. Lockman (1984) found that a basic ability to detour around a barrier is present in 12-month-old infants. By testing infants longitudinally starting at age 8 months, Lockman identified a sequence of improvements in spatial perception:

- Infants first learn to retrieve an object hidden behind a cloth; they become aware that objects still exist even if behind a barrier.
- Some weeks after developing the ability just described, infants demonstrate they can reach around a barrier to obtain their goal.
- Infants demonstrate they can move themselves around a barrier to obtain their goal. On the average, several weeks pass between success in reaching around a barrier and success in traveling around it.
- Most infants can successfully detour around an opaque barrier before a transparent barrier. Transparent barriers initially puzzle infants because visual and kinesthetic (tactile) cues conflict.

McKenzie and Bigelow (1986) further demonstrated that infants become more efficient by taking the shortest path around a barrier (see Figure 6.6), and that they could better adapt to a relocated barrier by 14 months of age. Hence, as infants grow older, they can perceive spatial relationships at a distance from their bodies. Keep in mind that these barrier tasks are relatively simple. Success with increasingly difficult routes in progressively larger spaces comes during early childhood (Hazen, 1982).

### Perception of Movement

The perception of movement in the environment, critical to motor skill performance, involves the ability to detect and track a moving object with your eyes. Newborns can briefly track horizontally moving objects; they continue to acquire tracking ability in other spatial

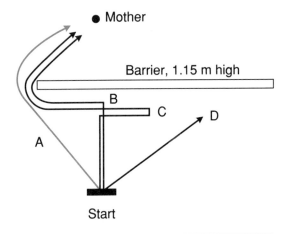

**Figure 6.6**   Room layout for a detour task. Infants can take the most efficient route (A) around a barrier to their mothers by 14 months of age. By this age they also can adapt when the barrier is relocated against the left wall. Younger infants usually take less efficient routes, such as approaching the barrier, then traveling along it (B), sometimes turning the wrong way and backtracking (C), or going to where the opening was before barrier relocation (D).
(Redrawn from McKenzie & Bigelow, 1986.)

paths at varying ages but in a fixed sequence—vertical, diagonal, then circular paths (Gallahue, 1983; Haith, 1966). Between ages 2 and 5 years, children improve in their eye-tracking abilities and their control of eye movements (Williams, 1983). Their tracking abilities improve even further; between the ages of 5 and 10, they can accurately follow moving objects (Haywood, 1977).

At present, our knowledge of the precise role accurate eye tracking plays in perceptual-motor skill performance is complicated by our additional ability to detect movement by peripheral vision. For example, a basketball player can determine a teammate's movement in order to judge where to throw a pass by either (a) following the player with movement of the eyes, or (b) fixing the eyes on another point and perceiving the player's movement with peripheral vision. The ability to perceive a moving object and move in response to it is well established by age 12, as demonstrated by children who made quick and accurate movement decisions similar to those of 20-year-olds (Williams, 1968, 1983).

## Visual Changes With Aging

We know that many perceptual processes involve judgments about visual stimuli from the environment. Once performers can make relatively accurate judgments, they maintain the ability to do so throughout adulthood and depend upon the integrity of their visual systems to deliver accurate information to the central nervous system. As a person ages, changes in the visual system occur naturally, and some conditions and diseases become more prevalent, especially in older adults. These changes may affect the quality of the visual information that reaches the central nervous system.

For example, the ability to see nearby images clearly decreases with aging, becoming clinically significant at around age 40. This condition is termed presbyopia (from *presbys* for "old man" and *ops* for "eye"). The resting diameter of the pupil also decreases with aging, reducing retinal illuminance (the amount of light reaching the retina) in a 60-year-old to one third that of a young adult. The lens yellows with age, further reducing the amount of illuminance reaching the eye, making glare a problem for older adults. Contrast sensitivity also declines with aging, and adaptation to the dark slows.

Some visual disturbances more prevalent in older adults include the following:

- Cataracts
- Glaucoma
- Age-related maculopathy

Cataracts are opaque areas in the lens. They prevent light rays from reaching the retina, thus blurring vision. In glaucoma, the internal pressure of the eye rises; this can eventually damage

the retina and cause loss of sight. Age-related maculopathy is a disease that affects the central area of the retina that provides detailed vision.

Although the visual system can function well for most of a person's adult life, especially with corrective lenses, changes in the eye itself may influence visual perception and, in turn, skill performance. For example, playing tennis at dusk can be difficult for an older adult with reduced retinal illuminance, which hinders visual judgments in dimly lit settings (Haywood & Trick, 1983). On the other hand, problems in depth perception appear to be related to visual acuity, and the individual may be able to correct acuity losses by wearing eyeglasses or contact lenses. In addition, older adults can wear polarized sunglasses to minimize the effects of glare. Active older adults can select settings that are well lit for indoor sports and that maximize the contrast between the background and the object of interest, such as a tennis ball.

Persons who work with children or older adults can look for certain signs that may indicate a visual problem. These include

- a lack of coordination in hand-eye tasks,
- squinting,
- under- or overreaching for objects, and
- unusual head movements to align one's gaze with a particular object.

Activity leaders should try to minimize the effect of visual problems on performance by making certain that activity areas are well lit and by maximizing the contrast between an object of attention (perhaps a ball) and its background.

---

Activity leaders should avoid creating environments that invite glare no matter what age group they work with, but this is a particular concern with older adults. Encourage performers to wear any corrective lenses prescribed for them, even though they often prefer not to wear their glasses for activities (Haywood & Trick, 1990).

---

Because vision provides so much of the perceptual information people need to perform skills successfully, efforts to enhance the visual information that the central nervous system receives should also enhance skill performance.

## Kinesthetic Development

The *kinesthetic* (proprioceptive or somatosensory) *system* is important to skill performance because it yields information about

- the relative position of the body parts to each other,
- the position of the body in space,
- an awareness of the body's movements, and
- the nature of objects with which the body comes in contact.

### Kinesthetic Sensation

Unlike in the visual system, which relies on just the eyes as sensory receptors, kinesthetic information comes from various types of receptors throughout the body (see Table 6.1). Muscle spindles, one type of receptor, are located among the muscle cells and gauge the degree of tension in a muscle. Golgi tendon organs function similarly to muscle spindles by responding to changes in muscle tension; these are found at the muscle-tendon junctions. The three types of joint receptors in the tissues of the joint capsule or the joint ligaments include the spray-type Ruffini endings, Golgi-type receptors, and modified Pacinian corpuscles. The spray endings signal direction, rate, and extent of joint movement plus steady position. The latter joint receptors give information about stationary joint position. All of these receptors are sometimes collectively termed *proprioceptors*.

Structures in the inner ear provide information about the position of the head. The semicircular canals house sensory receptors for rotational movements judging acceleration or

**Table 6.1  The Kinesthetic Receptors and Their Locations**

| Kinesthetic receptor | Location |
|---|---|
| Muscle spindles | Muscles |
| Golgi tendon organs | Muscle-tendon junctions |
| Joint receptors<br>  Spray-type Ruffini<br>  endings<br>  Golgi-type<br>  receptors<br>  Modified Pacinian<br>  corpuscles | Joint capsule and ligaments |
| Vestibular semicircular canals | Inner ear |
| Utricle and saccule | Inner ear |
| Cutaneous receptors | Skin and underlying tissues |

deceleration of the head. The utricle and saccule house receptors for linear movements. These provide information about body position relative to gravity. These structures are collectively referred to as the *vestibular apparatus*.

Finally, the cutaneous receptors in the skin and underlying tissues provide information about touch, temperature, pain, and pressure (Dickinson, 1974). Some of the cutaneous receptors respond to mechanical stimulation, some to thermal and pain stimulation, and others to bending of the hair or pressure on the skin.

### Development of Kinesthetic Receptors

Recall from chapter 3 that many reflexes are stimulated through kinesthetic receptors. Therefore, the onset of a reflex indicates that the kinesthetic receptor involved is functioning. The first prenatal reflex that can be elicited is opposite-side neck flexion through tactile stimulation around the mouth at just 7.5 weeks after conception. Thus we know that cutaneous receptors are present and functioning around the mouth at this early prenatal age.

Researchers have used tactile stimulation to other body parts to determine that cutaneous receptor development proceeds in an oral, genital-anal, palmar, and plantar (sole of foot) sequence. This developmental sequence follows the cephalocaudal and proximodistal growth directions we discussed in chapter 2. By 12.5 prenatal weeks, cutaneous receptors are developing in the hands, as are the muscle spindle receptors in the biceps brachii muscle of the upper arm. We know, too, that the vestibular apparatus is anatomically complete at approximately 9 to 12 weeks of prenatal life. During the 4th to 6th prenatal months, cutaneous receptors for touch and pressure continue to develop, as do muscle spindles, Golgi tendon organs, and joint receptors. Perhaps these receptors function long before birth, but a fetus's sensitivity to temperature via cutaneous receptors is unrefined, and pain sensitivity is poorly developed.

---

The functional status of the vestibular apparatus before birth is unclear, but we have seen that the righting reflexes appear around the 2nd postnatal month (Timiras, 1972). Therefore, the system for kinesthetic sensation is functional early in life.

---

## Kinesthetic Perception

As was the case with vision, an individual can process kinesthetic sensations early in life, but improvements in kinesthetic perception continue throughout childhood. The major aspects of kinesthetic perception are perception of tactile location, multiple tactile points, objects, the body itself, limb movements, spatial orientation, and direction. Balance, too, relies on kinesthetic (as well as visual) sensation. We will discuss how these aspects of kinesthetic per-

ception develop, noting that our knowledge in some areas remains limited.

### Tactile Localization

*Tactile localization* is your ability to identify (without looking) a spot on your body that has just been touched. Four-year-olds are less accurate than 6- to 8-year-olds in locating a touch on the hands and forearms. Performance on this type of task does not improve significantly between ages 6 and 8 years (Ayres, 1972; Temple et al., 1979). Based on this limited data, then, the perception of tactile localization on the hands and arms seems relatively mature by age 5.

### Multiple Tactile Points

One type of *tactile point perception* involves discriminating between two points touching the skin in close proximity simultaneously (see Figure 6.7). Threshold (the smallest gap detectable) discriminations vary with different areas of the body, but we do not know if they vary with age (Van Duyne, 1973; Williams, 1983).

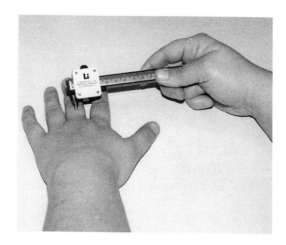

**Figure 6.7** Tactile point perception includes accurate judgment of the number of simultaneous touches on the skin. As two points get closer and closer, it is difficult to discriminate between a single touch and two touches.

Ayres (1966), however, reported that only half of a group of 5-year-olds could consistently discriminate a touch on different fingers, though average performance improved through 7.5 years of age (the oldest age tested).

### Perception of Objects

Recognizing unseen objects and their characteristics by feeling them with the hands is another aspect of kinesthetic perception. In infants, such manipulation is often more accidental than purposeful. By age 4 an average child can handle objects purposefully, a 5-year-old can explore the object's major features. Manual exploration becomes systematic, that is, it follows a plan, at about age 6 (Van Duyne, 1973), and in the next two years, haptic (cutaneous) memory and object recognition also improve (Northman & Black, 1976). Research by Temple et al. (1979) indicates that children also increase their speed of tactile recognition during this time.

### Perception of the Body (Body Awareness)

To carry out everyday activities as well as perform complex skills, you need a sense of the body, its various parts, and its dimensions. One aspect of *body awareness* is the identification of body parts. As children get older, more of them can label the major body parts correctly (DeOreo & Williams, 1980), and they can name more detailed body parts (Cratty, 1979). The rate at which an individual child learns body part labels is largely a function of the amount of time parents or other adults spend practicing with the child. Probably two-thirds of 6-year-olds can identify the major body parts, and mistakes are rare in all normally developing children after age 9.

Children also need a sense of the body's spatial dimensions, such as up and down. They usually master the up-down dimension first, followed by front-back, and finally side. A high percentage of 2.5- to 3-year-olds can place an object in front of or behind their bodies, but more of them have difficulty placing an object in front of or behind something else. By about age 4, most children can do the latter task as well as place an object to the side of something (Kuczaj & Maratsos, 1975).

**Laterality.**    Although children typically master up-down and front-back awareness before age 3, they develop an understanding that the body has two distinct sides at approximately 4 to 5 years of age (Hecaen & de Ajuriaguerra, 1964). We call this side awareness *laterality*. The child comes to realize that, even though his two hands, two legs, and so on are the same size and shape, he can position them differently and move them independently. Eventually, the child is able to discriminate right and left sides— that is, to label or identify these dimensions.

An age-related improvement in the ability to make right-left discriminations occurs between age 4 or 5 and age 10, with most children responding almost perfectly by age 10 (Ayres, 1969; Swanson & Benton, 1955; Williams, 1973). But children can be taught to label right-left at younger ages, too, even as young as 5 (Hecaen & de Ajuriaguerra, 1964). Young children also have difficulty executing a task when a limb must cross the midline of the body, such as writing on a chalkboard from left to right. This ability improves between ages 4 and 10, but some 10-year-olds still have difficulty with such tasks (Ayres, 1969; Williams, 1973).

**Lateral Dominance.**    *Lateral dominance* is the preferential use of one of the hands, feet, or eyes. If the favored hand, foot, and eye are on the same side of the body, the dominance is termed pure; otherwise, it is mixed. Lateral dominance emerges during early childhood, but exact ages are difficult to pinpoint. In certain situations children might find it more convenient to use their nonpreferred limb, and they do so (Connolly & Elliot, 1972). Adolescents and adults, in contrast, typically use their dominant limb even if it is more awkward and less efficient in a given situation. Hand preferences, though, are evident even in infants (see Table 6.2). Infants younger than 3 months grasp objects longer, make a fist longer, and are more active with one hand than the other (Hawn & Harris, 1983; Michel & Goodwin, 1979; Michel & Harkins, 1986). These asymmetries are not consistently predictive of adult hand dominance (Michel, 1983, 1988) but might be linked to it because the asymmetries tend to follow orientation. Infants who prefer to turn their heads to the right seem to prefer reaching with their right hands, and vice versa. These self-generating experiences possibly facilitate eye-hand coordination of one hand more than the other (Bushnell, 1985; Michel, 1988).

When infants begin to reach after 3 months, they also demonstrate a hand preference (Hawn & Harris, 1983). Unimanual manipulation appears at approximately 5 months, and by 7 months infants show a preference for manipulating with a particular hand (Ramsey, 1980). Approximately 1 month after bimanual manipulation first appears, a hand preference is evident, even as both hands hold an object (Ramsey, Campos, & Fenson, 1979). Infants

typically prefer the same hand in both unimanual and bimanual handling; that is, they use either the right or the left hand in both types of manipulation (Ramsey, 1980).

Although some children might change their hand preference, in most cases the hand a child prefers emerges in early childhood, most often by age 4, and remains stable during childhood (Sinclair, 1971).

Researchers have provided several theories to explain the emergence of lateral dominance. The most popular of these links lateral dominance to dominance of a cerebral (brain) hemisphere or cortical lateralization; that is, a right-sided person has a dominant left hemisphere, and vice versa. The cerebral hemispheres are structurally different and assume the control of different functions; thus there is much diversity of function.

The perceptual-motor theory of Doman and Delacato suggests that pure lateral dominance is necessary for proper neurological organization (Delacato, 1966)—they believe the same side of the brain should dominate use of the hands, feet, and eyes. Further, individuals with mixed dominance could anticipate problems in perceptual-motor performance, reading, speech, and other cognitive abilities. Other investigators have criticized this theory, however, because they failed to find a similar significant relationship between pure lateral dominance and perceptual-motor performance, perceptual judgments, or cognitive performance (Horine, 1968; Sabatino & Becker, 1971; Williams, 1973).

It is also possible that the asymmetrical use of one hand that is linked to head orientation in early infancy plays a role in the emergence of hand dominance. The early experiences an infant obtains in using one hand more than the other might facilitate later skill acquisition with

**Table 6.2 Infant Hand Preferences**

| Nature of hand preference | Approximate age |
| --- | --- |
| Fisting and longer grasps | Before 3 months |
| Unimanual reaching | After 3 months |
| Unimanual manipulation | 7 months |
| Bimanual manipulation | Within 1 month of emergence of unimanual manipulation |
| Hand dominance | By 4 years |

the preferred hand (Michel, 1988). We need more research, especially longitudinal, to help us better understand whether specialization of the cerebral hemispheres alone brings about limb dominance, or whether experiences facilitate the dominant use of one limb or the other and the brain hemispheres have equal potential to dominate.

### Limb Movements

You can assess a child's perception of the extent of movement at a joint by asking the child to accurately reproduce a limb movement or to relocate a limb position without looking. Children improve in this task between ages 5 and 8, with little improvement noted after age 8 (Ayres, 1972; Williams, 1983).

### Spatial Orientation

Kinesthetic spatial orientation involves perception of the body's location and orientation in space independent of vision. Temple et al. (1979) tested this perception by asking children to walk a straight line while blindfolded, and then measuring their deviation from the straight path. Performance improved between 6 and 8 years of age, the latter being the oldest age group included in the study. Because these were the only children tested, we need investigations of spatial orientation over a wider age range.

### Perception of Direction

*Directionality*, the ability to project the body's spatial dimensions into surrounding space, is often linked to laterality, an awareness of the body's two distinct sides. Children with a poor sense of laterality typically have poor directionality as well. Although this relationship seems intuitively logical, deficiencies in laterality are not known to cause deficiencies in directionality (Kephart, 1964).

Individuals obtain information for directional judgments through vision, so these judgments rely on integration of visual and kinesthetic information. Long and Looft (1972) suggested that children improve their sense of directionality between ages 6 and 12. By age 8, children typically can use body references to indicate direction. They are able to say correctly both "The ball is on my right" and "The ball is to the right of the bat." At age 9, children can change the latter statement to "The ball is to the left of the bat" when they walk around to the opposite side of the objects. They can identify right and left for a person opposite them. Improvements in directional references such as these continue through age 12. Long and Looft noted that some refinement of directionality must take place in adolescence, because many 12-year-olds are unable to transpose left and right from a new perspective, such as when looking into a mirror.

## Kinesthetic Changes With Aging

We know very little about how aging affects the kinesthetic receptors themselves, but researchers have identified age-related changes in kinesthetic perception. Some, but not all, older adults lose cutaneous sensitivity, vibratory sensitivity, and sensitivity to temperature and pain (Kenshalo, 1977). Older adults experience some impairment in judging the direction and amount of passive lower limb movements (in which someone else positions the limb) (Laidlaw & Hamilton, 1937). However, they remain fairly accurate in judging muscle tension produced by differing weights (Landahl & Birren, 1959).

## Auditory Development

Although it is not as important to skill performance as vision or kinesthesis, auditory information is still valuable for accurate performance. People often use sounds as critical cues to initiate or time their movements. Just as with the other senses, we must distinguish between auditory sensation (merely hearing sound) and auditory perception (actually judging sound). We will first consider auditory sensation, beginning with prenatal ear development.

## Auditory Sensation

The external ear, the middle ear, and the cochlea of the inner ear are involved in hearing. The inner ear develops first and is close to adult form by the 3rd prenatal month. By midfetal life, the external ear and middle ear are formed (Timiras, 1972). Fetuses reportedly respond to loud sounds, but perhaps this response is actually to tactile stimuli, that is, vibrations (Kidd & Kidd, 1966).

A newborn's hearing is imperfect, partly because of the gelatinous tissue filling the inner ear. This material is reabsorbed during the first postnatal week so that hearing improves rapidly (Timiras, 1972; Hecox, 1975). By 3 months, infants hear low-frequency sounds (500 to 1,000 Hz) very well but do not hear high-frequency sounds (4,000 Hz) quite as well. Because human speech generally is under 5,000 Hz, this level of hearing permits the infant to sense speech; the infant can hear low- to mid-pitched voices better than high-pitched voices. By 6 months infants have adultlike hearing, even of high-frequency sounds (Spetner & Olsho, 1990). Auditory acuity improves through childhood and adolescence, but these might be attributed, at least in part, to improvements in attentional level and ability to follow directions on auditory assessment tests (Kidd & Kidd, 1966).

## Auditory Perception

In addition to hearing sound, children must learn to judge the characteristics of the various sounds they hear. Some aspects of auditory perception include perception of the following:

- Location
- Differences in similar sounds
- Patterns
- Auditory figure-and-ground

These are similar to aspects of perception in the other senses.

### Location

Children must perceive the direction from which a sound comes so that they can connect the sound with its source (see Figure 6.8). Infants as young as 4 to 6 months old are able to turn their heads in the general direction of a nearby sound. They can localize distant noises at 11 to 12 months and continue to improve so that by age 3 years, they can localize the general direction of even distant sounds (Dekaban, 1970). However, more detailed aspects of localization, such as threshold levels and

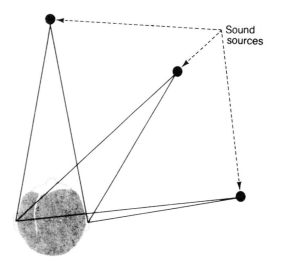

Sound sources

**Figure 6.8** Sound localization. The more a sound deviates from the straight-ahead position, the greater the time difference in the arrival of the sound at each ear.
(From *A Primer of Infant Development* by T.G.R. Bower, 1977, San Francisco: W.H. Freeman. Copyright 1977 by W.H. Freeman. Reprinted by permission.)

localization of multiple sources, have not been examined in children.

### Perception of Differences

Tasks requiring children to distinguish two sounds similar in pitch, loudness, or speech sound (for example, *d* and *t*, or *b* and *p*) are termed *discrimination tasks* . Infants as young as 1 to 4 months can discriminate basic speech sounds (Doty, 1974), but children between 3 and 5 years old experience increasing accuracy in recognizing differences in sounds (DiSimoni, 1975). Temple et al. (1979) found a further improvement in auditory discrimination between 6 and 8 years, as did Birch (1976) between 7 and 10 years with an auditory matching task. A similar trend apparently exists for discrimination of pitch (Kidd & Kidd, 1966). In general, it appears that by 8 to 10 years of age, children have greatly improved their ability to detect differences in similar sounds, but they continue to refine their auditory discrimination skills until they are at least 13.

### Patterns

For speech and music to be more than just noises, individuals must perceive relationships among sounds. Of course, we perceive patterns in other senses. *Visual pattern perception* has long interested developmentalists, but only recently has *auditory pattern perception* received attention.

Auditory patterns are nonrandom, temporally (time) ordered sound sequences. Three properties of sound give rise to auditory patterns:

1. Time
2. Intensity
3. Frequency (Morrongiello, 1988)

Speech and music have a temporal pattern, an intensity (loudness/softness) pattern, and a frequency (high pitch/low pitch) pattern simultaneously. Developmentalists usually study one characteristic at a time.

Infants as young as 2 to 3 months old react to changes in the temporal pattern of a tone sequence, showing that they perceive temporal patterns (Demany, McKenzie, & Vurpillot, 1977). Young infants, though, perceive only pattern changes involving the number of groups of tones; for example, changing 9 tones from three groups of 3 to two groups, one of 5 and one of 4 (Morrongiello, 1984). At 12 months infants can perceive changes in the number of groups and the number of tones in each group (see Figure 6.9). So by the end of the 1st year, infants can perceive sound on the basis of temporal pattern, which is probably a prerequisite for language development.

Infants between 5 and 11 months can discriminate intensity changes for vowels in a syllable (Bull, Eilers, & Oller, 1984), but we know little else about intensity perception in infants.

Infants younger than 6 months can discriminate frequency relationships in a simple, short sequence. Not until the end of their 1st year, though, can infants perceive frequency relationships among the tones in a long, complex sequence (Morrongiello, 1986; Trehub, Bull, & Thorpe, 1984). The same is true of speech

Nine tones in 3 groups of 3 tones:

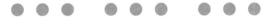

Changing the number of groups:

Changing the number of tones in each group:

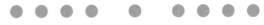

**Figure 6.9**    Auditory stimulus presented to infants. Young infants can detect a change in the number of groups from what is familiar to them, but not until they are 12 months old can they detect changes in both the number of groups and the number of tones in a group. Time between tones in a group was 0.2 s and between groups was 0.6 s.
(Based on Morrongiello, 1988.)

patterns. Infants under 6 months can discriminate short sequences of syllables for frequency, but not long sequences (Trehub, 1973, cited in Morrongiello, 1988). So young infants can perceive frequency patterns that are short and simple. As they grow older, they can perceive increasingly longer and more complex patterns. Children between 4 and 6 years can discriminate the frequency features of six-tone melodies played at normal speed (Morrongiello, Trehub, Thorpe, & Capodilupo, 1985). Slowing down the melody makes perception more difficult, and children at this age still have difficulty with these slowed melodies.

Infants progress rapidly in auditory pattern perception during their 1st year. These advances probably are prerequisites to language development. Preschool children make further progress in perceiving patterns in increasingly longer and more complex contexts.

What systems might limit the development of auditory pattern perception? Obviously, the auditory system must be developed. As mentioned earlier, auditory sensation is quite mature within days of birth. The sensory cortex of the brain, though, is still maturing rapidly over the first few years of life. With continuing development it probably permits conceptualization of patterns and identity of transformed patterns (Morrongiello, 1988)—for example, the same rhythmic pattern played at different tempos. Cognition also must advance, because to perceive patterns an individual must be able to remember and process information, especially long and complex sequences. We will discuss these topics further in chapter 8, but for now you should recognize that advances in cognitive processing occur when an infant is 6 to 7 months old.

Additionally, the environment in which infants develop might "tune" the developing auditory system to recognize certain features of language and music. In this way, we might learn to prefer the perceptual patterns prevalent in our native language and the music of our culture (Morrongiello, 1988).

## Auditory Figure-and-Ground

Often a person must attend to certain sounds while ignoring other, irrelevant sounds in the background. For example, try listening to someone talk to you on the telephone (figure sounds) while your stereo is playing and several people in your room are talking (ground sounds). Young infants can detect sounds amid ambient noise (Morrongiello & Clifton, 1984), but we know little else about the development of this important aspect of auditory perception. Some children have more difficulty than others separating auditory figures from the background. We would benefit from more research on the processes underlying these differences.

## Auditory Changes With Aging

More older adults than younger adults suffer a loss of hearing sensitivity, but the source of this loss varies among individuals. Loss of hearing in older adults is termed presbycusis (from presbys for "old man" and akousis for "hearing"). Some hearing loss might be due to physiologic degeneration. Various tissues involved in hearing can deteriorate, including the bones of the inner ear, the sensory neural cells in the ear, and the neural cells of the central nervous system involved in hearing. Often, hearing loss results from lifelong exposure to environmental noise (Timiras, 1972). Older persons who have avoided exposure to high levels of noise show much less hearing loss than others, especially those living or working in industrial environments. We know that extreme environmental noise, such as listening to loud music on stereo headsets, can lead to early hearing loss.

The *absolute threshold* (the quietest sound that a person can sense at least half the time) for hearing pure tones and speech increases in older adults, meaning that sounds must be louder for older adults than young adults. *Differential thresholds* (the closest that two sounds can be for a person to distinguish them from one another at least 75% of the time) also increase for pitch and speech discrimination (Corso, 1977). As a person ages, the ability to hear high-frequency sounds is particularly affected. One result is that older adults cannot hear certain consonant sounds well; they might report that they hear someone talking but cannot understand the message.

Older adults are at a distinct disadvantage in adverse listening situations, too. This might be due to a loss of central nervous system auditory neurons, which slows conduction of neural impulses from the ear to the brain.

Beyond these changes in hearing we know little about changes in auditory perception as people age, but as with vision, the perceptual process relies on clear and accurate sensations. Whatever factors affect hearing might also affect auditory perception. Fortunately, most older adults do not experience a hearing impairment before their 70s or 80s. Most, but not all, can benefit from hearing aids, which amplify sound. If the source of hearing loss is deterioration of central nervous system neurons, amplification does not help.

## REVIEW 6.1

From our discussions, it is clear that the visual, kinesthetic, and auditory systems function at an early age and continue to improve throughout infancy and childhood. By the time children are 8 to 12 years old, aspects of their visual perception have developed to near-adult levels. Kinesthetic perception typically develops to near-adult levels by about age 8, somewhat earlier than visual perception, although this generalization is based on limited research.

Young children can perceive the location of sound, and by age 10 they perform at near-adult levels on many auditory discrimination tasks. Refinement of auditory skills continues through the early teens. Some aspects of auditory perception have not been studied with children. In general, though, children between the ages of 8 and 12 approach adult levels of per-

formance on many perceptual tasks, with only small refinements in perceptual skills yet to be made.

It is clear that some aspects of perceptual development are not well documented and that further research is needed. We know little, too, about the cause of changes in the perceptual processes as people age, but we do know that the results of these decremental changes in the sensory systems reduce the quality of the sensory information reaching the central nervous system, thereby affecting motor skill performance.

## INTERSENSORY INTEGRATION

Think for a moment about the softball infielder we talked about earlier in this chapter. The player saw and heard the bat hitting the ball. The experience was sensed by two separate sensory systems, vision and audition. Concept 6.1 focused on the developmental improvements that occur within such individual sensory systems—that is, *intrasensory development*. In playing softball, an infielder must combine perceptions from individual sensory-perceptual systems to make more complex judgments. We term this aspect of perception *intersensory integration*. The player integrates information from two or more senses to accurately judge the ball's path.

You can find many examples of intersensory integration in skilled performance. A gymnast on a narrow balance beam integrates visual and kinesthetic information to perform stunts. A dancer integrates musical sounds with visual and kinesthetic information to present a dance, and so on. Intersensory integration is necessary for nearly all skilled performances.

If you have ever watched a young child's first attempts to hop and clap in time with music, you know that intersensory integration is not fully functional early in life. A young child cannot well integrate the kinesthetic input from clapping with the beat of the music to assist the timing of the hop. How does the ability to simultaneously use information from many senses develop?

### CONCEPT 6.2

Intersensory integration improves during childhood.

## Levels of Integration

Developmentalists generally accept that intersensory integration, sometimes termed *cross-modal functioning*, is partially functional at birth and improves as a child grows and develops. We can categorize this developmental process of intersensory integration into three levels:

1. The first level is the *automatic integration* of basic sensory stimuli, a process inherent to the functioning of the subcortical brain. Neural impulses arising from the registration of a stimulus in two or more senses converge at one location in the brain. Automatic integration is probably functional at birth or very early in infancy.
2. The second level involves the integration of a particular stimulus or the features of a stimulus when it is experienced in two different senses. For example, a child who first touches a building block but does not see it later recognizes the block upon seeing it, even without touching it.
3. The highest level involves the transfer of concepts across sense modalities (Williams, 1983). Adults can transfer the concept of "soft" across vision, kin-

esthesis, and hearing. You might first encounter "soft" tactually, but you can also report that objects look soft, or you can describe a sound as soft. An individual attains these latter two levels of integration through the experiences of infancy and childhood.

It is tempting to think that intersensory integration follows intrasensory development—that visual or kinesthetic sensation and perception are refined first, then sensory integration develops. In fact, the development of intra- and intersensory integration is closely linked. Some evidence suggests that even very young infants can interact with their environment through two senses concurrently. For example, Aronson and Rosenbloom (1971) had infants 30 to 55 days old watch their mothers while their voices were projected either normally or from a displaced location. The infants became visibly agitated when their mothers' voices came from a displaced location. Spelke's (1979) research demonstrated that 3- to 4-month-old infants, when shown two movies side by side, spent more time watching the movie for which the proper soundtrack was played. At a very young age, then, children are uncomfortable with discrepancies between two senses, such as vision and hearing, indicating that they are capable of the first level of integration, the automatic integration of basic sensory stimuli.

Intersensory integration at the second level seems to emerge in the second half of the infant's 1st year. Brown and Gottfried (1986) found no evidence that 1-, 3-, and 5-month-olds could integrate shapes across vision and kinesthesis, but many have reported transfer of shape in infants older than 6 months (Bushnell, 1982, 1986; Rose, Gottfried, & Bridger, 1981). It is likely that intrasensory discrimination precedes intersensory integration (Brown & Gottfried, 1986). Keep in mind, though, that infants' performance on intersensory integration tasks depends on many things, including their exploratory abilities and attentional tendencies (Bushnell, 1986). It is also difficult for researchers to design studies of infants so young. Our knowledge of infant behavior is limited by our research techniques.

It is misleading to emphasize the perceptual development of one sense system independent of other systems. Auerbach and Sperling (1974) argue that a single common dimension underlies perception when a person uses two or more sensory systems. For example, we can localize an object through vision and through hearing. Rather than possessing a "visual direction" or an "auditory direction," we judge direction through a common directional dimension, not by perceiving the stimuli as different events first, then integrating them in a second step. J.J. Gibson (1979) also suggested that perceptual systems perceive not only objects or events, but also the usages they permit the observer. For example, small objects can be picked up, whereas very large objects cannot. Even infants detect the properties of objects in their environment as a consequence of exploring that environment (Walker-Andrews & E.J. Gibson, 1986).

---

*The many experiences that contribute to a child's perceptual development are typically intersensory; thus, it is more accurate to view intrasensory refinement and intersensory integration as interrelated processes.*

---

## The Development of Sensory Integration

Researchers typically study sensory integration by pairing two sensory-perceptual systems. They expose a child to an object or stimulus first in one system, then the other.

### Visual-Kinesthetic Integration

Because sensory refinement and integration are interrelated processes, we will base our dis-

cussion of the course of development in sensory integration on visual-kinesthetic, visual-auditory, and auditory-kinesthetic integration. Goodnow (1971a) conducted a series of experimental studies of sensory integration in children. In an initial study involving visual and kinesthetic integration, Goodnow presented five shapes (Greek and Russian letters) by either sight or feel to three age groups (5.0 to 5.5-year-olds, 5.6- to 6.8-year-olds, and 9.0- to 10.0-year-olds). She then presented these five shapes with five new ones, again by sight or feel, and challenged the children to identify the familiar shapes. Four presentation patterns were possible:

1. Visual presentation–visual recognition (V-V)
2. Kinesthetic presentation–kinesthetic recognition (K-K)
3. Visual presentation–kinesthetic recognition (V-K)
4. Kinesthetic presentation–visual recognition (K-V)

The judgments the children had to make represent the second level of sensory integration—the integration of the features of stimulus information. Goodnow found that children, especially the youngest ones, had more difficulty in the K-K pattern than in the V-V pattern. This performance discrepancy narrowed in the older age groups. The K-V task proved more difficult for the children than the V-K task. Goodnow noted that the scores of the youngest group in the kinesthetic conditions were extremely variable. This study and others, using similar tasks and different age groups, lead us to the conclusion that visual-kinesthetic integration improves as children grow older. When the kinesthetic task involves active manipulation of an object, 5-year-olds can recognize the shapes relatively well, but slight improvement continues until age 8. If passive movements are involved, performance is not as advanced, and improvements continue through age 11 (Williams, 1983).

## Visual-Auditory Integration

Goodnow (1971b) also examined visual-auditory integration. She presented an auditory-visual task by tapping out a sequence (* ***) and then asking children to write the sequence, using dots to picture where the taps occurred. She could reverse this auditory-visual (A-V) task by asking children to tap out a pictured sequence (V-A). Children around age 5 did not perform the A-V sequence as well as children at age 7. A trend toward improved performance on the V-A sequence was also found in children between ages 6.9 and 8.5 years. The result of this experiment and similar studies with other groups indicates that visual and auditory integration improves between ages 5 and 12 (Williams, 1983). Young children find A-V tasks more difficult than V-A tasks, but this difference diminishes after age 7 (Rudel & Teuber, 1971).

## Auditory-Kinesthetic Integration

The amount of research conducted on auditory-kinesthetic integration is small compared with the amount involving vision. Temple et al. (1979) included the Witeba Test of Auditory-Tactile Integration in a test battery administered to 6- and 8-year-olds. In this test, an experimenter twice tells a child the name of an object or shape. The child then feels a number of objects or shapes, attempting to select the one that matches the auditory label. The investigators found that 8-year-olds performed this task much better than 6-year-olds.

This experimental method is based on children understanding the label given the object or shape. Possibly, this age difference resulted from younger children's misunderstanding or not remembering the auditory label in addition to, or instead of, their auditory-kinesthetic integration ability. Based on this limited data, we can conclude that auditory-kinesthetic integration improves in childhood.

In summary, then, sensory integration improves in childhood, and the accuracy of children's performance depends on the order of sensory presentation. Presenting the visual pattern or object first yields better performance than auditory-first presentation.

## Spatial-Temporal Integration

Another aspect of integration involves the spatial-temporal characteristics of the task to be performed. Recall Goodnow's second experiment. When children viewed the dot pattern, they were dealing with a spatial stimulus. When they listened to an auditory pattern, they were attending to a temporal (time) stimulus. Sterritt, Martin, and Rudnick (1971) devised nine tasks that varied the number of sensory integrations to be made as well as the type of integration, including spatial-temporal characteristics—for example, the child must integrate a short pause between two tones (temporal) with a short space between two dots (spatial). They presented the nine tasks to 6-year-olds. The easiest task for the children was the V-V spatial (intrasensory) task. Children had intermediate difficulty with those tasks requiring them to integrate visual spatial stimuli and visual or auditory-temporal stimuli. The children found integration of two temporal patterns difficult, whether the task was intra- or intersensory. While progressing in intersensory integration, then, children also improve their ability to integrate spatial and temporal stimuli as well as to integrate two sets of temporal stimuli.

## Refinements in Adolescence

Difficult or subtle aspects of intersensory integration might continue to develop during adolescence. Botuck and Turkewitz (1990) studied auditory-visual and temporal-spatial integration in 7-, 13-, and 17-year-olds. The 7-year-olds found intrasensory matching much easier than intersensory matching, whereas the 13-year-olds could match spatial with temporal patterns across the visual and auditory systems as well as within the sensory systems. The 17-year-olds did not score significantly higher than the 13-year-olds, but they handled the matching tasks equally well whether the visual or auditory pattern was presented first. In contrast, the younger groups made more errors when the auditory pattern came first. Adolescents, then, may continue to refine intersensory integration.

## REVIEW 6.2

Infants have a limited ability to integrate basic sensory stimuli, but children attain higher levels of sensory integration. Improvements in intersensory integration are closely linked to intrasensory development. Children also learn to integrate sensory stimuli along a spatial-temporal dimension. They first master spatial-spatial integration tasks, followed by mixed spatial and temporal tasks, and finally temporal-temporal tasks. It is possible that improvement in intersensory integration is linked to cognitive development, because the experimental methods researchers use to study integration often rely on an understanding of labels or memory of a previously presented object or shape. Subtle refinements in intersensory integration continue through adolescence.

## BALANCE

Balance is an example of a motor response that depends on the integration of stimuli from the visual and kinesthetic systems. Vision tells you how your body is positioned relative to the environment. Kinesthetic input from your body's proprioceptors tells you how your limbs and body parts are positioned relative to each other.

Whenever you must maintain your balance, a stream of sensory information must be integrated in the central nervous system, and your muscles constantly activate or relax as needed.

You must maintain balance in an almost infinite number of situations. Sometimes you balance when stationary (static balance), and sometimes when moving (dynamic balance). You are called upon to balance on a variety of body parts, not just your two feet. Think of all the body parts on which gymnasts must balance in their various events. Sometimes you need to balance on surfaces other than the ground, such as a ladder. You might even have to balance without all the information you would like—for example, when you have to walk in the dark.

Movement scientists find that performance levels on various types of balancing tasks are specific to the task (Drowatzky & Zuccato, 1967). Balance is not a general ability, but many specific abilities. A person can perform one type of balance task well but may perform another type at only an average level. For this reason, the course of balance development is best related to the specific balance task used to assess performance.

**CONCEPT 6.3**

Balance improves throughout childhood and adolescence; however, a loss of balance ability in an older adult can lead to injury.

## The Development of Balance

Strong evidence indicates that balance performance improves as children advance from 3 to 19 years of age (Bachman, 1961; DeOreo & Wade, 1971; Espenschade, 1947; Espenschade, Dable, & Schoendube, 1953; Seils, 1951; Winterhalter, 1974). The exact pattern of improvement depends largely on the assessment task. On some balance tasks, the average performance of a group of children does not change significantly from year to year, but improvement is steady over a number of years (DeOreo & Wade, 1971); on other tasks there is significant improvement each year. Despite this general trend, some researchers have noted instances of no improvement or even decline in performance scores (Bachman, 1961; Espenschade, 1947; Espenschade et al., 1953). No definitive explanation is available for these findings, but that may be partly because researchers predominantly use quantitative rather than qualitative assessments of balance. It is possible that at certain ages and on certain tasks, children attempt more efficient movement patterns with a resulting, presumably temporary, decline in quantitative score. For example, DeOreo (1971) noted that young children could attempt to walk a balance beam with either a shuffle step, a mark-time pattern (the rear foot placed alongside the lead foot), or a more mature alternate-step pattern. A child first changing from an easier shuffle step to a more difficult alternate-step pattern may lose balance and step off the beam sooner than when using a shuffle step. With more practice, though, the child will travel the beam longer and faster.

Children, then, can be expected to make both qualitative and quantitative improvements in balance performance.

## Early Reliance on Vision

It is also possible that using a dynamic systems perspective can help us explain the development of posture and balance, including the regressions and plateaus in performance. For example, we can study the role of vision, proprioception and vestibular stimulation, and their integration in balance. We can also relate to balance the effects of neuromuscular and biomechanical changes that accompany physical growth. Developmentalists have used this perspective recently to study posture and balance, even in 2-month-old infants. Often, they use a "moving room" technique, in which infants sit on a stationary platform while the walls and ceiling surrounding them move and researchers measure the responses of the infants' muscles with an electromyograph (EMG). If infants are sensitive to visual information, they will adjust their heads, reacting as if their bodies are swaying even though their kinesthetic receptors do not register movement. Two-month-olds make this response (Pope, 1984). By 6 months, infants are less susceptible to the moving room effect, but they demonstrate the effect again at the onset of sitting alone and standing alone (Butterworth & Hicks, 1977; Lee & Aronson, 1974).

Another technique is to place infants sitting or standing on a movable platform that is moved unexpectedly (see Figures 6.10 and

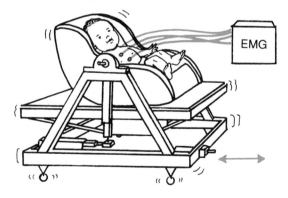

Figure 6.10 An infant seated on a platform that can be unexpectedly moved forward or backward. EMG responses of the posture muscles are recorded.
(Reprinted by permission from Woollacott, Debu, & Shumway-Cook, 1987.)

6.11). Researchers record EMG measurements of the infants' posture and balance muscles. Seated infants 4 to 6 months old make appropriate responses to being thrown off balance only about 60% of the time when they can view the room. But when opaque goggles are placed over the infants' eyes, they always make the appropriate response (Woollacott, Debu, & Mowatt, 1987). By 8 months, infants make the appropriate response with or without vision. These two types of studies indicate that young infants rely heavily on visual information for balancing, even though their proprioceptive and vestibular systems can regularly mediate the proper postural response to being thrown off balance.

When infants who have just begun standing are placed in the moving room, they often sway, stagger, or fall, unlike adults who can keep their balance (Lee & Aronson, 1974).

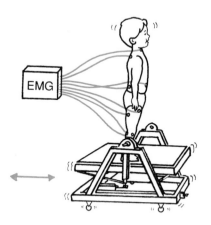

**Figure 6.11** A child standing on a movable platform with electrodes positioned to record the posture and balance muscles' response to a sudden movement.
(Reprinted by permission from Debu, Woollacott, & Mowatt. 1988.)

This again indicates a reliance on visual information for balance. The moving room effect diminishes in children after their 1st year of standing. Newly standing children take longer to use their postural muscles when thrown off balance and sway more before attaining stability than adults (Forrsberg & Nashner, 1982). These responses improve, particularly in the lower body, but children 4 to 6 years old seem to regress (Shumway-Cook & Woollacott, 1985; Woollacott et al., 1987). During this time children again take longer to respond and vary greatly in the way they respond, although they sway less. Possibly, children at this age are starting to rely more on kinesthetic systems and less on vision. In addition, they might be refining their integration of sensory information from the various sensory systems (Woollacott, Shumway-Cook, & Williams, 1989). Children 7 to 10 years old generally show adultlike postural responses (Shumway-Cook & Woollacott, 1985).

### Biomechanical Factors

Woollacott et al. (1987) found little evidence that balance differences between children and adults resulted from biomechanical factors, namely the physical growth in childhood that changes limb and trunk proportions and masses. Therefore, children's regressions and plateaus in balance performance seem to be associated with changes in the nervous system, specifically shifts in the child's reliance on specific sensory systems and the integration of the sensory systems. Further, Bertenthal and Bai (1989) associated postural responses to movement of various parts of the moving room over the 1st year and hypothesized that improvements are also driven by infants engaging in new tasks. For example, the onset of crawling might sensitize infants to movement in different parts of the visual field.

Movement contributes to developmental advances along with the development of various systems.

## Balance Changes With Aging

Older adults experience a decline in the ability to balance. Those over 60 sway more than younger adults when standing upright, especially if they are in a leaning position (Hasselkus & Shambes, 1975; Hellebrandt & Braun, 1939; Sheldon, 1963). Age-related changes in balance also occur when older adults stand on a movable platform that is momentarily shifted, simulating a slippery surface. Compared to young adults, slightly more time passes before an older adult's leg muscles respond to maintain balance, and sometimes the upper leg muscles respond first instead of the lower leg muscles as in young adults. The strength of the muscles' response is more variable from time to time in older adults (Woollacott, Shumway-Cook, & Nashner, 1982, 1986).

Woollacott (1986) studied the reaction of older adults when a movable platform tipped forward or back. Half the older adults she observed lost their balance the first time, but these adults learned to keep their balance after a few more tries. So older adults are more liable to fall on a slippery surface than young adults but are capable of improving their stability with practice.

Falls by older adults are a significant concern. In fact, falls are the leading cause of accidental death for people over 75 years old. A common result of falling, especially among those older adults with osteoporosis, is fracture of the spine, hip (pelvis or femur), or wrist. Complications of such a fracture can result in death. Even when older adults recover, they experience heavy health care costs, a period of inactivity,

and dependence on others. A fear of falling again can make them change their lifestyles or be overly cautious in subsequent activities.

Age-related changes in balance ability could be related to a variety of changes in the body's systems, especially the nervous system. As mentioned previously, some older adults experience changes in the kinesthetic receptors, and these changes might be more extreme in the lower limbs than in the upper ones. Vision changes, as well as those that occur in the vestibular receptors and nerves in adults over 75, might also place the older adult at a disadvantage (Bergstrom, 1973; Johnsson & Hawkins, 1972; Rosenhall & Rubin, 1975). A decrease in fast-twitch muscle fibers or a loss of strength could hamper an older adult's quick response to changes in stability, as might arthritic conditions in the joints. Whether the decrements noted result from increased perceptual thresholds, changes in the peripheral nerves, changes in the musculoskeletal system, or changes within the central nervous system remains unclear (Timiras, 1972).

## REVIEW 6.3

The motor responses we make to maintain our posture and balance are excellent examples of movements based on integrated sensory information. Both vision and kinesthesis provide information for balancing but during infancy and early childhood we sometimes rely more on visual information than kinesthetic information. By age 10 preadolescents make adultlike postural responses. Performance on various balance tasks improves throughout childhood and adolescence although the timing of these improvements depends on the type, static or dynamic, and the nature of the task.

Falls can be especially dangerous for older adults. Because it takes longer for older adults to respond to a loss of balance, they fall on slippery surfaces more often than young adults. Changes in the body with aging can decrease balance ability, but one research study demonstrated that older adults can improve in keeping their balance with practice.

## PERCEPTUAL-MOTOR EXPERIENCE

Our discussion of intrasensory development, intersensory integration, and balance revealed that infancy and early and middle childhood are times of rapid improvement in perceptual-motor activities. Adults make perceptual judgments so routinely that they often do not realize how much change infants and children undergo. Nor do adults realize the role motor activity plays in the development of perceptual processes. Developmentalists are now taking greater interest in the role of early motor activity in an individual's overall development.

It is likely that active movement through the environment is vital to the integration of perceptions and purposeful movements. Much of the evidence for the importance of movement, though, comes from animal studies. Developmentalists obviously cannot withhold from humans any experience that even possibly is part of normal development. So researchers cannot implement the ideal research study wherein they deprive a group of individuals of movement and compare them to a group given the opportunity to move. Reports of such studies are available for animals and contribute to our knowledge.

In addition, researchers can study infants and children whose motor experiences vary through naturally occurring circumstances. For example, some parents use baby walkers, which allow infants to move through their environment at an earlier age than they can move by themselves, and some parents do not.

Let us consider the information available on the importance of early motor experience from both human and animal research, then review the types of activities that comprise a perceptual-motor activity program for children.

> **CONCEPT 6.4**
> Early motor experience is important to perceptual-motor development.

## Perceptual-Motor Theories

The exact nature of the relationship between perception and motor activity has been elusive for developmentalists. So too has the nature of the relationship between perception and cognition, and therefore the relationship among all three—perception, cognition, and motor activity. In the late 1950s, 1960s, and early 1970s several developmentalists hypothesized the nature of this three-way relationship. Currently, these hypotheses are considered invalid, but knowing them helps us appreciate the complexity of this relationship. Additionally, the work of this era yielded screening tools and activity programs that still are useful. Let us learn from the history of perceptual-motor theories.

### Motor Activity and Cognition

Perception is important to cognition. As a simple demonstration, consider a child learning to read or to add two-digit numbers. The form of letters and numbers, their orientation in space (such as *d* or *b*), and the direction of processing them (left to right in reading, but right to left in adding) are just a few aspects of perception that children must master before they can perform these cognitive activities. Is there a link, then, between perceptual-motor functioning and cognitive functioning?

The perceptual-motor theories proposed around the 1960s suggested the two are directly linked. One assumption was that educators could identify deficiencies in cognitive functioning (typically reading) due to faulty perceptual judgments by administering perceptual-motor test batteries and remedy them by training a child on perceptual-motor activities requiring those specific perceptual judgments. Among these theories is the neurological organization theory of Delacato (1959, 1966), the physiological optics program of Getman (1952, 1963) (see Cratty, 1979, for a review of these two programs), the visual perception tests and the program of Frostig, Lefever, and Whittlesey (1966), the sensory-integration tests of Ayres (1972), the movigenics theory of Barsch (1965), and the perceptual-motor theory of Kephart (1971). Of course, the value of such programs rests on the assumption that perceptual-motor functioning and cognitive functioning are indeed linked. Let us use one of the more popular theories, that of Kephart, to examine the hypothesized nature of this link.

## Kephart's Theory

Newell C. Kephart, a clinical psychologist, proposed that perception and cognition develop from a motor base, in that a child must establish motor "generalizations" to reach full intellectual growth. Kephart emphasized the generalizations of posture and balance, laterality, locomotion, contact, receipt and propulsion, and body image. He outlined seven developmental stages that represent increasingly efficient information processing strategies. A child who does not learn the stages sequentially and completely will experience deficiencies in later learning at higher levels.

In Kephart's view, normal children proceed automatically through these stages, but a child who learns slowly either does not progress through the sequence or is markedly delayed (Kephart, 1971). Any child who skipped a stage or left it uncompleted must be returned to that stage and, through training, subsequently moved through the remaining stages. Develop-

mentally delayed children, then, require supplementary experiences to enhance their development. Kephart further suggested that providing perceptual-motor activities for all children, especially preschoolers, decreases the likelihood that children will leave a stage incomplete or skip a stage entirely.

Kephart's (1971) training program for slow learners included perceptual-motor, perceptual-motor matching, ocular control, chalkboard training, and form-perception activities. He presented the skills in a hierarchy, with the gross-motor activities trained first, followed by fine-motor skills. Eye-hand coordination, eye movement control, and perceptual monitoring of motor activities are highlighted.

To summarize Kephart's program, we might outline the assumptions he made in his theory, survey, and training program. First, Kephart assumed that perception and cognition are linked by a common motor base. Certain motor generalizations are necessary for a child to attain full intellectual functioning. Slow learners are those who have not proceeded through the developmental stages in the proper time frame. These children may be restored to the normal course of development by a training program of perceptual-motor activities. Kephart also assumed that developmental problems may be forestalled by early (preschool) training in perceptual-motor activities.

## Critiques of Kephart's Theory

The foundation of Kephart's theory is the perception-cognition link through a motor base. Strong evidence of a perceptual-motor/cognitive link is lacking. Most studies have reported little or no relationship among perceptual-motor development, perception, and cognition (Williams, 1983). The behavioral study undertaken by Belka and Williams (cited in Williams, 1983) is an example. These investigators tested two subdomains of perceptual-motor behavior, gross and fine, on 63 children, ages 5, 6, and 7. They included two subdomains of perception: vision and audition. A standardized test appropriate for each age level measured cognitive behavior. Belka and Williams found perceptual-motor behavior and perceptual behavior to be related only in the younger groups, indicating that the close link between the two domains might diminish with age. Perception and cognition were related at all ages. In contrast, relationships between perceptual-motor and cognitive behavior were low and significant only at age 6. Belka and Williams could predict the cognitive performances of kindergarten children from their perceptual-motor development, but not those of older children. This study and similar ones indicate that the perceptual-motor/cognitive link is indirect, if it exists at all. Hence, Kephart's basic theoretical assumption of a perceptual-motor/cognitive link has no strong experimental support.

Kephart advocated a perceptual-motor training program for slow learners who have normal intelligence but are a year of more behind their peers in achievement (delayed in cognitive development). Slow learners often display sensory-perceptual judgments appropriate for younger children (Williams, 1983). The same is true of performance on perceptual-motor tasks. Although this may indicate that delayed development in several domains is related, it is still not strong evidence of a direct link between perceptual-motor and cognitive functioning. Without such evidence, we have little reason to assume that perceptual-motor training improves cognitive functioning.

Indeed, little research evidence shows that visual-motor training like Kephart recommended improves performance. Goodman and Hamill (1973) reviewed 16 well-designed experimental studies on this topic and found that the overwhelming majority failed to show that children improved their readiness skills, intelligence, achievement, language, or even visual-motor skills after receiving visual-motor skill training. Therefore, not enough empirical evidence exists to support the hypotheses proposed during this era, of which Kephart's is a classic example.

## Sensitive Periods in Perceptual Development

Although the research does not strongly support remediation of cognitive deficiencies through perceptual-motor activities, there are indications that sensitive periods for perceptual development exist. It is important that individuals have experience moving in their environment during these periods. Perceptual deficiencies that result from lack of experience could later manifest themselves in both motor and cognitive performance. Let us look at the support for sensitive periods in perceptual development.

### Self-Produced Locomotion

Consider first the well-known animal study of Held and Hein (1963). These researchers deprived some newborn kittens of motor activity while permitting others to move. They kept visual experience identical for all the kittens by placing them in pairs in a merry-go-round apparatus. One of the pair was harnessed but could walk around (active kitten) whereas the other was restricted to riding in a gondola (passive kitten; see Figure 6.12). The passive kittens later failed to accurately judge depth perception and failed to exhibit paw placing or eye blinking when an object approached. Evidently, in animals self-produced movement is related to the development of behavior requiring visual perception. There also is evidence of more brain growth and more efficient nervous system functioning in young animals when researchers provided them extra perceptual-motor stimulation (Williams, 1986).

As mentioned earlier, visual cliff studies seem to indicate that depth perception is present from very early in life. Alternatively, an infant's avoidance of heights might develop during the second half of the 1st year as a result of self-produced locomotor experience. Bertenthal, Campos, and Barrett (1984) found that pre-locomotor infants given artificial locomotor experience by use of a baby walker (a seat in a frame on wheels) responded to heights whereas other infants the same age did not. Additionally, one infant whose locomotor skills were delayed as a result of a heavy cast did not respond to the visual cliff until self-produced

## The Purdue PMS

Kephart and a colleague, Eugene C. Roach, authored a screening test, the Purdue Perceptual-Motor Survey (PMS), to help educators identify children whose perceptual-motor abilities are insufficient for them to acquire academic skills (Roach & Kephart, 1966). It is doubtful that the survey is the best method of identifying children with academic deficiencies, because, as we just discussed, the perceptual-motor/cognitive link cannot be substantiated. On the other hand, the Purdue PMS may be useful in identifying children with perceptual-motor deficiencies.

The Purdue PMS is intended for boys and girls ages 6 to 10 and includes 22 items, each scored on a 4-point scale for a maximum score of 88. The survey items are divided into five categories:

1. Balance and posture
2. Body image and differentiation
3. Perceptual-motor match
4. Ocular control
5. Form perception

The balance and posture category includes walking on a board, jumping, hopping, and skipping. Body image activities consist of a range of tests, including identifying body parts, imitating movements, moving specified arms or legs as directed, and traveling an obstacle course. It also includes a measure of strength. Perceptual-motor match consists of chalkboard drawing and rhythmic writing, and ocular control consists of pursuit and convergent eye movements. In the form perception category, the child draws geometric forms. The authors provide adequate directions and scoring criteria for the survey, and the test requires a minimum of special equipment. It is easy to administer, but the tester should be trained in giving the tests.

Educators who want survey scores to be meaningful need average scores or norms for comparison. Roach and Kephart gathered and reported normative data based on 200 children, but all were from one school. Although the children came from six different socioeconomic groups, it is not clear whether the range available in this one school represented all the socioeconomic groups that might be given the survey.

Any test or survey of this type also should yield a reliable score—that is, a child taking the test more than once should score the same each time. The authors estimated this test characteristic by retesting a number of participants and correlating their two scores. The test-retest reliability reported for the Purdue PMS is .946, a high correlation. The authors also correlated the scores of the normative group with their teachers' ratings to establish validity, the ability of a test to measure what it is intended to measure, and obtained an estimated concurrent validity of .654. This moderate correlation was considered acceptable by the authors. The survey does need further standardization and cross-validation (Buros, 1972), but trained administrators can use it successfully to screen children for perceptual-motor deficiencies.

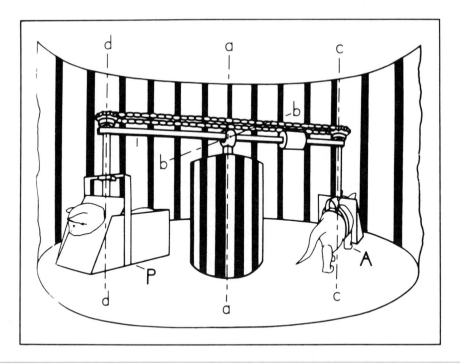

**Figure 6.12**   The apparatus Held and Hein used for equating motion and consequent visual feedback for an actively moving (A) and a passively moved (P) animal.
(Reprinted by permission from Held & Hein, 1963.)

locomotion began. Finally, many more infants who averaged 41 days of creeping experience avoided the visual cliff than infants with 11 days of experience, even at identical ages.

---

Self-produced locomotion appears to facilitate development of depth perception.

---

Kermoian and Campos (1988) also investigated the link between infants' self-produced locomotion and their perception of spatial relationships by studying the infants' strategies in searching for objects. They gave infants a set of progressively more difficult searching tasks (called "object permanence tasks"), ranging from retrieving a half-hidden object to retrieving objects under one of several cloths after the passage of time. Three groups of 8.5-month-old infants performed the tasks:

1. Prelocomotor infants
2. Prelocomotor infants with walker experience
3. Locomotor (creeping) infants

The more locomotor experience infants had, the better they scored (see Figure 6.13). Locomotor experiences also appear to facilitate development of an infant's spatial perceptions.

How might locomotor experience facilitate perceptual development? Greenough, Black, & Wallace (1987) hypothesized that an excess number of synapses (connections) among neurons initially form. With continued development some survive but others do not. Those connections activated by sensory and motor experience survive. Disuse leads to loss of connections. Synaptic proliferation prepares an organism for experience, presumably the experiences common to all members of a species. Therefore, undergoing the experiences during

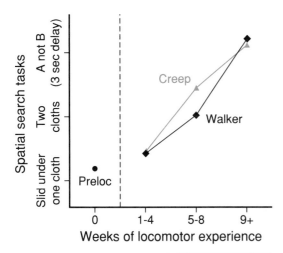

**Figure 6.13** Performance on spatial search tasks improves with locomotor experience compared to no experience and with weeks of locomotor experience. No difference exists between infants whose locomotor experience comes from creeping (hands and knees) or an infant walker. All infants, including the prelocomotor infants, were 8.5 months old.
(Reprinted by permission from Kermoian & Campos, 1988.)

the sensitive period of development promotes survival of the synaptic connections.

The Greenough et al. hypothesis certainly needs much experimental verification, but it provides a plausible explanation for the effect of self-produced locomotion on perceptual development (Bertenthal & Campos, 1987). Even if perceptual-motor activities cannot remediate perceptual-cognitive deficiencies, perceptual-motor experiences might be critical to normal perceptual development in infants and young children. The failure of the perceptual-motor theories and programs of the 1950s and 1960s to provide a vehicle for cognitive remediation should not diminish the importance of perceptual-motor experiences to overall development. Certainly a lack of emphasis on or deprivation of such experience puts an individual at risk of deficient perceptual development.

## The Perception-Action Perspective

The perception-action perspective outlined in chapter 1 provides us insight to the importance of motor activity. Note that from this perspective, perception and motor activity are inseparable. The development of perception is intertwined with individuals' actions in their environment: You do not perceive a long list of object characteristics and subject them to calculations in your brain. Instead, you perceive directly what the objects in your environment afford or permit you to do. The activities any object affords are a combination of its functional utility and your own capabilities. For example, a set of stairs with an 8-in. (20.3 cm) rise between steps does not afford an 18-month-old alternate-step climbing, as it does an adult. A 24-in. (61.0 cm) rise does not afford the average adult alternate-step climbing. As you grow and develop, your perception of affordances might change as your action capabilities change, even though an object's physical properties remain the same. Taking action, then, is a critically important aspect of development of the perception-action system.

Because we perceive affordances rather than object characteristics, individuals must be sensitive to the scale of their bodies. In our stair-climbing example, perhaps individuals must be sensitive to their leg length to judge the "climbability" of any set of stairs. Warren (1984) tested this notion with adults and found that individuals perceived stairs with a riser height of more than 88% to 89% of their leg length to be "unclimbable" with alternate stepping. This model did not apply to older adults, whose affordances for stair climbing related more to strength and flexibility than to leg length (Konczak, Meuwssen, & Cress, 1988, cited in Konczak, 1990). Nor did the model apply to infants and toddlers. Infants in a study chose smaller step heights than toddlers (see Figure 6.14), but no anthropometric measurements related to the choice of step height (Ulrich, Thelen, & Niles, 1990).

Obviously, individuals may use many types of body scales, and the important scales may change throughout life. Perhaps changes in a person's various body systems influence which scale she or he uses. We need continued research to determine the reference scales individuals use for particular tasks. Yet, according to the perception-action perspective, not only do a person's perceptions influence actions; actions also impact perceptions.

---

Our sensitivity to body scaling has implications for skill instruction. For example, if a child cannot swing a big, heavy adult-sized racket with one hand, the child cannot use adult technique. Either the racket must be scaled down to fit the child, or the child might need to use two hands to swing the racket.

---

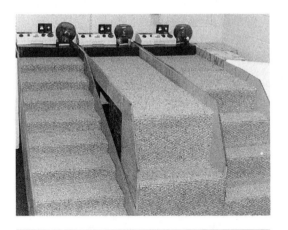

Figure 6.14 Infants might choose a set of steps depending on whether the step height affords them climbing. This in turn might depend on their body size; affordability is related to some individual body scale. For example, the middle set of stairs might be too high to afford climbing by infants with short arms and legs. Either set of side stairs would afford infants climbing, and infants are as likely to choose one as the other. The researchers placed the same kind of toys at the top of each set of steps as a motivation for climbing. (Photo provided by B.D. Ulrich of Indiana University.)

# Perceptual-Motor Activities

If indeed young children are sensitive to the deprivation of motor activity, they need perceptual-motor experiences to optimize their development. It is also apparent that such experiences are vital if children are to later master skills in exercise, sport, and dance performance. Realizing this, most educators include perceptual-motor activities in the regular physical education, music, and early childhood curricula. These activities expose children to a wide range of stimuli and give them opportunities to explore and practice perceptual-motor responses. As a result, children gradually master their physical environments and become increasingly confident in their abilities.

We will review some of the typical perceptual-motor activities that comprise perceptual-motor programs, organized by the perceptual system targeted in the activity. We will also review balance activities. Note that some activities require intersensory integration.

## Visual Perception

Visual-motor activities require children to match a visual shape with movement, manipulate objects they can see, and move appropriately for certain distances and spaces.

### Figure-and-Ground Perception

In many catching and striking skills, the performer must attend to a ball approaching from a confusing, multicolored background. Children eventually need practice with such perceptual displays, but early in their learning they will benefit from a simpler display. For example, educators should provide balls and backgrounds of contrasting solid colors when possible. They can gradually lessen the contrast between ball and background or make the background more complex as a child acquires skill.

## Distance and Depth Perception

Children should also refine their distance and depth perception. Recall that depth perception is related to visual acuity. If children have great difficulty judging depth, educators should refer them to an eye-care specialist for examination.

Children can practice fine judgments of depth and distance in many ways. You might set up a throwing task, placing targets at varying distances and challenging the children to judge the distance to each target and gauge their throw accordingly. This activity involves kinesthesis, too, because children must learn to vary the force of their throws.

## Pattern and Form Perception

One aspect of visual space orientation is form perception, or the ability to recognize forms and shapes regardless of their orientation, size, color, and so on. Many teachers use geometric shapes as targets for tossing beanbags or balls or challenge children to travel along various geometric shapes taped to the floor. In this way children experience the shapes in many orientations and sizes and learn to match a name to the shape.

Children also benefit from practice with pattern perception, the appreciation that objects they can see are arranged in a pattern. Teachers can arrange various items such as hoops or cones in a pattern, then ask children to reproduce that pattern with their own hoops or cones.

## Spatial Awareness

It is often necessary to make judgments about space based on visual information. A simple form of this perception is to locate objects in space. A more difficult task is to view a space and judge whether your body can fit through it. Children practice this visual-kinesthetic task when they climb on playground equipment. You can make the openings in the apparatus in geometric shapes to involve form perception.

## Kinesthetic Perception

Kinesthetic-motor activities help children develop an awareness of the body and environment as distinct, label body parts, and identify directions for both the body and the surrounding space.

## Tactile Discrimination

Touch is an important aspect of kinesthetic perception and is related to accurate body awareness. Children need experience in localizing touches and in discriminating multiple touches and varied surfaces. Teachers often vary the texture of the surfaces that children contact. It is also fun and valuable to play games in which you challenge blindfolded children to identify or match objects and textures.

## Spatial Dimensions

Educators often focus much attention on laterality and left-right discrimination in perceptual-motor programs, but awareness of other body dimensions is equally important. These dimensions include the following:

- Up-down
- Front-back
- Side

Many activities involve spatial dimensions. One of the most enjoyable activities for children is a lummi stick routine to music wherein they hold two short sticks and tap them in front, in back, and to the side of the body in rhythmical patterns.

## Body Awareness

Body awareness or body image is an important aspect of kinesthesis. Recall that body awareness involves perception of the locations and names of the body parts, their relation to one another (including joint position), and movement of specific body parts. Children can practice touching and naming body parts on cue ("touch your wrist," "touch your heel to your knee"), forming various shapes such as letters and numbers with their bodies, and moving a body part on cue ("shake your foot").

### Crossing the Body's Midline

Many motor skills require alternate patterns of movement on the right and left sides of the body (skipping, swimming) or movements of the limbs from one side, across the body's midline, to the other side (batting). Simple activities in which children can practice crossing the midline include connecting dots placed to the child's right and left on a chalkboard. Basic skills such as skipping and striking also demand alternate patterns or crossing the midline.

### Laterality

Laterality is an awareness that the body has two distinct sides. A popular activity for practicing left-and-right side movements is "angels in the snow." Ask children to lie on their backs and move two limbs in an arc along the floor. Vary the combinations to include same-side and opposite-side pairs. Doing this in the snow or sand produces the outline of an angel. You can also challenge children to make symmetrical and nonsymmetrical shapes. Children can practice left-right discriminations in many ways. Simple rhythmic activities often require them to step or hop on a particular foot.

### Lateral Dominance

For most of us, use of one of our hands, feet, and eyes is primary and the other is secondary, or supportive. In most activity programs, teachers allow children to learn skills first with their preferred limb. Eventually they prompt children to attempt skills with the other limb. In many sports, it is desirable to master some skills with both limbs. Kicking in soccer and dribbling in basketball are two examples.

### Directionality

Directionality is an aspect of directional awareness that is often linked to laterality. It refers to the ability to project the body's spatial dimensions into surrounding space. Teachers can help children practice directionality by cueing them to place objects in relation to their bodies (i.e., "put the hoop in front of you, now over you, now to your left side"). Eventually, they can practice relationships between objects ("place the hoop behind the chair"). Cueing children to move in a particular direction gives them practice as well.

When children are still unsure of left and right, remind them of the appropriate label by identifying their right or left hand or foot. Marching and other rhythmic activities offer many opportunities to move in various directions.

## Auditory Perception

Auditory-motor activities promote the location, discrimination, and identification of sounds, sometimes amid background noise.

### Auditory Localization

The ability to listen for auditory cues and identify the source of a sound is important in everyday life as well as in motor performance. For example, when crossing a busy street, a person uses sound to help locate traffic. Many traditional games have a listening component, such as Mother, May I?, Red Light, and Simon Says. Children can practice locating a sound by playing such games as Where Is the Bell? (Gallahue, 1982): One child leaves the room while you give another child a jingle bell small enough to conceal in his hand. The group forms a circle, and everyone shakes their fists above their heads when the child returns. The child must locate the classmate with the bell.

### Auditory Discrimination and Figure-and-Ground Perception

Discrimination and auditory figure-and-ground perception involve paying attention to one specific sound amid a background of varied sounds. Children enjoy practicing sound discrimination when you challenge them to change movement directions on a sound cue. You may tap a drum softly, and the children must change the direction they are traveling every time you play a loud beat. You could also play music and periodically sound a bell as a signal. This activity also involves directionality.

## Balance

Among the elements of the kinesthetic system are the vestibular apparatus and receptors in the head and neck muscles, tendons, and joints. Sensations from these receptors and from our vision provide information important to our sense of balance, an integral part of most skill performance. Balance is specific to the environmental situation (i.e., whether you are stationary or moving, elevated or on the ground, have eyes open or closed, are supported by one, two, or more body parts, etc.) rather than general for all balance tasks. For this reason it is important for children to experience a wide range of balancing tasks. Vary the activities, including stationary and moving skills, experiences at different elevations (on the floor and on apparatus), and balancing on different body parts and with the eyes open and closed.

## REVIEW 6.4

Infants and children undergo rapid improvement in perception and in matching movements to perceptions. Animal research and human studies indicate that during this period individuals might be sensitive to the deprivation of motor activity. If so, educators should include perceptual-motor activities in early childhood education programs. Such programs should include motor activities that emphasize visual perception, kinesthetic perception, auditory perception, and the integration of these perceptual systems, as well as balance activities.

The exact nature of the relationship among perception, motor activity, and cognition, which often depends on accurate perceptions, is elusive. Developmentalists of the past hypothesized the nature of the relationship, but today the need for more research and more comprehensive theories still exists.

## SUMMARY

Early childhood is a particularly important period of intrasensory development and intersensory integration. Refinements in perceptual abilities continue until at least age 12 for vision, 8 for kinesthesis, and 10 for audition. Intersensory integration parallels intrasensory development, and subtle refinements in integration continue through adolescence. We know little about changes in perception in older adults, but the sensory receptors often undergo age-related changes.

Balance requires intersensory integration and improves throughout childhood and adolescence. In balancing, children progress from an early reliance on visual information to better use of kinesthetic information. Age-related changes in balance in older adults include slower responses to changes in stability, making older adults more susceptible than younger adults to falling on slippery surfaces.

Motor experiences appear to play an important role in perceptual-motor development in infants and young children, but no evidence exists that perceptual-motor activities can remediate delays or deficiencies in cognitive development. Perceptual-motor activities are a part of most early childhood curricula.

## Key Terms

accommodation
auditory pattern perception
body awareness
constancy scaling
contrast sensitivity
cross-modal functioning
depth perception
differential threshold
directionality

discrimination tasks
figure-and-ground perception
intersensory integration
kinesthetic system
lateral dominance
laterality
perception
perceptual-motor
perceptual size constancy
proprioceptors
retinal disparity
sensation
spatial orientation
tactile localization
tactile point perception
vestibular apparatus
visual pattern perception
whole-part perception

## Discussion Questions

1. What is the difference between sensation and perception? Give an example of an improvement in visual sensation and of an improvement in visual perception.
2. Discuss the changes in visual sensation and in visual perception that occur during childhood.
3. Discuss the changes in kinesthetic sensation and in kinesthetic perception that occur during childhood.
4. Discuss the changes in auditory sensation and in auditory perception that occur during childhood.
5. Does intersensory integration precede, parallel, or follow intrasensory development? Give examples of intersensory integration tasks.

6. Describe the changes that occur in the visual, kinesthetic, and auditory receptors in older adults.
7. On what perceptual system do young children seem to rely for balance information? How does this change during childhood?
8. What changes in various body systems might lead to a higher frequency of falls in older adults?
9. What evidence is there that infants and young children might be sensitive to the deprivation of motor experience?
10. Describe some visual-motor, kinesthetic-motor, auditory-motor, and balance activities appropriate for early childhood education programs.

## Suggested Readings

Corbin, C.B. (1980). *A textbook of motor development* (2nd ed.). Dubuque, IA: Brown.

Konczak, J. (1990). Toward an ecological theory of motor development: The relevance of the Gibsonian approach to vision for motor development research. In J.E. Clark & J.H. Humphrey (Eds.), *Advances in motor development research* (Vol. 3, pp. 201-224). New York: AMS Press.

Williams, H. (1986). The development of sensory-motor function in young children. In V. Seefeldt (Ed.), *Physical activity and well-being* (pp. 104-122). Reston, VA: American Alliance for Health, Physical Education, Recreation and Dance.

# Chapter 7

# Physical Fitness
# Through the Life Span

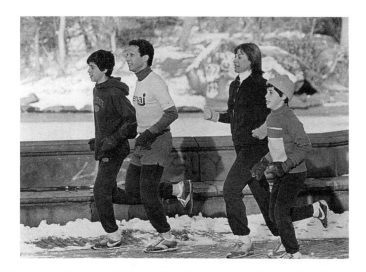

*Physical fitness* is a multifaceted quality. It is made up of several factors, or components, such as endurance and strength. A person who is fit in one component is not necessarily fit in another. For example, an individual may be very strong but not very flexible. The components of fitness that we will discuss in detail are the following:

1. Cardiorespiratory endurance
2. Strength
3. Flexibility
4. Body composition

Some writers describe additional components of fitness, such as agility and power, but the four mentioned here are the essential components. Potentially, a person can improve physical fitness through a systematic program of exercise aimed at these four components. Our discussion of the fitness components begins with endurance for vigorous activity.

## THE DEVELOPMENT OF CARDIORESPIRATORY ENDURANCE

Of all the fitness components, *cardiorespiratory endurance* has the greatest implications for lifelong health, but its development in children is surrounded by many myths. For many years, experts thought that children's cardiovascular and respiratory systems limited their capacity for extended work. Even though a misinterpretation of blood vessel size, as mentioned in chapter 2, contributed to this view and was quickly discovered, the myth persisted for decades (Karpovich, 1937, 1991). In addition, many parents and teachers feel that children automatically get enough exercise to become and remain fit, and consequently they do not believe that it is necessary to promote

vigorous exercise for children. Studies conducted in recent years (Bailey, 1976; Gilliam, Katch, Thorland, & Weltman, 1977; Simons-Morton et al., 1990) tend to counter this view by showing that the sedentary lifestyle that many of today's adults have adopted has spilled over to the lives of their children. A high percentage of children and teens already exhibit one or more of the risk factors for coronary heart disease, and children in poor physical condition are likely to maintain that status throughout their adult lives. Educators and exercise leaders must thoroughly understand cardiorespiratory endurance development and potential so that they can challenge children to attain an appropriate level of fitness for vigorous activity.

Our discussion of endurance begins with the body's basic physiological adaptations to exercise. Keep in mind that an individual's performance on endurance tests reflects a variety of factors. For example, people with good neuromuscular coordination can move more efficiently and are likely to perform longer than those less coordinated. Some tests require participants to maintain or match a cadence, and this might be difficult for young children. Cultural factors influence performance too, because a person's culture sometimes dictates whether vigorous physical activity for endurance and all-out effort is socially acceptable.

Realizing that factors such as these play a role in the measurement of endurance, we now focus on those factors that directly influence endurance. We will review the body's basic physiological responses to increased demand of vigorous activity and the changes in these responses that occur as a person grows. We will also discuss the changes that tend to occur with aging and how they affect an older adult's capacity for prolonged activity.

> **CONCEPT 7.1**
> An individual's response to the demands of endurance activities improves with physical growth and with training.

# Physiological Responses to Short-Term Exercise

Vigorous physical activity can be a short burst of intense exercise, a long period of submaximal or maximal work, or a combination of these. Our bodies meet the demands of brief, intense activity and longer, more moderate activity with different physiological responses. During a brief period (10 sec) of intense activity, the body responds by depleting local reserves of oxygen and phosphate compounds and by breaking down glycogen (energy reserves) to lactic acid, creating a deficit of oxygen that must eventually be replenished. These are anaerobic

(without oxygen) systems. The rate at which a person's body can meet this demand for short-term, intense activity is called *anaerobic power*, and the maximum oxygen deficit that a person can tolerate is called *anaerobic capacity*.

As the period of exercise demand grows longer, the anaerobic systems contribute less to the body's response. Respiration and circulation increase to bring oxygen to the muscles. Ninety seconds into an exercise bout, anaerobic and aerobic (with oxygen) energy systems contribute about equally. After 3 min, aerobic processes meet the demands of exercise. First let's examine anaerobic performance.

## Assessing Anaerobic Performance

You can measure anaerobic performance with short-duration tasks. The Quebec 10-sec and the Wingate 30-sec all-out rides on a bicycle ergometer and the Margaria step-running test are common laboratory tests that provide scores in total work output, mean power, or peak power. Total work output indicates how much work an individual can do in the 10- or 30-second time period. In contrast, *power* indicates the rate at which individuals can produce energy—that is, the work they can do within a specific time. Mean power is the average power individuals achieve during the 10- or 30-sec period, whereas peak power is the highest rate they achieve. The 50-yd dash and sprinting a flight of stairs are common field tests. Participants must be willing and able to give an all-out effort. At any age, anaerobic performance is related to

- body size, particularly fat-free muscle mass and muscle size;
- the ability to resist acidosis as lactic acid accumulates in the muscles;
- the rate of phosphate compound resynthesis; and
- quick mobilization of oxygen delivery systems.

Some of these factors change as a person grows (Malina & Bouchard, 1991).

## Developmental Changes in Anaerobic Performance

Young children have smaller absolute quantities of energy reserves than adults because they have less muscle mass (Eriksson, 1978; Shephard, 1982). Therefore, children attain less absolute anaerobic power output. As children grow, their muscle mass increases, as does the phosphate concentrations and glycogen content in their muscle tissue, and they develop a higher tolerance of lactic acid concentrations. So anaerobic power improves steadily as a person ages (Inbar & Bar-Or, 1986). Total work output scores improve over the entire adolescent period for boys, but only until puberty in girls, perhaps reflecting the patterns of muscle growth in the sexes (see Figure 7.1a and b). Accounting for differences in muscle mass, though, apparently does not eliminate entirely the differences in anaerobic performance that favor boys (Van Praagh, Fellmann, Bedu, Falgairette, & Coudert, 1990). Not all of the difference between children and adults is attributable to body size, either. When we divide anaerobic performance scores by body weight, scores still improve with age. Undoubtedly, better coordination and skill contribute to improved performance as children grow older.

## Anaerobic Training

Preadolescent and adolescent boys can improve their anaerobic capacity through training on anaerobic activities (Grodjinovsky, Inbar, Dotan, & Bar-Or, 1980; Rotstein, Dotan, Bar-Or, & Tenenbaum, 1986). When young adolescent boys receive this conditioning, their muscle concentrations of phosphates and glycogen increase and their rate of glycogen use improves, therefore improving anaerobic capacity (Eriksson, 1972). Little research has examined girls.

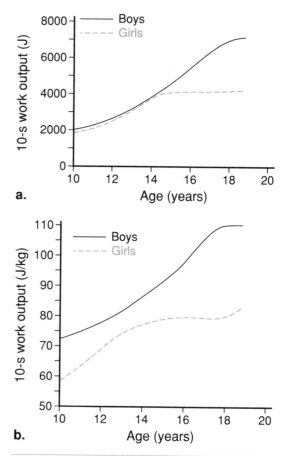

**Figure 7.1**　Anaerobic performance. Figure (a) shows the change in total work output (measured in Joules) on a 10-sec, all-out bicycle ergometer ride with advancing age. C. Bouchard and J.A. Simoneau (unpublished data) measured a cross-sectional group of French Canadian youth on this task. When anaerobic performance scores are divided by body weight, as in Figure (b), scores still improve with age.
(Reprinted by permission from Malina & Bouchard, 1991.)

## Anaerobic Performance in Older Adults

Once individuals attain adult body size, their anaerobic performance remains stable throughout young adulthood (Inbar & Bar-Or, 1986). Any improvement in anaerobic power and capacity is achieved through training alone. It is not clear, however, whether anaerobic power and capacity necessarily decline as adults grow older. View with caution indications that anaerobic power and capacity are significantly lower in 65-year-olds than in 25-year-olds, because such results could reflect in part the older adults' reluctance or inability to undergo an all-out effort in anaerobic tests such as sprinting up a flight of stairs (Shephard, 1978b). Yet any loss of muscle mass in older adults is likely to affect their anaerobic performance, and a lack of training in anaerobic tasks to maintain conditioning logically would affect their performance.

## Physiological Responses to Prolonged Exercise

How do our bodies sustain submaximal physical activity for prolonged periods? Unlike with short-term exercise, the energy for prolonged exercise is derived from the oxidative breakdown of food stores in addition to the local reserves depleted in the first few minutes of exercise. The rate at which we meet this long-term oxygen demand is termed *aerobic power*, whereas the total energy available is termed *aerobic capacity*.

Sustained, prolonged activity depends on the transportation of sufficient oxygen to the working muscles for longer periods. Heart and respiratory rates, cardiac output, and oxygen uptake increase to deliver the oxygen needed for prolonged activity. Increased respiratory rate brings more oxygen to the lungs, making it available for diffusion into the bloodstream. Cardiac output (the amount of blood pumped into the circulatory system) increases to allow more oxygen to reach the muscles. The body achieves this increased cardiac output through increased heart rate or increased stroke volume. Changes in stroke volume during exercise are relatively small, but one of the benefits of training is greater initial stroke volume.

The limiting factor to continued vigorous activity is the heart's ability to pump enough blood

to meet the working muscles' oxygen needs. When individuals engage in very heavy activity, their heart rate rises throughout the session until exhaustion ends the activity. When they stop vigorous activity, their heart rate drops quickly for 2 to 3 min, then more gradually for a time related to the duration and intensity of the activity.

This description is necessarily a brief summary of the physiological responses to exercise. You can find a more detailed treatment in exercise physiology textbooks.

### Assessing Aerobic Performance

You can use several methods to assess a person's physiological responses to sustained activity. A common measure of fitness for endurance activities is *maximum oxygen consumption* or peak oxygen uptake, the maximum volume of oxygen that the body can consume per minute (Heyward, 1991; Zwiren, 1989). The more efficiently a person's body uses oxygen (that is, consumes less oxygen for the same amount of work performed), the more fit the individual.

In a test assessing maximum oxygen consumption, you can measure or estimate the actual amount of oxygen consumed during activity. This score is also expressed as oxygen consumed per minute per kilogram of body weight. Maximum oxygen consumption is a common measure of endurance in studies of children and older adults because you can estimate it from an exercise period of limited length and intensity (a submaximal test), thus avoiding the need for an exercise bout to exhaustion (a maximal test). Also, direct measures of oxygen use require more sophisticated and expensive equipment than that needed for estimates from submaximal tests. Cycling on an ergometer or walking or running on a treadmill is usually the type of graded exercise used in both submaximal and maximal tests.

Measurements of aerobic power and capacity tend to be specific to the task performed (cycling, running, etc.), so use caution in comparing scores on different tasks. Young children have difficulty keeping a cadence during bicycle ergometer tests. They are also more likely than adults to make unnecessary movements during testing.

Another measure of physiological response to prolonged exercise is that of maximal *working capacity*, which means the highest work or exercise load that a person can tolerate before reaching exhaustion (Adams, 1973). Because this test requires maximal effort, it may be difficult to motivate individuals to work to exhaustion, and, though unlikely, the possibility of heart attack exists during such a test. For this reason you may not want to ask children or older adults to exercise to exhaustion. Estimating working capacity from submaximal working capacity tests remains the preferred procedure for assessing these groups.

Other measures of endurance fitness are less common. For example, you can measure maximal cardiac output directly, but this test is difficult to administer because it requires intubation (inserting a tube into the body). Measuring an individual's electrocardiograph changes during exercise is of interest when studying adults (Heyward, 1991), but it does not apply very well to most children because its main purpose is to identify impaired heart function.

---

The most appropriate measures of endurance fitness in children and older adults for research purposes remain maximum oxygen consumption for changes in aerobic power and adaptations to submaximal exercise efforts for changes in aerobic capacity.

---

Several research investigators attempted to identify field tests for children that estimate endurance nearly as reliably as when measured in a laboratory. Such field tests allow educators to measure aerobic performance without laboratory equipment. They compared maximum oxygen consumption scores from laboratory tests with performance in 800 m, 1,200 m, and 1,600 m runs for 83 children in grades 1, 2, and 3. Performance on the 1,600 m run was a better predictor of maximum oxygen consumption for both boys and girls than performance on the 800 m or 1,200 m runs. An average velocity score on the 1,600 m run had a slightly higher correlation with maximum oxygen consumption than a total time score. We can conclude that a 1,600 m run is a better field test of endurance in children than shorter runs. This test proved to have a high test-retest reliability (Krahenbuhl, Pangrazi, Petersen, Burkett, & Schneider, 1978), but researchers still need to determine the validity of such running tests (Safrit, 1990).

## Developmental Changes in Aerobic Performance

How do children respond physiologically to prolonged activity? Children tend to have *hypokinetic circulation* (Bar-Or, Shephard, & Allen, 1971); that is, their cardiac output is less than an adult's. You'll recall that cardiac output is the product of stroke volume and heart rate. Children have a smaller stroke volume than adults, reflecting their smaller hearts. Children compensate in part with higher heart rates than adults at a given level of exercise, but their cardiac output is still somewhat lower than an adult's. Children also have lower blood hemoglobin concentrations than do adults. Hemoglobin concentration is related to the blood's ability to carry oxygen.

You might assume that these two factors, the hypokinetic circulation and low hemoglobin concentration, result in an oxygen transport system that is less efficient in children than in adults. However, children's ability to extract relatively more of the oxygen circulating to the active muscles compared to adults (Malina & Bouchard, 1991; Shephard, 1982) seems to compensate for these factors. The result is a comparatively effective oxygen transport system. Children also mobilize their aerobic systems faster than adults (Bar-Or, 1983, p. 15).

Children do have a lower tolerance for extended periods of exercise than adults, ostensibly the result of smaller glycogen stores. When their glycogen stores are exhausted, performance is limited. As children grow, their hypokinetic circulation is gradually reduced as the following changes occur:

- Heart size increases.
- Hemoglobin concentration increases.
- Oxygen-extraction ability decreases to adult levels.

Both longitudinal and cross-sectional studies demonstrate that absolute maximum oxygen consumption increases linearly in children from age 4 until late adolescence in boys and until age 12 or 13 in girls (Mirwald & Bailey, 1986; Shuleva, Hunter, Hester, & Dunaway, 1990). Figure 7.2 pictures this trend between ages 6 and about 16 years. Boys and girls are similar in maximum oxygen consumption until about age 12, although boys have a slightly higher average. The strong relationship between absolute maximum oxygen consumption and lean body mass explains most of the improvement and the gender-related difference. In fact, the picture is quite different if we express maximum oxygen consumption in relative rather than absolute terms, dividing it by body weight, lean body weight, or another body dimension. As Figure 7.2a and b show, maximum oxygen consumption relative to body weight stays about the same through childhood and adolescence in boys. It declines in girls, probably because adipose tissue is increasing. When maximum oxygen consumption is related to fat-free mass, scores show a slight decline during and after puberty, and gender differences remain.

So body weight appears to grow slightly faster than maximum oxygen consumption increases around puberty (Malina & Bouchard, 1991). Maximum oxygen consumption might depend somewhat on maturity, in addition to

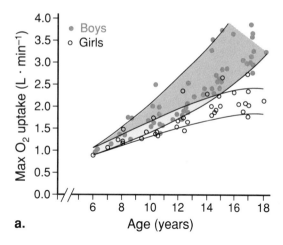

a.

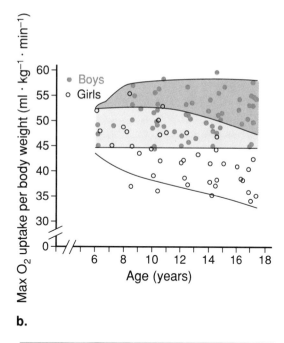

b.

**Figure 7.2** The relationship between maximum oxygen consumption and age. In Figure (a), absolute scores are plotted. In Figure (b), maximum oxygen consumption values relative to kilogram of body weight are plotted. The boys' scores are centered in the shaded area; the girls' scores in the white area.

(Reprinted by permission from Bar-Or, 1983.)

body size, because comparisons of maximum oxygen consumption to age show a relationship in adolescents who vary in age but are identical in size (Sprynarova & Reisenauer, 1978). Two adolescents identical in size could differ in maximum oxygen consumption if one is more physiologically mature than the other.

Even though maximum oxygen consumption is the best single measurement of endurance, it might not predict running performance in children as well as it does in adults. Running test performance relates more to anaerobic measures in children than in adults. In addition, children's ventilatory mechanisms, lower aerobic reserves, and mechanical inefficiencies affect their endurance fitness. Use caution in inferring maximum oxygen consumption level from children's running performance.

It is important that you recognize the relationship between children's increasing body size and their improving ability to sustain exercise during growth. With body growth come increases in heart and stroke volume, total hemoglobin, and lean body mass. These factors foster improved cardiac output and, subsequently, exercise capacity and absolute maximum oxygen consumption. Recalling how children vary in size despite their chronological age, you can see that evaluations of exercise capacity among children should relate to body size rather than age alone. In the past, educators frequently based evaluation only on age.

---

Although we expect average exercise capacity and average body size of groups of children and adolescents to increase with age, exercise capacity follows maturation rate and warrants individual consideration.

---

In children, body size also is a far better predictor of endurance than the child's sex. After puberty, though, boys on the average attain a considerable edge over girls in absolute maximum oxygen consumption and have the potential to retain this edge throughout life. Several factors contribute to this gender difference. One is body composition. The average man gains more lean body mass and less adipose tissue during adolescence than the average woman. Interestingly, women are similar to men in maximum oxygen consumption per kilogram of fat-free body mass, but when adipose tissue is included, women have a lower maximum oxygen consumption. Another factor in gender differences in oxygen consumption is women's tendency to have lower hemoglobin concentrations than men (Åstrand, 1976).

By the time he reaches late adolescence, then, the average male has an edge over the average female in both oxygen consumption and working capacity (see Table 7.1). Keep in mind that environmental factors, especially training, influence the endurance capacities of individual men and women throughout their lives. So it would not be surprising to find that an active woman has a higher maximum oxygen consumption than a sedentary man.

## Aerobic Performance in Older Adults

We reach our peak maximum oxygen consumption in young adulthood. How well does a person maintain this fitness component into middle and older adulthood? Some information on this topic is available, but it remains difficult to separate the inevitable consequences of aging from those brought about by lower levels of activity. Accordingly, information based on group averages or general tendencies reflects that middle-aged and older adults lead increasingly more sedentary lifestyles. Such information does not reflect the performance of those who remain active. Keeping this in mind, we now review the structural and functional changes in the cardiovascular and respiratory systems as people age.

### Structural Cardiorespiratory Changes

The major structural changes a nondiseased heart undergoes as an adult ages include a pro-

**Table 7.1    The Physical Working Capacity at Heart Rate of 170 of Canadian Schoolchildren**

| | Boys | | Girls | |
| --- | --- | --- | --- | --- |
| Age (year) | Absolute value (watts) | Relative value (watts · kg$^{-1}$) | Absolute value (watts) | Relative value (watts · kg$^{-1}$) |
| 7 | 50 | 1.96 | 39 | 1.57 |
| 8 | 57 | 2.08 | 47 | 1.74 |
| 9 | 63 | 2.08 | 50 | 1.68 |
| 10 | 70 | 2.09 | 55 | 1.66 |
| 11 | 81 | 2.16 | 59 | 1.65 |
| 12 | 90 | 2.18 | 68 | 1.62 |
| 13 | 107 | 2.28 | 74 | 1.50 |
| 14 | 119 | 2.26 | 71 | 1.39 |
| 15 | 121 | 2.10 | 73 | 1.35 |
| 16 | 139 | 2.20 | 75 | 1.39 |
| 17 | 143 | 2.18 | 78 | 1.39 |

*Note.* Based on data of Howell & MacNab (1966). Measurements made in school classrooms, without habituation of subjects. Readings would probably be up to 10% higher, given climatic control (20° to 22° C) and some familiarization with experimental procedures. Measurements are in watts (1 watt = 6 kg m/min) and watts per kilogram of body weight. Reprinted by permission from Shephard, 1982.

gressive loss of cardiac muscle, loss of elasticity in cardiac muscle fibers (Harrison, Dixon, Russell, Bidwai, & Coleman, 1964), and fibrotic changes in the valves (Pomerance, 1965). The major blood vessels also lose elasticity. It remains unclear whether these changes are unavoidable in aging or reflect a chronic lack of oxygen. The consequences of these structural changes in the heart and blood vessels are numerous.

## Functional Cardiorespiratory Changes

Whereas resting heart rate values of older adults are comparable to those of young adults, the maximum achievable heart rate with physical exertion gradually declines with aging. The decline is not as great as experts once thought. A 65-year-old man can attain a maximum rate of 170 beats a minute, for example, compared with 200+ beats a minute for children and young adults (Shephard, 1978a, 1981). Decreased maximum heart rate may be the major factor in reduced maximum oxygen consumption with aging (Hagburg et al., 1985). A lower responsiveness to sympathetic stimulation of the heart muscle could cause this decrease (Stamford, 1988).

The stroke volume of older adults may or may not decline with aging; research studies have yielded both results (see Stamford, 1988 for a review). Asymptomatic *ischemic heart disease* (affecting blood supply to the heart) may account for the equivocal results. Investigators using rigorous screening for heart disease may find no decrease in stroke volume, whereas researchers whose studies include participants with undetected disease may find a decrease. If coronary disease is associated with decreased stroke volume, then older adults with disease will logically have a decreased cardiac output during exercise resulting from both their decreased maximum heart rate and their decreased stroke volume.

Active older adults maintain heart volumes well (Davies, 1972). In a few cases very active older adults maintain excellent physiological functioning. For example, Clarence DeMar ran 12 miles a day throughout his life and competed in marathons at age 65. The autopsy performed after his death from cancer at age 70 showed well-developed cardiac muscle, normal valves, and coronary arteries two to three times the size normally seen (Brandfonbrener, Landowne, & Shock, 1955).

Older adults reach their peak cardiac output at a lower intensity of work than do younger adults (Brandfonbrener et al., 1955; Shephard, 1978a). Their more rigid arteries resist the volume of blood the heart pumps into them. This resistance is even greater if the adult has *atherosclerosis*, the buildup of plaque on the artery walls. In turn, this resistance raises resting pulse pressure (the difference between systolic and diastolic blood pressure) and systolic blood pressure. Whether blood pressure increases or decreases during exercise also depends on the health of the cardiac muscle fibers and their ability to tolerate an increased work load. During vigorous activity, older adults typically exhibit higher blood pressure than younger adults (Julius, Amery, Whitlock, & Conway, 1967; Sheffield & Roitman, 1973), but some postcoronary patients cannot sustain systolic blood pressure as their work load increases (Shephard, 1979).

Pulmonary function may also limit older adults' physiological responses to vigorous exercise. One of the important pulmonary function measurements is *vital capacity*, the maximum volume of air the lungs can expel following maximal inspiration. A large vital capacity reflects a large inspiratory capacity of the lungs and results in better alveolar ventilation. Because the greatest part of oxygen diffusion to the capillaries takes place at the alveoli (see Figure 7.3), better alveolar ventilation contributes to increased amounts of oxygen circulating in the blood and reaching the working muscles.

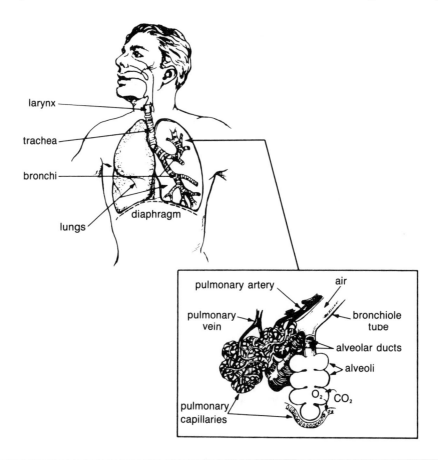

**Figure 7.3** The respiratory system. Oxygen diffusion to the capillaries takes place at the alveoli, enlarged on the right.
(Reprinted by permission from Sharkey, 1984.)

A person's vital capacity tends to increase with training. A sufficient number of capillaries in the lungs optimizes oxygen diffusion as well. Therefore, a decreased vital capacity or decreased number of lung capillaries detracts from vigorous physical performance. A decreased vital capacity with aging is well established (Norris, Shock, Landowne, & Falzone, 1956; Shephard, 1978b), as is a reduced number of capillaries in the lungs (Reid, 1967).

The decrease in vital capacity with aging probably relates to a loss of elasticity in tissues of the lungs and chest wall (Turner, Mead, & Wohl, 1968). These pulmonary changes, though, are more dramatic in smokers than in nonsmokers.

The end result of these cardiac and pulmonary changes is that maximum exercise capacity and maximum oxygen consumption (whether absolute or relative to body weight) decline as an adult ages, and the recovery period following vigorous activity lengthens. The results of both longitudinal (filled circles) and cross-sectional (open circles) studies are plotted in Figure 7.4. A decline with advancing age is evident. Adipose tissue gain, muscle tissue loss, and inactivity all influence this decline. In addition, a lifetime of negative environmental factors such as smoking or poor nutrition can contribute to or accelerate the changes. In contrast, a lifetime of exposure to positive environmental factors such as healthful exercise can better maintain endurance levels.

Evidence exists (Dehn & Bruce, 1972; Drinkwater, Horvath, & Wells, 1975; Kasch & Wallace, 1976; Shephard, 1978b; Smith & Serfass, 1981) that these changes are not as dramatic in older adults who remain active as in those who become sedentary. Figure 7.4b pictures a steeper incline in maximum oxygen consumption in inactive (dotted line) than in active (solid line) adults with advancing age.

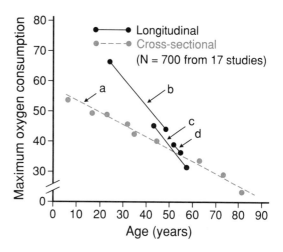

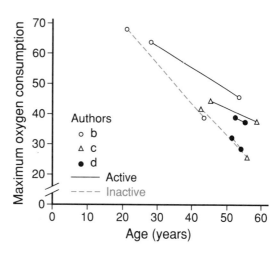

Figure 7.4 Maximum oxygen consumption declines as a person ages. As seen in Graph A, both cross-sectional studies (open circles) and longitudinal studies (solid circles) show declines in adulthood. Graph B shows that the decline is not as rapid in active adults. The dotted lines represent the change in inactive adults and the solid lines the change in active adults.
(Reprinted by permission from Stamford, 1988; redrawn from Dehn & Bruce, 1972; data plotted are from: (a) Dehn & Bruce, 1972, (b) Dill et al., 1967, (c) Hollmann, 1965, all cited in Dehn & Bruce, and (d) Dehn & Bruce.)

Vigorous training can even keep maximum oxygen consumption steady for a time in older adults (Kasch & Wallace, 1976). People who would like to maintain as much endurance as possible throughout their lives should stop smoking, eat properly, and follow an appropriate exercise program designed for endurance.

## Endurance Training

You may already know that adults who engage in vigorous activity 20 min or longer at least three times a week can improve their cardiorespiratory endurance. Such training results in a decrease in heart rate for a given submaximal exercise intensity (as the body becomes more efficient in transporting oxygen) and increases in heart volume, stroke volume, blood volume, and total hemoglobin. The result is greater working or exercise capacity (Adams, 1973).

### Training Effect in Children

Can children experience the same training effect as adults? Educators are interested in whether children can improve their endurance with proper training. Before discussing research results we should consider several factors.

The result of aerobic training is typically an improvement in whatever measure of aerobic power is used, most often maximum oxygen consumption. Recall that maximum oxygen consumption improves as a child grows, related to the increase in muscle mass. Therefore, the change associated with training occurs in the same direction as that associated with growth. Researchers must be able to separate the increase associated with growth from any increase resulting from training.

In chapter 2 we saw that children mature at different rates. Researchers also must assess maturation level when testing participants between 9 and 16 years old. Comparing a group that contains many early maturers with a group

that contains many late maturers certainly can bias an investigation of training effects. In fact, one research group noted that when they sought to compare "inactive" and "active" groups of children, late maturers more often fell into the inactive category (Mirwald, Bailey, Cameron, & Rasmussen, 1981).

---

At the very least, training studies of children should use a control group to document changes with growth and assess maturation.

---

Studies of prepubescent children fail to provide strong evidence of an aerobic training effect. Of seven studies comparing a training group to a control group (see Figure 7.5), three found a significant increase in maximum oxygen consumption by the training group over the control group, and four found no significant difference after training. In a few longitudinal studies, training did not result in differences between active and inactive groups until the children reached peak height velocity (Kobayashi et al., 1978; Mirwald et al., 1981; Rutenfranz, 1986). In other words, activity was not associated with a higher maximum oxygen consumption in preadolescents (beyond the increase due to growth), but it was in adolescents.

Several factors might contribute to these equivocal findings. The length and intensity of training varied across studies. If children are active on a daily basis, possibly only intense, long-term training will yield a difference between a training group and a control group. The cross-sectional studies might have compared groups with unequal proportions of early and late maturers. Finally, it is possible that maximum oxygen consumption is not a good measurement of aerobic fitness in prepubescent children (Rowland, 1989a). Some researchers suggest that other measurements, specifically anaerobic threshold (when lactic acid production in the blood exceeds its elimi-

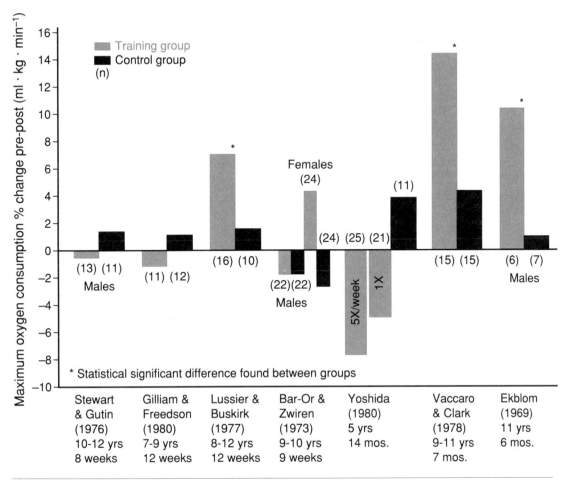

**Figure 7.5**    Change in maximum oxygen consumption with training of prepubescent children. The three bars marked with an asterisk (*) indicate studies finding a significant improvement over the control group. The other four studies found no differences after training.
(Graph data from Sady, 1986; reprinted by permission from Zwiren, 1989.)

nation) and ventilatory anaerobic threshold (when ventilation increases dramatically), are better indicators of cardiorespiratory endurance in children, but more research is needed on this topic (Washington, 1989). Even so, it appears that prepubescent children do not respond to aerobic training in the same way that pubescent children, adolescents, and adults do. Almost no information is available on whether the adult formulas used for target heart rate

zones in training and adult frequency guidelines apply to children (Rowland, 1989b).

In contrast, adolescents after puberty respond to aerobic training much like adults. Heart size and volume, total blood volume, total hemoglobin, stroke volume, and maximal cardiac output all increase in adolescents who receive training (Ekblom, 1969; Eriksson & Koch, 1973; Koch & Rocker, 1977; Lengyel & Gyarfas, 1979), whereas submaximal heart rate for a given level of exercise decreases (Brown, Harrower, & Deeter, 1972). Kobayashi et al. (1978) found a 15.8% increase in aerobic power with training between ages 14 and 17.

### Training Programs for Children

We cannot discuss training methods in detail in this text, but you should keep some concerns regarding training children in mind. To improve endurance, training programs must be sufficiently long and intense, but if they are too demanding, they may harm young children. What is a safe level of training duration and intensity for children?

One of the principles trainers follow is that of *progressively overloading* the body, meaning that the intensity or duration of each exercise bout gradually increases over several weeks or months. This is a valuable principle in programming for children. Teachers should begin by asking their students to exercise at a level that is comfortable for them. With this level as a baseline, they can design an individualized program that gradually increases the exercise challenge for each child.

---

A constant threat to a well-planned training program is the pressure that adults can place on children. Children might try to exercise at an intensity above what is reasonable for them, just to please a parent, win a valuable prize, or gain prestige among classmates. Educators must minimize such pressures, enabling children to stop their activity if they become overly fatigued.

---

Children need special supervision when exercising in hot and humid conditions. In moderate conditions, children's bodies adequately regulate their temperature. In extreme heat, above 45° C, children's bodies cannot dissipate heat as well as adults' bodies do and they dehydrate rapidly. A variety of factors contribute

to this difference. Compared to adults, children have

- a larger surface area for their body mass,
- a limited sweating capacity,
- lower blood volume, and
- lower cardiac output than adults (see Bar-Or, 1989b for a review).

A few investigators found that boys are able to acclimate to exercising in the heat, but the process takes longer for prepubescent boys than for older boys (Inbar, 1978; Wagner, Robinson, Tzankoff, & Marino, 1972). No information is available on girls.

---

Children typically feel dizzy, faint, or nauseated when suffering heat stress, so educators should be alert for children reporting these symptoms.

---

### Training Programs for Older Adults

Appropriate training can improve endurance in children and young adults, but can older adults achieve the same effect in light of the structural and functional changes they undergo? The answer is yes, older adults can significantly increase their maximum oxygen consumption with a good training program (Shephard, 1978b), even if they have undertaken little training earlier in their lives (Stamford, 1973). The mechanisms for this improvement are unclear and need further research (Ehsani, 1987). The guiding principle in designing training programs for older adults as well as for children is the gradual increase in exercise intensity and duration. Low training intensity can be very effective for older adults early in their exercise program. A more extensive discussion of these improvements and training regimens for older adults is available in Shephard (1978b).

### Long-Term Training Effects

Despite the body's favorable response to training at any age, the question arises as to whether active youths have an advantage over their sedentary counterparts in maintaining endurance into older adulthood. Ideally, researchers would assess this aspect of fitness through long-term longitudinal studies; however, the difficulties involved in obtaining longitudinal data (expense and subject attrition) make such research nearly nonexistent.

In the absence of such research, consider a cross-sectional study conducted by Saltin and Grimby (1968) that measured the maximal oxygen consumption of three groups of men between ages 50 and 59. The men in the first group had been nonathletes in their youth; those in the second group were former athletes but were now sedentary; and the men in the third group had been athletes and still maintained active lifestyles as older adults. The investigators had to rely on self-reports (rather than laboratory data) to determine the men's activity levels in youth. Even so, measures of maximum oxygen consumption yielded average values of 30, 38, and 53 ml/min/kg body weight for the nonathletes, sedentary former athletes, and active adults, respectively.

Despite the limitations of this single study, the evidence suggests that regular activity in childhood has positive lifelong benefits. Nevertheless, the most important factor in endurance is the individual's current activity level. At all ages, the capacity for prolonged, vigorous work tends to be transitory. A person maintains (or improves) endurance if he is currently training for endurance; conversely, endurance capacity decreases when individuals discontinue their training programs.

## Effects of Disease on Working Capacity

Teachers and coaches must keep in mind that some diseases reduce an individual's working capacity. A detailed discussion of diseases and working capacity is beyond the scope of this text, but a brief overview can sensitize those new to the field to the potential effects of diseases.

Diseases that could reduce working capacity fall into the categories of cardiovascular, pulmonary, infectious, and neuromuscular. The cardiovascular diseases that reduce children's working capacity, usually by reducing cardiac output (Bar-Or, 1988), include cyanotic congenital heart disease (affecting oxygenation of the blood) and valvular disease (affecting the valves in the heart). However, most children with congenital heart disease who survive infancy can eventually perform exercise at near-normal levels.

Whether a child with a cardiovascular disease must refrain from physical activity depends upon the particular disease involved (Shephard, 1982). For children and adults, exercise is often an important part of therapy programs, even following surgery. Controlled exercise can strengthen the cardiovascular system, whereas continued inactivity weakens it. Educators and parents should not be overly protective but should carefully implement any program a child's physician has prescribed.

A number of cardiovascular diseases may also affect exercise performance in older adults. Among them are the following:

- *Arteriosclerosis* (hardening of the arteries)
- Atherosclerosis (formation of lipid deposits in the arteries)
- Ischemic heart disease (affecting the oxygen supply to the heart tissues as a result of reduced blood supply)
- Peripheral vascular disease (affecting circulation)

People who suffer from such diseases must be carefully monitored during physical activity. Although inactivity probably contributed to the onset of these diseases, engaging in overly stressful activity after the disease is established could lead to cardiac failure.

Rehabilitation programs often use exercise following a heart attack. The major benefits of exercise are increased cardiac output, decreased blood pressure, and decreased blood lipids. To be effective, rehabilitative exercise programs must be vigorous enough to create improvement without placing the participant at risk. Those who design and lead rehabilitative programs should follow some important guidelines. These include establishing a safe entry level into the program, gradually increasing intensity, monitoring each participant individually, and working closely with a physician or exercise physiologist.

Two pulmonary diseases that reduce children's working capacity are severe asthma (breathing difficulty due to temporary bronchial constriction) and cystic fibrosis (an exocrine gland disorder resulting in pancreatic insufficiency, chronic pulmonary disease, and excessive loss of salt). Asthmatic children can vary in the amount of their functional impairment. Some children show little effect, especially during periods of remission. Others must rely on a closely supervised drug therapy program. Sometimes even light exercise can induce an asthma attack (Shephard, 1982). Yet many asthmatics who participate in training programs demonstrate improved lung function, improved working capacity, reduced amounts of adipose tissue (Walker, 1965), and a reduced incidence of exercise-induced asthma (see Lemanske & Henke, 1989, for a review). Because exercise is not harmful to asthmatics, educators should encourage children, with their physician's approval, to participate in physical activity as a necessary means to maintain cardiorespiratory fitness. Educators should be alert to the symptoms of wheezing, coughing, and shortness of breath and be prepared to follow therapy programs the child's physician recommends.

Cystic fibrosis affects children's response to exercise as well as their normal growth and development through a secondary lack of nutrients (Shephard, 1982). Yet most cystic fibrosis patients are capable of some exercise, and in some patients regular exercise might benefit the respiratory muscles (see Cerny & Armitage, 1989, for a review).

Among the respiratory diseases that affect older adults are chronic bronchitis and emphysema. Chronic bronchitis is characterized by a recurrent cough, lasting at least 3 months in two successive years. Emphysema involves abnormal enlargement of the terminal air spaces in the lungs. In both of these *obstructive lung diseases*, much of the oxygen the affected person breathes in during exercise is used by the respiratory muscles themselves. As a result, an unusually high proportion of muscular effort elsewhere in the body is carried out anaerobically.

Infectious diseases, such as influenza, infectious mononucleosis, and chicken pox, generally reduce an individual's working capacity (Adams, 1973) but to varying degrees. It is important for a teacher or coach to keep this in mind when monitoring performance. Athletes who want to maintain their peak efficiency may expect to adhere to training schedules and performance levels even when they are ill, but this is an impractical goal.

Some neuromuscular diseases do not affect a person's physiological responses to exercise directly, but they contribute to inefficient and uncoordinated performance. Inefficient movement can reduce working capacity because the body expends energy on unnecessary movements. Muscular dystrophy is an example of a condition that has both a direct and an indirect effect on exercise performance. It affects cardiac function directly while it reduces muscle strength; thus it increases the metabolic "cost" of activity compared to individuals without the disease (Eston et al., 1989).

---

Clearly, diseases affect a person's exercise performance in varying ways. This makes cooperation and communication imperative among teachers and coaches, medical personnel, parents (when children are involved), and the participant. Activity may be beneficial in many cases, but it must never place the participant at increased risk. Those involved in the participant's exercise program, then, must plan the limits of activity carefully, set expectations accordingly, and monitor the participant closely.

---

## REVIEW 7.1

Endurance for vigorous activities improves as the body grows. In addition, an individual can increase endurance after puberty by training, although the effects are transitory. A person must maintain training to preserve higher levels of endurance. After the adolescent growth spurt, gender differences in working capacity are apparent. Although the cause of these differences is still open to discussion, body size, body composition, and hemoglobin levels are at least partially responsible. Due to societal norms and expectations, some individuals, especially women and older adults, feel that all-out physical endurance efforts are inappropriate. These attitudes are changing, but complete acceptance will take many years; adults of today are products of their upbringing, and they in turn tend to raise their children in the manner in which they were raised.

Some cardiovascular, pulmonary, infectious, and neuromuscular diseases reduce endurance at any age, so educators must work closely with the affected individual, parents (if appropriate), and medical personnel to plan appropriate endurance activities.

## THE DEVELOPMENT OF STRENGTH

As we review how muscle strength improves with training, recall our earlier discussion of muscle growth in concept 2.3. We know that muscle mass follows a sigmoid growth pattern and that this growth is largely due to an increase in muscle fiber diameter. But what about gains in muscle strength, or the ability to exert force? Strength tends to improve as muscle mass increases. Consider a pair of twins, a boy and a girl, age 10. Do their strength gains simply follow their gains in muscle mass, or can they improve strength beyond that which accompanies muscle growth?

First, consider that the amount of isometric force a muscle group exerts depends on the fibers activated and on leverage. Further, the fibers activated depend on both the cross-sectional area of the muscle and the degree of coordination in activating the fibers—that is, the nervous system's pattern and timing in innervating the various motor units to bring about the desired movement. The cross-sectional area of muscle increases with growth so that strength increases as muscles grow. But does coordination of contractile effort improve at the same pace as muscle mass increases?

We must answer this question before we can describe the development of muscle strength in the twins. We know from our earlier discussion that gender differences exist in the growth of muscle mass. What implications do these differences have for the twins' strength development? Could they be given an appropriate training program to increase their strength beyond what they would typically acquire with growth? If so, how might such training influence the maintenance or improvement of their strength when they are adults?

## Assessing Strength

In strength assessments, individuals typically exert maximum force against resistance. They might actually move their limbs, as in an isotonic (constant resistance) or isokinetic (constant speed of movement) test, or they might exert force against an immovable resistance, as in an isometric test. Researchers report the muscle group, such as knee flexors or elbow extensors, used in the assessment; for isometric tests, they also report the angle of the joint in degrees as force is exerted. The latter is necessary because a muscle group can exert different levels of force at different joint angles. When individuals are asked to move their limbs, researchers report the speed of movement, usually in degrees per second.

A device commonly used in strength testing is a spring-loaded dynamometer; individuals are usually asked to compress a handle on the dynamometer as exertion is registered. When an individual is given an isometric test, a tensiometer, placed on a cable between the immovable resistance and the handle (or bar) against which the individual pulls, registers the force of exertion. Both dynamometers and tensiometers usually measure in Newtons, a measurement unit for force.

## Developmental Changes in Strength

Strength increases as children and adolescents grow older (see Table 7.2). To find out if strength development exactly parallels muscle mass development, consider the age at which individuals reach peak gains in muscle mass and strength. In chapter 2 we noted that peak gain (the peak in the velocity curve) indicates the point of the fastest increase. If strength development directly follows muscle mass development, the peak gain in strength would coincide with the peak gain in muscle mass. Teachers and coaches then could predict children's strength levels by measuring their muscle mass, which in turn they could estimate from weight measurements or by subtracting a child's estimated fat weight from body weight.

But several studies indicate that these peak gains do not coincide with each other. For example, Stolz and Stolz (1951) found that boys on the average reach their peak gain in strength approximately 6 to 9 months after their peak weight velocity and 1.6 years after their peak height velocity. Carron and Bailey (1974) generally confirmed this trend, finding that maximum gains in overall, upper body, and lower body strength occurred about 1 year after peak height and peak weight velocity in boys. Only one study examined strength development in girls with this method. Jones (1947) concluded that girls reach their peak growth rate at 12.5 years on average, but they reach their near-adult levels of strength in a thrusting movement (pushing a dynamometer held in front of the chest with two hands) at 13.5 to 14.0 years. These limited data on girls are consistent with the findings for boys.

Keep in mind that peak weight velocity is not necessarily equivalent to peak growth in muscle mass, because increasing body weight could reflect an increase in fat weight as well as muscle weight. Tanner (1962), however, indicates that if peak weight and peak muscle mass velocity do not coincide, peak muscle mass velocity occurs *before* peak weight velocity. This widens the gap between peak muscle mass velocity and peak strength gain and lends support to the theory that muscles grow first in size and then in strength. Tanner (1962) suggests that this sequence probably results from the effects of adrenocortical and testicular hormones on the protein structure and enzyme systems of the muscle fibers.

Another way to examine muscle growth and strength development is to relate measures of muscle strength to various body sizes in children and determine whether strength increases at the same rate as body size. Asmussen and Heeboll-Nielsen (1955, 1956) took this approach in studying Danish children between ages 7 and 16. They assumed that body height could represent changes in body size, including

**Table 7.2  Development of Isometric Muscle Force (Newtons) in Selected Urban Populations**

| Sample | Age | | | | | |
|---|---|---|---|---|---|---|
| | 8 | 10 | 12 | 14 | 16 | 18 |
| Handgrip force | | | | | | |
| Boys | 146 | 192 | 240 | 348 | 491 | 527 |
| Girls | 134 | 168 | 226 | 291 | 343 | 343 |
| Elbow flexion force (right arm) | | | | | *† | |
| Boys | 128 | 164 | 216 | 301 | 344 | — |
| Girls | 114 | 149 | 192 | 176 | 217 | — |
| Elbow extension force (right arm) | | | | | *† | |
| Boys | 113 | 142 | 173 | 253 | 292 | — |
| Girls | 97 | 123 | 164 | 160 | 178 | — |
| Knee extension force (right leg) | | | | | *† | |
| Boys | 235 | 310 | 375 | 504 | 535 | — |
| Girls | 228 | 308 | 372 | 363 | 383 | — |
| Leg lift force (dynamometer) | | | | | *† | |
| Boys | 649 | 952 | 1275 | 1627 | 1906 | — |
| Girls | 577 | 903 | 1158 | 1014 | 1173 | — |
| Back lift force (dynamometer) | | | | | *† | |
| Boys | 360 | 476 | 644 | 889 | 959 | — |
| Girls | 318 | 421 | 574 | 607 | 633 | — |

*Based on data accumulated by Shephard (1978b) for handgrip and on unpublished results of Howell et al. (1968) for other muscle groups.

†In the sample of Howell, Loiselle, and Lucas (1966), final column is for children one year older than the previous category (i.e., 15.6 years). Reproduced with permission from Shephard, R.J., *Physical Activity and Growth* (p. 104). Copyright 1982 by Yearbook Medical Publishers, Inc., Chicago.

body weight; body weight is proportional to the body height raised to the third power in this age group. Asmussen and Heeb-oll-Nielsen showed this was approximately true for their sample of Danish boys and girls. Because height measures could represent body size, they grouped the children into height categories by 10 cm intervals and measured them for isometric strength (exertion of force against immovable resistance). Successive height groups demonstrated increasing muscle strength, but at a rate greater than that of their height increase.

Asmussen and Heeboll-Nielsen also divided boys of the same height into two age groups, one younger and one older by approximately 1-1/2 years. The older group showed greater arm and leg strength by about 5% to 10% per year of age. This experiment demonstrates that strength is not related to muscle size alone. As children mature, some factor other than muscle growth contributes to improved strength. This factor most likely is improved coordination of muscle fiber recruitment, that is, increased skill in using the muscles to exert force.

The studies mentioned thus far typically measured isometric strength directly, with a cable tensiometer or a dynamometer. The benefit of measuring strength with this equipment is that the effects of skill, practice, and experience are minimized. Yet these factors do influence the performance of sport skills. For this reason studies of functional muscle strength development are also useful. Functional strength tasks have a skill component as well as a strength component.

Two skills that involve *functional muscle strength* are vertical jumping and sprinting. Practice and experience as well as leg strength influence children's performance on both tasks. Asmussen and Heeboll-Nielsen (1955, 1956) measured performance on these two skills in successive height groups of Danish children. They found that functional muscle strength, like isometric strength, increased at a faster rate than one would anticipate from muscle growth alone. Further, the rate of functional muscle strength gain was even greater than that of *isometric strength*, emphasizing again the role of improved coordination and skill in improved muscle strength as children mature.

## Gender Differences

Boys and girls have similar strength levels until they are about 13 years old, although boys are very slightly stronger than girls of the same height during childhood (Asmussen, 1973). You'll remember from chapter 2 that boys gain more muscle mass in adolescence than girls, largely as a result of higher androgen secretion levels. In fact, boys undergo a spurt of increased strength at about age 13 that corresponds to increased secretion of androgens. It is not surprising, then, that on the average men are stronger than women. Women can produce only 60% to 80% of the force that men can exert, although we can attribute most of these differences to differences in arm and shoulder

strength rather than trunk or leg strength (Asmussen, 1973).

The average difference in body or muscle size accounts for only half of the difference in strength between men and women, so other factors must contribute as well. Cultural norms probably play a role in the sex differences in strength. For example, Shephard (1982) noted the effect of repeating strength measures on "naive" boys and girls (that is, boys and girls who have never been tested for strength). Whereas the boys showed no tendency to improve over three visits, the girls improved on each subsequent visit in almost every case and improved significantly on two of the eight strength measures (see Table 7.3). Although we could attribute this effect to learning, it is possible that the task gained acceptability to the girls as they became more familiar with it. Do not discount motivation as a major factor in strength measurement. Certainly, if Shephard had recorded only the first set of scores, he would have concluded that the gender differences in strength were much greater than if he compared the third set of scores.

Recent research has hinted that gender differences exist in muscle fiber composition; that is, men and women do not have the same proportions of Type I (slow-twitch) and Type II (fast-twitch) muscle fibers. If so, we might attribute part of the gender differences in strength to muscle fiber composition, because indications from animal studies show that muscle composition is related to isometric strength (see Komi, 1984, for a review). Such research is limited, and continued investigation is necessary to confirm any relationship between gender differences in strength and muscle composition.

## Strength in Older Adults

Typically, men attain their maximal levels of strength when they are young adults and women attain theirs in adolescence, although

**Table 7.3  Effect of Test Repetition on Measurements of Isometric Muscle Force (Results for 52 "Naive" Children 9 Years of Age, Tested at Intervals of 2 to 3 Days)**

| | Muscle force (newtons) | | | | | |
| | Boys | | | Girls | | |
| Measurement | Visit 1 | Visit 2 | Visit 3 | Visit 1 | Visit 2 | Visit 3 |
|---|---|---|---|---|---|---|
| Tensiometer technique (Clarke, 1966) | | | | | | |
|  Elbow flexion | 195 | 192 | 201 | 174 | 177 | 186 |
|  Shoulder flexion | 120 | 120 | 120 | 101 | 101 | 104 |
|  Hip flexion | 218 | 219 | 206 | 187 | 204 | 208 |
|  Knee flexion | 174 | 180 | 172 | 158 | 159 | 164 |
|  Knee extension | 209 | 203 | 191 | 208 | 213 | 214 |
| Dynamometer readings | | | | | | |
|  Handgrip (Stoelting) | 159 | 148 | 150 | 131 | 124 | 130 |
|  Leg extension (Mathews) | 1330 | 1490 | 1410 | 967 | 1380 | 1484† |
|  Back extension (Mathews) | 529 | 598 | 602 | 378 | 521 | 547† |

Note. Based on data of Shephard et al. (1977).

†A statistically significant and important learning effect was observed in the two tests using the dynamometer of Mathews (1963).

Reprinted by permission from Shephard, 1982.

cultural norms may influence the latter generalization. Strength levels then plateau until approximately age 50 when they begin to decline. The loss of strength is significant after adults reach their mid-60s (Shock & Norris, 1970). In their 50s the loss is typically 18% to 20% (Shephard, 1978b), but after age 65 losses as high as 45% are reported (Murray, Gardner, Mollinger, & Sepic, 1980). Both isometric strength, the ability to exert force against immovable resistance, and *dynamic strength*, the ability to exert force against movable resistance, decline. The loss is particularly noticeable in the muscles of the upper leg.

Just as with the development of strength in young people, it is interesting to consider whether the decline of muscle mass parallels the decline of strength in older adults. Recall from chapter 2 that adults lose muscle mass as they age; they can lose as much as 50% of

their young adult level. This loss occurs through decreases in both the number and size of muscle fibers (*atrophy*), especially Type II fibers, but the molecular mechanism of this loss is presently unclear.

Yet this loss of muscle volume might not be as large as the loss of strength. Young, Stokes, and Crowe (1985) found a 39% loss of strength but only a 25% loss in cross-sectional area in the quadriceps muscles of older men compared to younger men. Aniansson, Hedberg, Henning, and Grimby (1986) documented a 10% to 22% strength loss (as illustrated in Figure 7.6), but a 6% muscle mass loss in the same muscle group over a 7-year span.

So muscle mass loss does not parallel strength loss. The proportionally greater loss of Type II than Type I muscle fibers could explain the discrepancy between muscle mass loss and strength loss, but further research on this

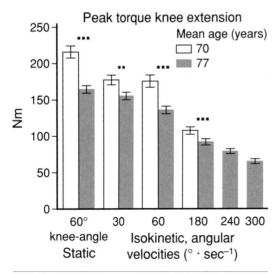

**Figure 7.6** Changes in strength with aging. The average force (torque measured in Newton-meters, Nm) exerted in a stationary knee position and at several speeds of knee extension decreased for 23 men over a 7-year interval. Changes are significant at the confidence levels of p <.01 (**) or p <.001 (***).
(Reprinted by permission from Aniansson, Hedberg, Henning, & Grimby, 1986.)

topic is necessary. As with so many other aspects of aging, it is impossible to distinguish based on current information whether older adults' loss of muscle mass and strength is inevitable or a reflection of reduced occupational duties, training, and activity levels.

## Strength Training

You already know that an adult can increase muscle strength with strength training. Drug-free strength training also results in a noticeable increase in muscle size, but only in post-pubescent men. In light of this, many educators questioned the effectiveness of strength training programs for prepubescent children. Recently, researchers have focused on this age

group, and we will now consider the findings of these studies.

### Prepubescent Children

An early study (Vrijens, 1978) failed to show much strength improvement when prepubescent children received strength training. But subsequent studies demonstrated decisively that boys and girls as young as 6 or 7 years old could increase their strength with a variety of resistance-training methods, including weights, pneumatic machines, hydraulic machines, and isometrics (Nielsen, Nielsen, Hansen, & Asmussen, 1980; Pfeiffer & Francis, 1986; Rohmert, 1968, cited in Bailey, Malina, & Rasmussen, 1978; Servedio et al., 1985; Sewall & Micheli, 1986; Weltman et al., 1986). Some of these results are shown in Figure 7.7. Pfeiffer and Francis (1986) compared the strength of 14 prepubescent boys to a control group before and after a 9-week, 3-day-a-week training program. The boys trained on a Universal machine and with free weights, completing three sets of 10 repetitions in each session. The young boys improved their strength significantly. In fact, they achieved a greater percentage increase than the pubescent and postpubescent boys Pfeiffer and Francis also tested (see Figure 7.8).

Several investigators found that increased muscle size did not accompany strength increase in prepubescents (Sale, 1989; Weltman et al., 1986). What accounts for the strength increase? Recall that strength is related to both muscle size and the central nervous system's ability to fully activate muscles. Improvement in prepubescents likely results from the children's improved ability to exert force in the intended direction as they are better able to activate the agonist (contracting) muscles and coordinate the antagonist (lengthening) muscles (Sale, 1989). These neural factors probably account for much of the initial strength gain when any age group of males or females begins training.

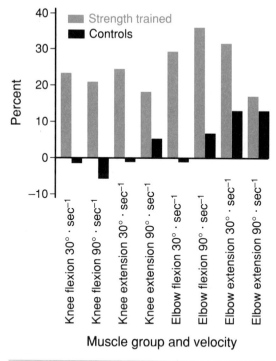

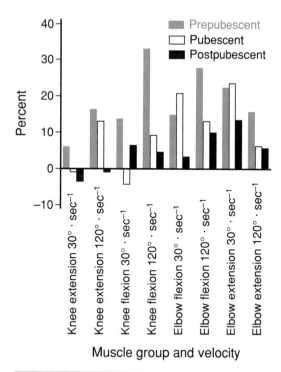

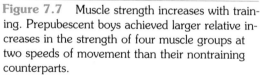

**Figure 7.7**   Muscle strength increases with training. Prepubescent boys achieved larger relative increases in the strength of four muscle groups at two speeds of movement than their nontraining counterparts.
(Reprinted by permission from Malina & Bouchard, 1991.)

**Figure 7.8**   Percentage increases in strength with training. Prepubescent boys generally achieved larger relative increases in the strength of four muscle groups at two speeds of movement with 9 weeks of training than pubescent or postpubescent boys.
(Reprinted by permission from Malina & Bouchard, 1991.)

Even if prepubescent children can improve their strength with training, some doubt that weight training is advisable for this age group. Children's bones are still growing and could be susceptible to injury at both traction and pressure epiphyses. Weight training potentially could cause a single traumatic injury or chronic injury from repeated lifts. Injury is significant when it occurs in a young child; it may threaten continued growth because it involves an epiphyseal growth plate in a weight-bearing bone. Also, some who work with children are concerned that a loss of flexibility may accompany strength training. Several studies found no damage to bones or muscles in training pre-

pubescents and recorded no injuries (Rians et al., 1987; Servedio et al., 1985; Sewall & Micheli, 1986). Neither did researchers find loss of flexibility (Rians et al., 1987; Servedio et al., 1985; Sewall & Micheli, 1986; Siegel, Camaione, & Manfredi, 1989). Yet all of the prepubescents in these studies were closely monitored; you must not overlook the importance of supervision. Do not have children attempt single maximal lifts. If close, individual supervision is impractical, children can gain strength with other training methods, such as using stretch tubing and self-supporting movements, that do not place the child at a high level of risk (Siegel et al., 1989).

Educators should be cautious in using weight training with young children and must adhere strictly to guidelines (see Sale, 1989).

## Adolescents

Developmentalists generally accept that strength training has beneficial effects for adolescents. In the study described earlier, Pfeiffer and Francis (1986) demonstrated that pubescent and postpubescent boys also improved their strength with the training previously described. Other training methods yield the same result, including isometric training (Nielsen et al., 1980) and *plyometric training* (Steben & Steben, 1981). Ikai (1967) demonstrated an improvement in muscle endurance with training in adolescents 12 to 15 years old. In this study, the criterion for muscle endurance (ability to exert submaximal force for extended periods) was the number of contractions completed at one-third maximal strength, performed at 1-sec intervals. Results indicated that the adolescents' gains in muscle endurance also were greater than those expected with adults.

After puberty, muscle hypertrophy can accompany regular strength training. Recall that due to hormonal differences adult men have far more muscle mass than adult women. Do the sexes also differ in their response to training? Cureton, Collins, Hill, and McElhannon (1988) placed young adult men and women on a weight-training program in which the resistance level was 70% to 90% of the individual's maximum. Both men and women gained strength, the level being identical in terms of percentage increase but greater for the men in terms of absolute increase for two of four tests. For example, both men and women might increase 5%, but if the men were stronger at the start, their increase was greater in absolute terms. Both men and women experienced muscle hypertrophy in their upper arms, again by

an identical percentage increase, although one measure yielded a greater absolute increase in men. After puberty, then, improved coordination in recruiting the muscle units needed to exert force and muscle hypertrophy response to strength training appears to be similar in men and women in relative terms. Muscle hypertrophy is more noticeable in men, in that a percentage increase of a larger muscle mass yields greater absolute dimensions.

Adolescents, as with children, should be closely supervised when using weight training to improve strength. Their bones are still growing, and they are susceptible to a variety of musculoskeletal injuries (Risser & Preston, 1989). Performing Olympic-style lifts in particular can bring about back injuries (Jesse, 1977). Any activity that could possibly limit the ability to be active throughout life is of doubtful benefit to youths. Educators may want to take a cautious approach by starting adolescents with light resistance and scheduling progression in small increments. Close supervision is warranted because adolescents are susceptible to peer pressure; they can be easily drawn into games of trying to outperform each other.

Often researchers have found that children and adolescents who participate regularly in sports are stronger than those who do not (Bailey et al., 1978). We could take this as proof that the training provided by sport participation develops strength. Keep in mind, though, that young athletes are often more mature than nonathletes, perhaps reflecting a self-selection process. Bigger, more mature children may experience more success in physical activities than other children and consequently pursue regular sport participation.

## Adults

Can adults prevent or reverse losses in muscle mass and strength through training? It appears that older adults can benefit by specific weight-training programs. Chapman, DeVries, and Swezey (1972) demonstrated a strength increase in older adults with training, although they trained only index finger strength. Moritani and DeVries (1980) compared five younger men (average age about 22) and five older men (average age about 70) on their potential for muscle hypertrophy with training. The participants trained three times a week for 8 weeks on two sets of 10 repetitions of elbow flexion against a weight level representing two-thirds of their maximum force. The investigators found that both groups increased in strength after the 8 weeks of training. Neural factors—that is, a gain in muscle activation level—alone seemed to be responsible for the increase in older men. The younger men improved in both improved muscle activation level and hypertrophy of the muscle.

On the other hand, several other investigators reported hypertrophy in older men as a result of training (Aniansson & Gustafson, 1981; Larsson, 1982). It is possible that a reduced rate of protein synthesis reduces the effects of training (Makrides, 1983), but more research on this process is required.

---

Many questions regarding strength training in older adults remain, especially with regard to preventing the loss of muscle mass, but it does seem that strength training yields improvement in strength at any age. However, older adults with osteoporosis (skeletal atrophy) or arthritis should begin training with light resistance.

---

## Predicting Strength

It would be useful if educators and coaches could predict which children will be capable of success in strength tasks when they reach late adolescence or early adulthood. This prediction is possible only if strength is stable throughout childhood and adolescence—that is, if the strongest children become the strongest adolescents, the weakest children remain the weakest adolescents, and so on. You can demonstrate the stability of any factor such as strength by measuring that factor in a child, measuring it again when that child reaches adolescence, and correlating the two scores. A high correlation, .80 to 1.0, indicates that children tend to retain their relative position in the group over the age span tested. Lower correlations indicate that some adolescents are relatively stronger or weaker than they were as children; therefore, you could not predict their strength accurately by their childhood score.

Researchers used this procedure in two studies. As early as 1920, Baldwin showed that measures of grip strength in 9- and 10-year-olds correlated with scores at 15 to 16 years of age by coefficients of only .65 for boys and .45 for girls. Rarick and Smoll (1967) confirmed low correlation coefficients for strength stability in the Wisconsin Growth Study by recording strength measures on 25 boys and 24 girls every year from age 7 to age 12 and then again at age 17. Although correlations between measures 1 or 2 years apart were sometimes high, only a few measures across the full 10-year span, 7 to 17 years, were above .50 (see Table 7.4). Strength in adolescence cannot be predicted accurately by childhood scores.

Several factors probably contribute to the futility of attempting to predict strength across the growing years, including motivation and the extent and intensity of participation. Undoubtedly, another factor is the variability in individual children's rates of maturation. A late-maturing, relatively weak 7-year-old might develop into one of the strongest 17-year-olds.

---

## REVIEW 7.2

We can now say that the twins mentioned at the beginning of this section will become

**Table 7.4　Age-to-Age Correlations of Strength Measures**

| Measures | Childhood | | | | | Childhood to Adolescence | | | | | |
|---|---|---|---|---|---|---|---|---|---|---|---|
| | 7 to 12 | 8 to 12 | 9 to 12 | 10 to 12 | 11 to 12 | 7 to 17 | 8 to 17 | 9 to 17 | 10 to 17 | 11 to 17 | 12 to 17 |
| **Boys** | | | | | | | | | | | |
| Wrist flexion | .375 | .550 | .163 | .486 | .533 | .378 | .493 | .327 | .434 | .244 | .419 |
| Elbow flexion | .279 | .628 | .825 | .807 | .733 | .235 | .193 | .602 | .446 | .618 | .634 |
| Shoulder med. rot. | .202 | .372 | .605 | .625 | .702 | .258 | .307 | .568 | .612 | .505 | .674 |
| Shoulder adduction | .523 | .491 | .315 | .550 | .676 | .491 | .418 | .485 | .566 | .681 | .662 |
| Hip flexion | .353 | .406 | .668 | .682 | .813 | .334 | .393 | .355 | .682 | .402 | .515 |
| Hip extension | .706 | .481 | .614 | .674 | .861 | .344 | .076 | .430 | .117 | .426 | .488 |
| Knee extension | .430 | .465 | .277 | .668 | .732 | .429 | .503 | .483 | .721 | .735 | .797 |
| Ankle extension | -.020 | .634 | .737 | .794 | .763 | .209 | .416 | .413 | .640 | .480 | .590 |
| **Girls** | | | | | | | | | | | |
| Wrist flexion | .361 | .406 | .553 | .640 | .655 | .387 | .013 | .454 | .473 | .436 | .457 |
| Elbow flexion | .367 | .627 | .592 | .763 | .770 | .566 | .308 | .336 | .473 | .350 | .114 |
| Shoulder med. rot. | .184 | .300 | .751 | .774 | .758 | .156 | -.152 | .327 | .276 | .496 | .372 |
| Shoulder adduction | .133 | .608 | .302 | .597 | .740 | .260 | .360 | .622 | .309 | .499 | .185 |
| Hip flexion | .477 | .512 | .774 | .898 | .890 | .506 | .366 | .530 | .655 | .666 | .712 |
| Hip extension | .636 | .512 | .665 | .769 | .796 | .336 | .394 | .595 | .523 | .378 | .575 |
| Knee extension | .763 | .722 | .661 | .651 | .754 | .673 | .508 | .730 | .756 | .641 | .646 |
| Ankle extension | .035 | .276 | .533 | .770 | .670 | .267 | .306 | .523 | .520 | .275 | .265 |

Reprinted by permission from Rarick & Smoll, 1967.

stronger as they grow, reflecting in part their growth in muscle mass, but that their strength will increase at a rate faster than that accounted for by muscle growth alone. This additional increase in strength is largely due to their improved coordination in recruiting the muscle units they need to exert force. Before age 13, the twins will follow a similar pattern of strength development, but after that point the male twin is likely to make more rapid gains than his sister. This gender difference results in part from the large increase in muscle mass in males caused by increased secretion of the androgen hormones. Also, cultural norms may prevent an adolescent girl both from participating in activities that build strength and from giving an all-out effort on strength tests.

The twins could improve their strength beyond those increases that accompany muscle growth and improved coordination by undergoing appropriate strength training. If they choose to participate in a weight-training program, their instructors must carefully monitor them to keep the risk of injury low. If close supervision of training is impractical, light weight resistance exercise is preferable to heavy weight resistance with children and young adolescents. After puberty, both twins can promote muscle hypertrophy through resistance training, although the result is far more noticeable in the male twin. We are likely to have only limited success in predicting the strength level of these twins as adolescents from their childhood strength measures.

Whether a lifelong exercise program promoting strength can forestall any loss of muscle tissue in older adults is yet to be thoroughly researched. But people at any age can improve their muscle strength with training. Muscle strength is important in the performance of many everyday skills as well as sport skills. Flexibility is also an important component of motor skill performance and is our next topic.

## THE DEVELOPMENT OF FLEXIBILITY

Flexibility, the ability to move joints through a full range of motion, often benefits maximal performance, whereas limited flexibility is a factor in sports injuries. Yet young athletes sometimes overlook this important aspect of physical fitness, emphasizing endurance and strength at the expense of flexibility. Exceptions to this generalization are dancers and gymnasts, who have long realized the importance of flexibility to their activities. One reason for young athletes' indifference toward flexibility is their assumption that young people are naturally supple and need no further flexibility training. Additionally, people typically view lack of flexibility as a problem only for older adults, whose movement limitations are more readily apparent. The scientific investigations summarized in the following discussion yield some surprising information concerning these misconceptions about flexibility.

> **CONCEPT 7.3**
> An individual's flexibility decreases without training, even during childhood and adolescence.

## Assessing Flexibility

An important characteristic of flexibility is its specificity; that is, a certain degree of flexibility is specific to each particular joint. For example, you can be relatively flexible at one joint and inflexible at another. This means that one or two flexibility measures cannot accurately represent your overall flexibility. Despite this, giving a battery of flexibility measures is often impractical, especially if you are assessing strength, endurance, and body composition all at the same time. Fitness test batteries such as Physical Best (American Alliance for Health,

Physical Education, Recreation and Dance, 1988), FITNESSGRAM (Institute for Aerobics Research, 1988), and that used in the National Children and Youth Fitness Study II (Ross, Pate, Delpy, Gold, & Svilar, 1987) employ a single representative flexibility measure. The *sit-and-reach test* (see Figure 7.9) was chosen because trunk and hip flexibility are thought to be important in the prevention and care of low back pain in adults (Hoeger, Hopkins, Button, & Palmer, 1990).

The range of motion possible at any joint depends on that joint's bone structure and the soft tissues' resistance to movement. The soft tissues include muscles, tendons, joint capsules, ligaments, and skin. Habitual use and exercise preserve the elastic nature of the soft tissues, whereas disuse is associated with a loss of elasticity. To improve poor flexibility, a person must move the joint regularly and systematically through an increasingly larger range of motion to modify the soft tissues. Athletes, then, tend to increase the flexibility of joints they use in

their sport, whereas laborers who spend much of their time in one posture may lose flexibility in some joints. It is likely that people who do not exercise fully lose flexibility because everyday activities rarely require them to move through a full range of motion. So at any age, flexibility reflects the normal range of movement to which an individual subjects specific joints.

---

The belief that flexibility is related to the length of one's limbs is incorrect.

---

## Developmental Changes in Flexibility

Earlier we discussed the improvement of endurance and strength as children grow older. Does this trend hold for flexibility? Some researchers have noted improvement in flexibility with age in young children, but unfortunately, most

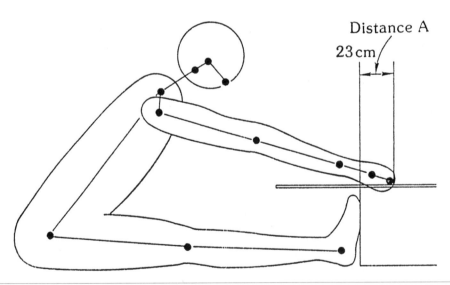

**Figure 7.9**  The sit-and-reach test. The individual sits with the feet against a box corresponding to the 23-cm point. Upon reaching forward as far as possible, the individual receives a score of 23 cm plus (Distance A above) or minus the distance reached.
(Reprinted by permission from Hoeger, Hopkins, Button, & Palmer, 1990.)

studies show a decline in flexibility. After reviewing the information available in 1975, Clarke concluded that boys tend to lose flexibility after age 10 and girls after age 12. For example, Hupprich and Sigerseth (1950) administered 12 flexibility measures to 300 girls, ages 6, 9, 12, 15, and 18 years. Most of the flexibility measures improved across the 6-, 9-, and 12-year-old groups but declined in the older groups (see Table 7.5). Krahenbuhl and Martin (1977) found that flexibility in both boys and girls declined between ages 10 and 14, but Milne, Seefeldt, and Reuschlein (1976) reported that 2nd-graders in their study already had poorer flexibility than kindergartners.

The sit-and-reach test has been used as the flexibility measure in several large studies of children and adolescents. Norms recently developed in the National Children and Youth Fitness II project (Ross et al., 1987) for children ages 6 to 9 reflect generally stable sit-and-reach performance during childhood. In an extensive cross-sectional study of Flemish girls 6 to 18 years old, the sit-and-reach scores of girls in the upper percentiles were stable until age 12, then improved. The scores of girls in the lower percentiles declined from 6 to 12 years, improved somewhat in midadolescence, then declined again at 17 and 18 (see Figure 7.10). The variability in sit-and-reach flexibility increased with successively older age groups (Simons et al., 1990).

Belgian boys measured longitudinally improved their sit-and-reach performance from 12 to 18 years of age at a rate of about 1 cm/yr, perhaps due in part to an increase in abdominal strength (Beunen et al., 1988). Generally, then, children maintain their sit-and-reach flexibility, whereas adolescents are able to improve their scores as they grow older. Some children and adolescents lose flexibility or improve very little, perhaps due to a lack of exercise and training.

Some researchers are concerned that the sit-and-reach test reflects body proportions as well as flexibility, because it measures flexibility relative to a point even with the feet. A small number of individuals with unusually long legs, short arms, or both are at a disadvantage. A modified sit-and-reach test corrects for limb length bias by measuring flexibility relative to an individual's fingertips when sitting straight up (Hoeger et al., 1990).

Girls as a group are usually more flexible than boys (Beunen et al., 1988; DiNucci, 1976; Phillips et al., 1955; Simons et al., 1990). This probably reflects that stretching exercises are more socially acceptable for girls than vigorous exercises, and that higher proportions of girls than boys participate in gymnastics and dance,

**Table 7.5 Average Range and Standard Deviations of Flexibility Measures (Degrees) of Girls**

| Age group (years) | N | Hip flexion-extension | Side trunk flexion-extension | Elbow flexion-extension | Shoulder |
|---|---|---|---|---|---|
| 6 | 50 | 121.3 ± 16.7 | 92.0 ± 14.0 | 156.0 ± 6.0 | 228.4 ± 12.9 |
| 9 | 50 | 126.5 ± 19.9 | 107.2 ± 18.1 | 157.3 ± 6.9 | 219.7 ± 11.0 |
| 12 | 50 | 139.1 ± 18.2 | 118.3 ± 20.4 | 157.4 ± 8.1 | 215.5 ± 12.0 |
| 15 | 50 | 126.9 ± 17.8 | 110.4 ± 18.8 | 155.7 ± 7.5 | 213.0 ± 11.9 |
| 18 | 100 | 128.6 ± 11.1 | 104.4 ± 18.0 | 151.3 ± 7.8 | 212.8 ± 12.0 |

Adapted by permission from Hupprich & Sigerseth, 1950.

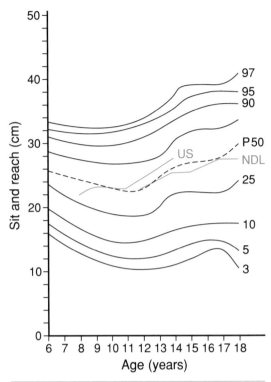

**Figure 7.10** Changes in sit-and-reach test performance over age. Flemish girls at the upper percentiles maintained their flexibility during childhood, then improved in adolescence. Girls at the lower percentiles declined with only slight improvement in midadolescence. The median scores of girls from the United States (U.S.) and Netherlands (NDL) are superimposed on the graph with bold lines.
(Redrawn from Bovend'eerdt et al., 1980, and Branta et al., 1984; reprinted by permission from Simons, Beunen, Renson, Claessens, Vanreusel, & Lefevre, 1990.)

muscle growth causes a measurable decline in flexibility.

Researchers, then, document both declines and improvements in flexibility during the growing years. Some changes might be particular to the joint or joints measured, but overall it is apparent that children and adolescents can lose their flexibility if they do not train to maintain or improve it. Flexibility becomes more variable within groups of adolescents, because some adolescents train and others abandon exercise programs and physical activities.

## Flexibility in Older Adults

Unfortunately, adolescence does not mark the end of a person's trend toward reduced flexibility. Boone and Azen (1979) obtained 28 flexibility measures of 109 males in age groups from 18 months to 54 years and found a steady decline throughout each period. For example, hip rotation range declined 15 degrees to 20 degrees in the early years and about 5 degrees in each decade of life thereafter. The greatest losses occurred in movements an individual does not habitually perform. Comparing adults older than 55 to younger people yields reduced flexibility scores for some, but not all, joint motions (Einkauf, Gohdes, Jensen, & Jewell, 1987; Germain & Blair, 1983; Murray, 1985; Sepic, Murray, Mollinger, Spurr, & Gardner, 1986; Smith & Walker, 1983; Walker, Sue, Miles-Elkousy, Ford, & Trevelyan, 1984).

Alexander, Ready, and Fougere-Mailey (1985) noted that the decline in flexibility is more significant after age 49 than before. Undoubtedly, one factor in the loss of flexibility is the limited range of motion required in everyday life. Individuals not engaged in sports, dance, or a regular exercise routine for flexibility seldom move through a full range of motion. Even those who participate in sports and dance may not move joints to their full extent, or they may exercise some but not all of the body's joints.

activities that emphasize flexibility. Participation in exercise programs emphasizing flexibility is a far better predictor of flexibility than gender.

It is possible that because the bones grow in length and then stimulate muscles to grow in length, a temporary loss of flexibility occurs during growth, especially early in adolescence (Micheli, 1984). It is not clear that the lag in

The trend toward declining flexibility represents the average state of fitness among representative groups of people. It does not indicate that everyone automatically loses flexibility. In fact, athletes, dancers, and others engaged in flexibility training usually maintain or improve their range of motion as they age.

## Flexibility Training

Developmentalists generally accept that a loss of flexibility is a characteristic of old age. Changes in the cartilage, ligaments, and tendons of the joints occur with aging, but no evidence exists that these changes are the cause of decreased flexibility (Adrian, 1981). In fact, most research links loss of flexibility in older adults to degenerative diseases of the tissues. Arthritis and osteoporosis contribute to both lost flexibility and lost stability in the joints.

Researchers generally agree that flexibility training can improve range of motion in the joints of young adults, and Munns (1981) demonstrated that older adults can also improve the range of motion in their joints with training. She formed two groups of 65- to 88-year-olds. One group served as a control, and the other

participated in a 1-hour program of exercise and dance three times a week for 12 weeks. The exercising group improved significantly over the control group in all six flexibility measures. Germain and Blair (1983) also documented improved shoulder flexibility in adults aged 20 to 60 who participated in a stretching program for shoulder flexion, and Raab, Agre, McAdam, and Smith (1988) found improvement in various joints in women over age 53 after an active (unassisted) and passive (assisted) stretching program.

Inactivity is certainly a major factor that may contribute to flexibility decline in old age. Fortunately, specific training can reverse a loss of flexibility, even in old age.

### REVIEW 7.3

The range of motion possible in a joint reflects a person's activity and training more than age, per se. Flexibility declines in the average adolescent and adult as a result of limited daily activity and lack of exercise. Flexibility training can bring about an improvement in the range of motion at any age.

## Assessing Fitness

Six physical fitness test batteries are widely used in the United States to test children. They are the following:

1. Physical Best (American Alliance for Health, Physical Education, Recreation and Dance, 1988)
2. FITNESSGRAM (Institute for Aerobics Research, 1987)
3. Fitness Test (Chrysler Fund—American Athletic Union, 1987)
4. Fit Youth Today (American Health and Fitness Foundation, 1986)
5. Presidential Physical Fitness Award Test (President's Council on Physical Fitness and Sports, 1987)
6. YMCA Youth Fitness Test (Franks, 1989)

*(continued)*

**Assessing Fitness** *(continued)*

These test batteries are health-related fitness tests because they emphasize testing components of physical fitness rather than motor performance, which includes a skill component. All of the batteries include a version of the sit-and-reach test to assess low back and hamstring (back thigh) flexibility and a version of a sit-up test to assess abdominal muscle strength and endurance. Most also include a version of a pull-up or flexed-arm hang to assess upper body muscle strength and endurance. All six have some measure of cardio-respiratory endurance, usually a 1-mile walk or run for time. Most contain a body composition assessment consisting of skinfold measurements, typically the sum of the triceps and calf skinfolds.

Of these six test batteries, the Physical Best, FITNESSGRAM, Fit Youth Today, and YMCA Youth Fitness Test emphasize criterion-referenced standards. The other two have normative-referenced standards. The criterion-referenced batteries seek to identify those children who meet a desirable level of fitness. This is accomplished through provision of a single standard for each age group and sex. For example, on the Physical Best Test, boys at age 9 must do 30 sit-ups in 1 min to meet the criterion; girls, 28 sit-ups. Children not meeting the criterion are prescribed exercises and activities to improve their abdominal strength and endurance. Therefore, an individual's performance is compared to a desirable fitness level, the level he or she needs for good health.

In contrast, individuals taking a normative-referenced test are compared to norms for their age and sex. Using this type of test, educators can identify individuals who are very fit. Yet our discussion of physical growth in chapter 2 and fitness development in this chapter demonstrates that comparisons based on chronological age overlook individual variation due to maturation rate. For example, you would expect a bigger, more mature 8-year-old to perform better on fitness tests than a smaller, less mature 8-year-old of the same sex, given equal experience, training, and motivation. Partly for this reason, criterion-referenced tests have become more popular than normative-referenced tests.

Although educators widely promote the use of these fitness tests today, the test batteries are not perfect. The criterion standards are a major concern for those who use the criterion-referenced tests. Little empirical evidence is available to tie criterion levels to good health. Most of the standards are derived from normative data and fall between the 25th and 50th percentiles (Plowman, 1992). As a result, the different test batteries often have differing criterion standards for the same test item. Concerns about normative-referenced tests include that some educators use them only to identify and reward children who perform at high levels, or administer them in a punitive manner.

No matter which type of test battery the schools employ, fitness testing should be only one component of a broader fitness-education curriculum. Educators should teach children health concepts and lead them to appreciate the role exercise plays in good health (Pate, 1989). Those who administer fitness tests, whether teachers or recreational leaders, should use an individual child's performance results to motivate that child toward higher levels of fitness. Most importantly, professionals who understand physical growth and its relationship to fitness development should help children and adolescents place their fitness test results into the wider context of their individual growth and maturation rates.

## BODY COMPOSITION

Your body mass can be divided into two types of tissue: *lean tissue* that includes muscle, bone, and organs; and fat or *adipose tissue*. The relative percentages of *lean body mass* and fat tissue that make up the body mass give a measure of body composition. Body composition is important for various reasons:

1. Higher proportions of lean body mass show a positive link to working capacity, and higher proportions of fat tissue show a negative link.
2. Excess fat weight adds to the work load whenever you move your body.
3. Excess fat can limit your range of motion.
4. Obesity places a person at risk of suffering coronary heart and artery disease, stroke, diabetes, and hypertension.

Body composition is also important because it can influence your feelings about yourself. Many societies value a lean body appearance. Obesity may contribute to a negative body concept and self-concept, thus making it difficult for an obese person to relate to others. Remember that everyone has some fat tissue, which is needed for insulation, protection, and energy storage. Women need a minimal level of fat tissue (approximately 12% of body weight) to support functions of pregnancy. Only excess fat weight is negatively related to fitness and health.

People can use two major environmental factors—diet and exercise—to manage the relative amounts of lean and adipose tissue in their bodies. An individual can consume too much food, resulting in excess fat storage. Because physical activity requires energy, the body uses calories from food for the activity rather than storing it as adipose tissue.

Maintaining body composition is in part a matter of balancing the calories you consume in your diet against your *metabolic rate* and amount of physical exertion. Your metabolic rate is the amount of energy you use in a given amount of time to keep your body functioning. Individuals vary; some use more calories than others do just to keep the body running. Your metabolic rate is under the control of various hormones, and you cannot easily alter it in the short term. In contrast, you can control your exercise level on a daily basis. The relationship between body composition and exercise, especially during the growing years, is the focus of the following discussion.

CONCEPT 7.4
Genetic and environmental factors, especially diet and exercise, affect body composition.

## Body Composition and Exercise: The Parizkova Studies

Fat tissue increases rapidly during two periods: the first 6 months after birth and again in early adolescence. In girls, this increase continues throughout adolescence, whereas in boys the gain stops and may even reverse for a time. Muscle tissue also grows rapidly in infants, followed by a steady period of increase during childhood, and it again increases rapidly during the adolescent growth spurt, more dramatically in boys than in girls. Either diet or exercise may alter this typical pattern. Overeating results in excess fat weight, and starvation can lead to levels of fat so low that the body obtains energy by muscle wasting (breaking down muscle tissue to use it as energy). Exercise burns calories, potentially altering a person's body composition, so the relationship between body composition and exercise deserves close attention.

In both cross-sectional and longitudinal studies, researchers have examined the relationship between exercise and body composition. Cross-sectional studies generally show that young athletes have lower proportions of body fat than more sedentary children (Parizkova, 1973). However, it is impossible to determine from a cross-sectional study whether an active lifestyle results in leanness. (It may be that leaner children find activity easier and adopt active lifestyles.) Longitudinal studies, then, are more valuable in the study of the interrelationships between activity levels and body composition, and wherever possible, we will discuss longitudinal information.

Parizkova conducted a series of studies on body composition and activity levels of boys and girls in Czechoslovakia. The first study was cross-sectional and was one of the few studies to examine very young children; the remainder of the studies were longitudinal. In the cross-sectional study, Wolanski and Parizkova (1976; cited in Parizkova, 1977) compared skinfold measures in two groups of children aged 2 to 5 years. One group of children attended special physical education classes with their parents, whereas the other group did not participate in any type of physical training program. Even at this young age, children in the physical education group had lower levels of subcutaneous fat. The following discussion focuses on Parizkova's longitudinal studies.

## Teenage Boys

An extensive longitudinal study of teenage boys (Parizkova, 1968, 1977) examined the same issue. Parizkova divided nearly 100 boys into four groups by activity level. The most active group of boys (Group I) were involved in basketball or track at least 6 hr a week. The least active group (Group IV) participated only in unorganized and unsystematic activity. The boys in the other two groups had intermediate activity levels.

Parizkova first tested the boys at an average age of 10.7 years and followed them in successive years until they were 14.7 years old. Over the 4 years, the children in the most active group significantly increased in body mass while their absolute level of fat weight remained the same; hence, the fat proportion of their total weight decreased. In contrast, the boys in the inactive group increased significantly in absolute fat weight. Interestingly, the two groups did not differ in amount of fat weight at the beginning of the study, but they did by the end. In the active group the increase in lean body mass alone accounted for the increase of body weight with growth (see Table 7.6). Physical activity had a beneficial effect on body composition in these boys.

Parizkova (1972) followed 41 of these boys for another 3 years, until they were 17.7 years old. The body composition trends of the first 4 years continued. The most active and least active groups differed in total weight by the time they reached age 16.7. The active group was heavier in total body weight because of the boys' greater lean body mass. The active boys had less total fat weight than the inactive boys, and their fat weight actually declined in some years. Parizkova determined that the groups did not differ in average skeletal age, so the body composition differences noted can be attributed not to maturational differences, but rather to activity level. He also noted that the boys maintained their relative position within the group in both distribution and absolute amount of subcutaneous fat. This means that the relative amount of fat weight and its pattern of distribution in the body was relatively stable over the years of the study.

Parizkova followed 16 of these 41 young men for another 6 years. Although this number was too small for a reliable analysis by activity level, Parizkova (1977) noted that percent body fat declined in the group until age 21.7 years,

**Table 7.6   Average Values and Standard Deviations (*M* and *SD*) of Relative Fat (%) and Absolute Lean Body Mass (kg LBM) of Groups With Different Activity Regimes**

| Group | | 1 1961 | | 2 1962 | | 3 1963 | | 4 1964 | | 5 1965 | |
|---|---|---|---|---|---|---|---|---|---|---|---|
| | | *M* | *SD* | *M* | *SD* | *M* | *SD* | *M* | *SD* | *M* | *SD* |
| I | % fat | 15.7 | 5.4 | 14.1 | 5.7 | 12.7 | 1.5 | 9.7 | 3.3 | 9.9 | 4.6 |
| | kg LBM | 31.6 | 3.3 | 35.0 | 3.8 | 40.4 | 5.4 | 45.5 | 6.8 | 54.4 | 7.1 |
| II | % fat | 15.5 | 5.6 | 13.5 | 5.9 | 12.4 | 4.7 | 11.4 | 4.1 | 12.5 | 4.1 |
| | kg LBM | 30.2 | 4.3 | 33.8 | 4.5 | 37.9 | 5.3 | 44.1 | 7.2 | 49.1 | 8.3 |
| III | % fat | 14.7 | 6.4 | 14.5 | 7.5 | 14.8 | 5.7 | 12.5 | 5.9 | 13.6 | 4.2 |
| | kg LBM | 31.0 | 3.1 | 34.1 | 3.4 | 37.3 | 3.6 | 43.9 | 5.1 | 49.7 | 5.4 |
| IV | % fat | 17.2 | 6.2 | 19.1 | 6.0 | 16.6 | 5.9 | 14.7 | 4.4 | 15.9 | 5.4 |
| | kg LBM | 31.4 | 3.3 | 33.8 | 3.9 | 37.8 | 4.6 | 43.8 | 6.3 | 49.6 | 6.6 |

*Note.* Subjects were groups of boys followed longitudinally during 5 years (from 10.7 to 14.7 years of age, 1961 to 1965, n = 96). Group I was most active and Group IV was least active.
Data from Parizkova, 1968a, 1968b; reprinted by permission from Parizkova, 1977.

then varied widely among individuals, probably reflecting changes in lifestyle. The Parizkova studies, then, indicate that physical activity has a favorable influence on boys' body composition during the growing years.

## Teenage Girls

The growth of adipose and lean muscle tissue differs dramatically between the sexes during adolescence when girls gain proportionately more fat than muscle compared to boys. Even so, the beneficial effect activity has on body composition found in boys also occurs in active girls. Over a span of 5 years Parizkova (1963, 1977) studied 32 girls who belonged to a gymnastics school and 45 girls who were not engaged in any type of training. The girls were first measured at the age of 12 or 13. The gymnasts had a regular yearly cycle of training in which they attended a rigorous camp in the summer, stopped training in the fall, and re-

sumed a heavy training schedule from October to December. These cycles are shown in Figure 7.11 as black bars; the higher the bar, the more intense the training. Measures of the girls' fat weight paralleled Parizkova's findings with boys: The gymnasts remained at the same level of subcutaneous fat during the 5 years, the total skinfold thickness showing no trend, even though it rose or fell for short periods of time. In contrast, the control group gained a significant amount of fat weight. Height and body weight trends in the two groups were similar throughout the 5 years, so the differences were truly in body composition.

The cyclic nature of the gymnasts' training schedule provided information about their weight and skinfold thicknesses as they progressed through the various training cycles. During periods of inactivity, the gymnasts gained in both total body weight and skinfold thickness (including subcutaneous fat tissue), but during training, the gymnasts increased in

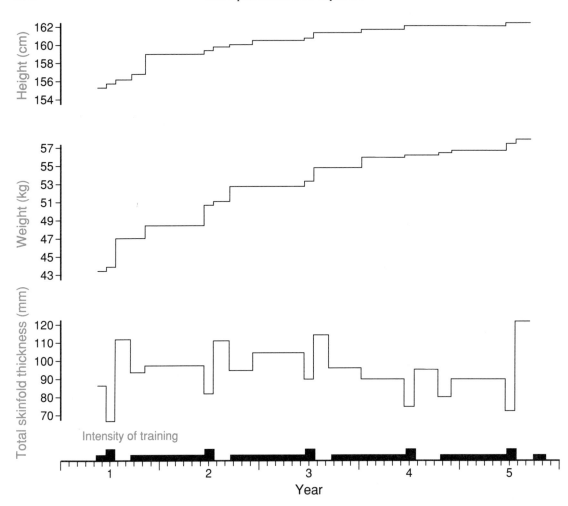

**Figure 7.11** Changes in height, weight, and subcutaneous fat (sum of 10 skinfold measurements) in a group of regularly training girl gymnasts (n = 11) during a 5-year period of varying intensity of training (see bottom scale).
(Data from Parizkova, 1963, 1965; reprinted by permission from Parizkova, 1977.)

total body weight while their skinfold thicknesses declined. (Note that in Figure 7.11, total skinfold thickness goes down when the intensity of training bar goes up, and total skinfold thickness goes up when training stops for a time. Total height and weight keeps increasing with age.) Therefore, their weight increases during the various activity periods resulted from changing ratios of fat and lean body weight. Parizkova also recorded the gymnasts' caloric intake and found that they consumed more calories during periods of intense training, but fat deposits declined and lean body mass increased.

## Comparing Adolescent Boys and Girls

Parizkova's longitudinal studies show the same general relationship between body composition and activity in both boys and girls, but they do not allow direct comparison of the sexes. So Parizkova (1973, 1977) simultaneously followed 12 boys and 12 girls engaged in swimming training from age 12 to age 16. At 12, the average height, weight, lean body mass, and fat weight of the two groups were about the same. Lean body mass values were higher for the swimmers than the average levels for teens not in training, probably reflecting the swimmers' previous training. By age 15, the boys were significantly taller, heavier, and leaner than the girls, but both sexes showed an increased proportion of lean body mass at the expense of fat weight over the 2 years of training. Although higher in percent fat than the boys, the girls did not gain as much fat as the typical nontraining adolescent girl. More research on this topic is necessary , especially to determine the length and intensity of training programs that have favorable results with girls. Tremblay, Despres, and Bouchard (1988) did not find a decline in fatness or a gain in lean body mass in girls after 15 weeks of intense training, although boys experienced significant changes in this time.

In summary, the Parizkova investigations show that involvement in training programs affects adolescents' body composition favorably. Limited information suggests that the body composition of preschool children also benefits from activity. Although children and adolescents who engage in active training exhibit the general growth trend of increased weight, this increase represents the addition of relatively more lean body mass and less fat weight than in their nontraining peers. A person's higher caloric intake during training evidently increases lean body mass rather than fat stores.

It is possible for a person to carry training to an extreme, so that the body cannot meet the energy required for continued growth. This condition mimics starvation and, as noted in chapter 2, can lead to loss of lean body mass and detrimental effects on growth (Lemon, 1989).

## Obesity in Children

There is a high incidence of *obesity* in industrialized countries, even among children, and many people become obese as they grow older. As we noted earlier, obesity is unfortunate from both medical and social viewpoints. This is particularly true for children. Obese children are likely to become obese adults at risk of heart disease, stroke, diabetes, and hypertension. In addition, the economy of obese children's physical work is poor: Their working capacity is low because their bodies require more energy just to move their excess fat weight (Vamberova et al., 1971; cited in Parizkova, 1977). During the years when an obese child is forming a self-concept, he or she must deal with negative feedback and evaluation from adults and peers alike (Allon, 1973; Dwyer & Mayer, 1973; Stunkard & Mendelson, 1967). Even children as young as 6 are aware of prejudice against obese people (Wadden & Stunkard, 1985). It is desirable for educators to intervene, when possible, and positively influence the factors contributing to a child's obesity.

### Decreased Caloric Intake

An individual can reduce obesity over time by lowering caloric intake, increasing activity to burn more calories, or a combination of the two. Increasing activity alone yields slow progress, because a 2-mile jog, for example, burns approximately 150 calories, and a deficit of 3,500 calories is needed to lose 1 lb of fat weight.

Which approach is best for obese children? Overeating in young children is probably rare (Mayer, 1968), and studies of the correlation between caloric intake and obesity fail to establish a relationship between the two in infants (Roberts, Savage, Coward, Chew, & Lucas, 1988; Rose & Mayer, 1968; Vobecky, Vobecky, Shapcott, & Demers, 1983) or adolescents (Rolland-Cachera & Bellisle, 1986). Yet reduced motor activity is a common characteristic of obese children (Bullen, Reed, & Mayer, 1964; Johnson, Burke, & Mayer, 1956; Roberts et al., 1988). For example, Stafanik, Heald, and Mayer (1959) noted that among 14 obese and 14 thin boys attending a summer camp, the obese boys consumed fewer calories but were also less active than the thin boys. Inactivity probably does not result from obesity, but rather precedes it (Parizkova, 1977).

Once children are overweight, they are trapped in a vicious cycle: An obese child must exert relatively greater effort for activity, making the activity less pleasurable and reducing the vigor of the child's participation (even when the activity consists of games or exercise); hence, the child burns fewer excess calories and remains overweight. Although no one has established a connection between caloric intake and obesity, current research is focused on the role of high-fat and high-sugar diets in obesity (see Oscai, 1989, p. 279 for a review). Perhaps the type of diet more than the total number of calories consumed has a greater influence on obesity. We would benefit from further research on this topic.

Adults who significantly reduce their caloric intake without exercising may lose lean body mass as well as fat weight (Parizkova, 1977). To prevent this loss of lean body tissue, simultaneous exercise and reduced caloric intake are most effective. In children, reducing caloric intake to 1,000 calories a day can temporarily slow down or even arrest growth (Vamberova, 1961; cited in Parizkova, 1977). Increasing the number of calories expended through increased activity permits a child to reduce weight while maintaining a safe level of caloric intake. Exercise, then, plays an essential role in weight reduction at any age, but particularly in children. As a goal, overweight individuals should avoid losing lean muscle tissue by engaging in vigorous exercise and controlling caloric intake rather than controlling calories alone.

The role of genetics in obesity is unclear. Separating genetic influence from a family's eating and activity habits is very difficult. Current research documents only a limited influence of genetic inheritance, and this affects internal fat more than subcutaneous fat (Bouchard, Perusse, LeBlanc, Tremblay, & Theriault, 1988). Individuals cannot choose their genetic inheritance, but they can control their activity levels.

## Increased Physical Activity

Parizkova, Stankova, Sprynarova, and Vamberova (1963; cited in Parizkova, 1977) demonstrated the effect of increasing obese children's activity level. They studied seven boys with an average age of 11.8 years during 7 weeks of a summer camp. The boys increased their activity levels and also controlled their caloric intake (1,700 calories a day). Over the summer the boys reduced their body weight an average of 11.4%, lost about 5 kg of fat weight, and raised their percentage of lean body mass from 69.9% to 75.9%. At the beginning of the summer, the boys' free fatty acid level (the usable fuel form of the triglyceride molecule, which the body must break down to metabolize fat) tended to decline during exercise and remain low during the subsequent rest period. By the end of the summer, their free fatty acid level increased significantly during the rest period. This change was probably due to the boys' improved ability to mobilize fat from its storage locations. The exercise program was thus effective in increasing the metabolic activity of adipose tissue.

Although Parizkova was able to report favorable results from such a summer program, follow-up studies (Parizkova, 1977) revealed a common problem. Most boys gained back much of the fat weight they lost during the summer when they returned to their home environments. The success of most intervention techniques depends on the child continuing to participate and receive family support. Education about nutrition and exercise is valuable for both children and their parents.

Some research indicates that the body forms new adipose tissue cells only during the prenatal and early postnatal months, and during adolescence (Hirsch & Knittle, 1970; Knittle & Hirsch, 1968). After adolescence, only the size of fat cells is variable. Research on this topic is limited, but if it is accurate, diet and exercise are particularly important for young persons during these sensitive periods. Animal studies suggest that regular vigorous exercise prevents the addition of excess fat cells during growth, perhaps making weight control easier later in life (Oscai, Babirak, Dubach, McGarr, & Spirakis, 1974).

## Body Composition in Older Adults

As we noted in chapter 2, average individuals usually experience an increase in total body weight in their adult years, reflecting fat accumulation, then a decrease after age 50, reflecting a decline in lean body weight rather than in fat weight. In older adults, loss of both bone and muscle tissue can mask adipose tissue gain. Other evidence suggests that such changes in body composition are not an inevitable consequence of aging. For example, Shephard (1978b) compiled data collected by Kavanagh and Shephard (1977), Pollock (1974), and Asano, Ogawa, and Furuta (1978) on older track participants, ages 40 to 70 and older. These participants exhibited no tendency for increasing weight or body fat with advancing age. Further, those older adults who still ran 30 to 40 miles a week showed no significant loss of lean body mass.

Saltin and Grimby (1968) similarly found no tendency among adults who regularly participated in orienteering events to gain fat weight, although they did lose body weight after age 45, presumably reflecting a decline in lean body mass. Heath, Hagberg, Ehsani, and Holloszy (1981) recorded similar levels of fat percent and lean body weight in young athletes and Masters athletes 50 to 72 years old. Apparently, maintaining endurance training as an adult has a favorable effect on body composition, although questions remain about the extent of lean body mass loss after the late 40s.

Can older adults who begin exercise programs bring about beneficial changes in body composition? Research conducted to answer this question is equivocal. Some researchers found little or no change in body weight, fat weight, or lean body mass in older adults who began training (Adams & DeVries, 1973; DeVries, 1970; Parizkova & Eiselt, 1968). On the contrary, Sidney, Shephard, and Harrison (1977) recorded significant losses of estimated percent body fat and subcutaneous fat in older adults after 14 weeks of endurance training. A smaller number of older adults in this study who continued to train for 1 year lost additional fat weight, but not body weight, which implies that an offsetting increase of lean body mass occurred. Obviously, further research is needed to resolve these conflicting findings.

## Avoiding Extremes

Traditionally, weight management was related more to the number of calories consumed than to what food was eaten. Now nutritionists give more attention to lowering fat intake. Low-fat diets are associated with ideal weight and reduced risk of heart disease. Adults appear to benefit from diets low in calories from fat. One might assume the same would be true for children, but is it really? Zealous parents, attempting to reduce their children's risk of future heart disease, can err in placing their children on a diet too low in fat. When foods are eliminated from the diet to keep the percentage of fat low, children may fail to get enough calories, protein, and such important nutrients as vitamin B12, niacin, and riboflavin. Because extremely low-fat diets don't satisfy hunger for long, children might compensate by eating high-sugar snacks. For example, in the Bogalusa Heart Study, children with low fat intakes consumed more sugar than those with higher fat intakes, in part because they consumed more beverages and candy (Nicklaus, Webber, Koschak, & Berenson, 1992). Parents and professionals must be careful to avoid extremes in children's diets. All three of the major foodstuffs,

- protein,
- carbohydrate, and
- fat,

are important to growth, and well-balanced meals also contain a balance of vitamins and minerals. While limiting the number of calories from fat is desirable, it is clear that an extremely low-fat diet could be harmful by limiting

- total calories,
- essential fatty acids,
- vitamins,
- minerals, and
- protein.

Until longitudinal research can assess the long-term effects of a very low-fat diet on children's growth and development, moderation is the most appropriate approach.

---

### REVIEW 7.4

Body composition is important for several health and social reasons, including its relation to physical fitness. Although body composition is controlled to an extent by genetic factors, the environmental factors of diet and exercise can greatly affect an individual's relative levels of fat and lean body mass. A person who wishes to change his or her body mass can manipulate both diet and exercise. People at any age can bring about favorable changes in body composition through regular, vigorous exercise. Specifically, lean body mass increases at the expense of fat weight. Because dramatic reductions in caloric intake alone can result in a loss of lean body mass in adults or in cessation of growth in children, exercise should be an important aspect of any weight-reduction program.

### SUMMARY

Children's capacity for exercise and physical activity typically improve as they grow older. This improvement is related to the greater endurance and increased strength that accompany an increase in body size, especially in lean body mass. A child's physical fitness is also improved through training. Educators should understand how the roles of growth and training combine in improving fitness. The fitness improvements associated with growth can mask the negative effects of a sedentary lifestyle in childhood and adolescence. Training definitely improves endurance after puberty and might improve it in childhood, although the childhood training levels necessary to obtain notable gains are not yet defined. Training improves strength, helps maintain flexibility, and has a favorable effect on body composition. A sound diet also contributes to healthy body composition.

Although gender differences in fitness are minimal in childhood, differences can be noted after puberty. Men add more muscle mass and less fat weight to their bodies in adolescence than women do, and, as a result, the average man has more absolute endurance and strength than the average woman. However, women who train regularly can be more fit than sedentary men. We should look beyond the stereotypical lifestyles of the sexes to fully comprehend the potential for fitness that can be achieved by both sexes through training.

The benefits of training continue in adulthood. In fact, many of the stereotypical characteristics of aging are minimized or forestalled in those with active lifestyles. Activities that promote endurance, strength, flexibility, and low body fat improve fitness at any age, whereas inactivity leads to a loss of fitness and a tendency toward increased fat tissue at any age. Some questions regarding the impact of an active lifestyle on life expectancy remain to be answered by research, but little doubt exists that good physical health and fitness improve the quality of life. Several myths about fitness—for example, that children are naturally fit, and that older adults necessarily lose fitness—are incorrect. Replacing these myths is the view that activity is desirable and beneficial throughout life.

## Key Terms

aerobic capacity
aerobic power
anaerobic capacity
anaerobic power
atrophy
cardiorespiratory endurance
hypokinetic circulation
lean body mass
maximum oxygen consumption
physical fitness
power
progressive overload
vital capacity
working capacity

## Discussion Questions

1. Which of the following aspects of physical fitness can prepubescent children improve with training: anaerobic endurance, aerobic endurance, strength, flexibility? Which can postpubescent adolescents improve with training?
2. Give an example of an anaerobic activity and an example of an aerobic activity.
3. How do anaerobic endurance and aerobic endurance change with growth?
4. How do anaerobic endurance and aerobic endurance change with aging?
5. How does the rate of increase in strength with growth compare to the rate of increase in muscle mass? How does the rate of decrease in strength and muscle mass compare in aging?
6. How does flexibility change with growth and with aging?
7. How does participation in regular physical activity affect body composition in children and adolescents?
8. What are the best weight-management strategies for obese children?

9. What are the gender differences in the development of endurance, strength, and flexibility in children and adolescents?
10. What fitness components can older adults improve with training?

## Suggested Readings

Bailey, D.A., Malina, R.M., & Rasmussen, R.L. (1978). The influence of exercise, physical activity, and athletic performance on the dynamics of human growth. In F. Falkner & J.M. Tanner (Eds.), *Human growth* (Vol. 2) (pp. 475-505). New York: Plenum.

Gisolfi, C.V., & Lamb, D.R. (Eds.) (1989). *Perspectives in exercise science and sports medicine, Volume 2: Youth, exercise, and sport*. Indianapolis: Benchmark.

Malina, R.M., & Bouchard, C. (1991). *Growth, maturation, and physical activity*. Champaign, IL: Human Kinetics.

Parizkova, J. (1977). *Body fat and physical fitness*. The Hague, Netherlands: Martinus Nijhoff B.V.

Rarick, G.L. (Ed.) (1973). *Physical activity: Human growth and development*. New York: Academic Press.

Rowland, T.W. (1990). *Exercise and children's health*. Champaign, IL: Human Kinetics.

Shephard, R.J. (1978). *Physical activity and aging*. Chicago: Year Book Medical.

Shephard, R.J. (1982). *Physical activity and growth*. Chicago: Year Book Medical.

Smith, E.L., & Serfass, R.C. (Eds.) (1981). *Exercise and aging: The scientific basis*. Hillside, NJ: Enslow.

Stamford, B.A. (1988). Exercise and the elderly. In K.B. Pandolf (Ed.), *Exercise and sport sciences reviews* (Vol. 16) (pp. 341-379). New York: Macmillan.

## Chapter 8

# Information Processing, Memory, and Knowledge Development

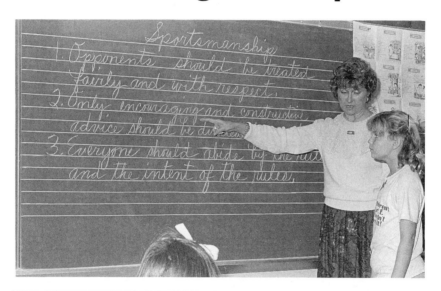

### CHAPTER CONCEPTS

**8.1**
We can study the perceptual-cognitive processes by using information processing models.

**8.2**
The amount of useful information that an individual can process increases during childhood to an optimal level in adulthood, but some decline is apparent in older adulthood.

**8.3**
Children use their memory systems more effectively as they mature, whereas older adults can experience memory deficits.

Information is critical to skill performance. How can you successfully throw a ball for distance, for example, without knowing what release angle is likely to produce a long throw? Or how can a basketball player successfully defend a pick without any prior experience with this offensive maneuver? Lack of knowledge can limit performance just as much as lack of strength or coordination. Age-related changes occur in *cognition*. The development of perceptual-cognitive systems influences motor development.

We will begin the discussion of perceptual-cognitive development with an example of a computerlike information processing model, then discuss age-related differences in various perceptual-cognitive processes from this perspective, and finally identify shortcomings and weaknesses in this perspective.

## INFORMATION PROCESSING PERSPECTIVE

We observed in chapter 1 that our current knowledge of the development of *perceptual-cognitive processes* is derived mostly from an information processing perspective. Scientists with this perspective model human brain functions after computers, so humans are said to process information in a series of steps, just as computers process data in a series of calculations. Movement scientists first studied the information processing steps in adults, then motor developmentalists studied children and older adults. As a result, age-related differences in the perceptual-cognitive processes were identified. The information processing perspective dominated the movement sciences in the 1970s and is still used today. The *dynamic systems* perspective has emerged recently to challenge some of the basic assumptions of the information processing perspective. However, there has been insufficient time for this new perspective to address all of the aspects of behavior explored from the information process-

ing perspective. Also, the information processing perspective yields valuable information about many aspects of motor behavior.

---

**CONCEPT 8.1**

We can study the perceptual-cognitive processes by using information processing models.

---

### Information Processing Models

Information processing models of the brain describe how information proceeds through various perceptual then cognitive steps and culminates with a decision to respond by moving the body in a particular way. These *perceptual-cognitive steps*, or components, are functional rather than structural; that is, they represent processes that appear to be involved in skill performance, based on either logical assessment of what must precede a skilled response or research investigations of these processes. They do not necessarily represent locations or centers in the nervous system. They are pictured to represent their proposed relationship to one another. Figure 8.1 is an example of such a model. Let's consider a single motor skill and follow the processing of information needed to perform this skill through the perceptual-cognitive steps.

## Using a Model to Analyze Information Processing

Imagine a basketball player who wants to pass to a teammate sprinting down the court. The passer's sensory receptors receive stimuli and transduce (convert) them to neural information:

- Kinesthetic stimuli regarding the passer's body orientation and limb position
- Light waves indicating the position and movement of the teammate and other players
- Sound waves generated by the players and fans

The passer holds this sensory input briefly in the *sensory register* component of memory. The player can selectively filter the sensory input and attend only to the information critical for the response. For example, the passer needs to attend to instructions from teammates and coaches but ignore crowd noises. He or she need not be passive but can orient the eyes, ears, and body to better receive relevant stimuli. The nervous system must *encode* the neural signals arising from environmental events, transforming them into an electrochemical form that can be processed or manipulated, then stored, in the brain. It is possible that the brain codes different types of information in different ways. For example, visual images might be coded differently from spoken words.

Next, the passer must integrate the signals from the various sensory systems. The sound of the teammate running down the court must be matched to the visual image of this event. This new perceptual information must now be interpreted and analyzed, in part by being compared to similar experiences. This requires the retrieval of memories from storage. Based on this analysis, the passer selects a response. It is unlikely that humans store a different motor response for each set of unique stimulus situations. Rather, the system generalizes. This generalization takes the form of a *schema*, a set of rules governing a class of situations. For example, the basketball player's previous experiences passing to a moving teammate result in a schema that allows him or her to project the receiver's position and select the appropriate throw.

These phases of information processing take place in a *channel*, or path of limited capacity. This means that the passer can deal with only a limited amount of information at one time. If the passer is inundated by too much information it will take too long for her to select a response. Of course, the situation may change by that time—for example, a defender may catch up with the teammate—and the selected response is now inappropriate. Skilled performers often overcome this limited capacity by grouping bits of information into patterns or categories. The passer might see the teammate's position and a defender's position as a relationship rather than as two individual paths that must both be projected to their future positions.

Once the player selects the response, it may be held in *choice delay*, if necessary, until the appropriate time for execution. The passer might wait until the receiver is far enough from a defender so that the ball is not intercepted. As the player executes the response, he or she compares it with the intended response. If the response is not being carried out as planned, some immediate correction is possible. The correction takes time, of course, so performers can correct only those movements that take longer than 500 msec. This information about the ongoing response is termed *internal feedback*. *External feedback* also is generated during and after the response—for example, seeing the receiver either catch the ball or miss it. Internal and external feedback are additional

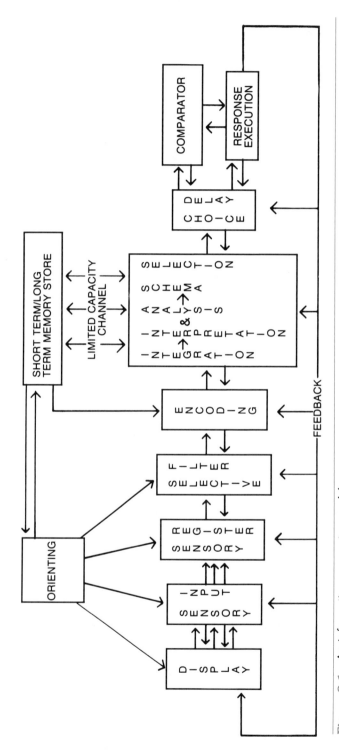

**Figure 8.1** An information processing model.
(Adapted by permission from Rothstein, 1977.)

input to the system. The response and its feedback are used to improve the schema for this class of skills. The player will benefit from this experience when a similar situation arises in the future.

---

## REVIEW 8.1

We can model perceptual-cognitive processes of the human brain after computers so that we can study the brain's step-by-step processing of information. This approach is derived from the information processing perspective, and it facilitates our studies. However, the new dynamic systems perspective challenges some aspects of this older perspective.

## INFORMATION PROCESSING CAPACITY

The preceding example of information processing serves as the background for an analysis of developmental factors in information processing. Although little is known about the development of some perceptual-cognitive processes, information available on others contributes to our understanding of the development and stability of skill learning and performance from early childhood through older adulthood.

---

### CONCEPT 8.2
The amount of useful information that an individual can process increases during childhood to an optimal level in adulthood, but some decline is apparent in older adulthood.

## Information Processing in Childhood

Age differences exist in the selective filtering and attention component of information processing. Young children seem less capable than adults of identifying relevant stimuli in the visual field and attending to them exclusive of irrelevant stimuli. For example, Smith, Kemler, and Aronfried (1975) found that children ages 5 and 6 attended to both relevant and irrelevant stimuli in a display. In contrast, older children, ages 7 and 8 years and 10 and 11 years, attended to more of the relevant stimuli, picking up irrelevant stimuli incidentally. Children up to age 12 also seem to weigh auditory stimuli too heavily compared with visual stimuli, diverting some of their attention away from critical visual information (Perelle, 1975).

Ross (1976) proposed that the development of attention occurs in three stages:

1. Infants and young children attend to one stimulus in the display exclusive of all others, termed the *overexclusive* mode.
2. In the next stage, the *overinclusive* mode, older children and preadolescents attend to many stimuli in the display, some of them irrelevant to the task at hand, as did the 5- and 6-year-olds of Smith et al. (1975).
3. Transition to the third stage, *selective attention*, is typically complete by age 12, so that adolescents can focus on the relevant stimuli even in complex displays.

Age differences in attention probably relate to age differences in experience. Whereas adolescents and adults know from past experience which stimuli are relevant to a particular response and which are not, children have more limited past experiences. Educators can assist children by pointing out the relevant stimuli in a task. Patterson and Mischel (1975) demonstrated that children can be taught to resist irrelevant cues, and Stratton (1978b) noted that children can acquire selective attention strategies. Is it helpful to have children learn in a sterile environment? Probably not, because children can actually benefit by learning a skill in the presence of irrelevant stimuli if those stimuli will be present during performance. As long as the irrelevant cues do not prevent them from learning the skill, children can learn to attend to the relevant stimuli and filter out irrelevant stimuli (Stratton, 1978a).

Children obviously become more efficient in processing increasingly larger amounts of information as they mature. We could attribute this to an increase in the child's limited capacity channel, but a variety of other factors can be involved as well (Rothstein, 1977). One might be children's improving ability to integrate information from the different sensory systems, as discussed in concept 6.2. Improved memory control processes, which we will discuss later in this chapter, might also contribute to improved information processing. The development of improved schemata and perhaps the development of *subroutines* for basic parts of complex tasks could also influence the efficiency.

Subroutines (the directions for basic components of more complex movement tasks) could be executed automatically, thus requiring little of the performer's attention and freeing it for attention to other factors. Whether an increased channel capacity or some of these other factors are involved, you can expect children to handle more information as they mature.

## The Use of Schemata

The earlier sketch of an information processing model included schemata, or generalized programs for executing a response. Think of performers as having programs consisting of commands for carrying out the many muscle contractions they need to make a motor response. A performer can apply a schema in

many ways, depending on the exact environmental conditions. A program based on the schema would designate which muscles contract and their order, force, and temporal pattern (Schmidt, 1977). When the performer executes this response, the initial conditions, intended response, feedback from this response, and movement outcome are related to one another. And for every such response made over time, the performer abstracts a relationship between the intended response (based on the initial conditions) and the movement outcome. The performer can generalize from his many individual experiences. Children have had few experiences from which to generalize. Their schemata, then, are not as accurate or as powerful as those of adults in adapting to a variety of initial conditions.

It follows that children benefit from practicing skills in a variety of conditions rather than in restricted settings where initial conditions are relatively constant. Two research teams support this reasoning. The first, Kerr and Booth (1977), divided children into two groups, both of which learned an underhand tossing task with their eyes closed. The groups had equal amounts of practice. One group practiced only at a distance of 3 ft, whereas the other practiced at both 2 ft and 4 ft. Therefore, one group practiced under more variable conditions than the other. The test was to execute the task at 3 ft. The variable-practice group outperformed the restricted-practice group, even though the latter group had practiced at the test distance.

Carson and Wiegand (1979) further demonstrated an advantage of variable practice: better retention of a motor skill. In this investigation preschoolers practiced tossing bean bags for accuracy under variable or restricted conditions. After 2 weeks the researchers tested the children on the task to determine how well they had retained their skill. The children who practiced in the highly variable situation retained their skill better than the others. Both of these studies indicated that though young children have less refined schemata than adolescents or adults, they are better able to form schemata for motor responses by practicing in variable conditions.

## Feedback

Movement scientists recognize that feedback is one of the most influential factors in skill performance. This is particularly true for children in the early stages of forming schemata for various skills. At the same time, it is clear that children often do not recognize the relevant stimuli amidst the *perceptual display* presented to them. You might expect, then, that children benefit from augmented feedback that a teacher provides, such as "You swung too late," and from hints on which aspects of the available feedback are particularly relevant, such as reminding children to feel for a level swing. Yet children cannot make use of too much information. For example, the teacher who says, "You stepped to the left instead of straight ahead, dropped your rear shoulder, swung too late, and did not follow through," probably has overwhelmed the child.

---

In teaching children, educators should provide information feedback but in a limited quantity for any single performance.

---

## Neuromuscular Control

Another aspect of performance that undergoes development is neuromuscular control, or the execution of muscular contractions in the proper patterns, sequence, and timing. Williams (1981) identified two age-related changes in neuromuscular control. The first is refinement of force production. Shambes (1976) found that when young children tried to maintain certain balance positions, they used more force than necessary and sometimes more muscle groups than necessary compared with skilled adults.

Because training produces changes in the timing of motor unit firing (contraction of a muscle fiber group), children probably learn to refine their force production through practice. Simard (1969) demonstrated that children as young as 3 and as old as 12 could be taught some degree of control in maintaining the activity of a motor unit. In addition, children undergo an age-related improvement in their ability to inhibit a muscle contraction, also a necessary aspect of skilled movement, because an opposing muscle group must be inhibited just before the prime muscles execute a movement. Gatev (1972) observed that infants up to 9 months old executed movements without well-defined inhibitory processes. Two- and 3-year-olds demonstrated improved but still immature inhibitory processes.

Therefore, it appears that the neuromuscular control phase of movement is not fully operational at birth but also undergoes a developmental process. It is likely that this aspect of performance is related to the development of improved response schemata. A variety of motor experiences, then, are of great value in helping children to refine their neuromuscular control.

## Speed of Processing Information

In addition to these developments in the component steps of information processing, the speed of processing increases as children mature. This is apparent in even the simplest of motor responses, a reaction-time task. Simple reaction time is the time between the onset of a stimulus (such as a light or buzzer) and the beginning of a movement (such as lifting a finger from a button). The maximum speed of this response increases from age 3 through adolescence (Wickens, 1974). An improvement with age also occurs in the time required to respond in continuous tracking (Pew & Rupp, 1971). In this type of task, children must continuously match their movement to a target. For example, a video game in which the player controls the image of a car with a joystick to keep the car on a curved road is a continuous tracking task. Factors considered to be *central processes* (processes of the central nervous system) appear responsible for the slower processing speed that children exhibit (Elliott, 1972). Attention is one such central process, and speed of the memory processes (discussed later in this chapter) is another.

The speed with which an individual can select motor responses is a function of age (Wickens, 1974). Clark (1982) demonstrated this by manipulating the spatial stimulus-response compatibility of a reaction-time task when testing 6-year-olds, 10-year-olds, and adults. In the compatible condition, participants pressed a key on the right if the right stimulus light came on and a key on the left if the left light came on. In the incompatible condition, participants pressed a key opposite the direction of the light. Spatial compatibility, then, affects the participant's response selection. Clark found that processing time decreased in the older groups tested in the incompatible condition.

Although these central factors of attention, memory, and response selection influence children's slower processing speeds, peripheral factors do not. For example, nerve impulse conduction speed in the peripheral nerves does not contribute substantially to the speed differences between children and adults.

---

Young children are able to process information faster as they mature because of improvements in central factors such as response selection and speed of the memory processes.

---

## Information Processing in Older Adults

Similar to young children, older adults exhibit limitations in the processing of information. These limitations are also apparently related to central processes. But researchers have found important differences between performers at opposite ends of the life span. For example, older adults do not exhibit declining performance in all types of skills. They undergo little change in their performance of single, discrete actions that can be planned in advance (Welford, 1977b) or on simple, continuous, and repetitive actions, such as alternately tapping two targets (Welford, Norris, & Shock, 1969). However, in actions requiring a series of different movements, especially when speed is important (Welford, 1977c), older adults show a large decrement in performance. The major limitations on older adults, then, seem to involve the decisions they base on perceptual information and the programming of movement sequences (Welford, 1980b). These are central rather than peripheral factors. Let's consider in more detail some of the central components of information processing that are affected by aging.

Older adults apparently learn new tasks, whether cognitive or motor, more slowly than younger adults. For example, rote learning of cognitive material is slower in older adults, because they need more repetitions to reach criterion—that is, to learn the material at a predesignated level. This may reflect the need for more time for the information to register in the long-term memory store. Similarly, older adults improve more slowly than younger adults in new motor skills, although they maintain well the skills they learned early in life (Szafran, 1951; Welford, 1980b).

Attentional factors also play a role in the performance limitations of older adults. Older adults perform their fastest on a reaction-time task when a warning signal is given a consistent time before the stimulus, but their slowest when the warning signal interval varies from trial to trial. This suggests that a fixed interval minimizes distraction by irrelevant associations (Birren, 1964). Rabbitt (1965) also demonstrated that older adults are hampered more than younger adults by the presence of irrelevant stimuli in a card-sorting task. In this task, participants are challenged to sort a stack of cards based on information given on the card face, such as the shape of a symbol or its color. If information on the card face is not relevant to the sorting task, older adults' performance suffers compared with that of younger adults.

Many older adults do not attend to critical stimuli as well as they did when younger and are more easily distracted. The cause of this decline in performance might be a lowered *signal-to-noise ratio* in the central nervous system (CNS). The neural impulses of the CNS take place against a background of random neural noise such that the effectiveness of a neural signal depends on the ratio between the signal strength and the background noise—the signal-to-noise ratio. As a person ages, signal levels within the CNS decrease because of changes in the sense organs, loss of brain cells, and factors affecting brain cell functioning, while at the same time, noise level increases (Crossman & Szafran, 1956; Welford, 1977a). Older adults can compensate for this lower signal-to-noise ratio if they are given extra time to complete a task, but if they must perform a series of movements or make a series of decisions rapidly, they are at a disadvantage.

Central factors also influence the slower speed of information processing in older adults. Researchers have consistently documented a slowing of reaction time with aging. Although a slight slowing of neural impulse conduction velocity is associated with aging, it is not great enough to account for the magnitude of lengthened reaction times. *Choice reaction time* slows in older adults even more than simple reaction time. In choice reaction-time tasks, a performer is challenged to respond to one of several signals with a particular response matched to each signal. (A *simple reaction-time* task consists of one signal and one response.) Making this task more complex by increasing the number of signals or designating responses that are less logical (pressing the left button in response to the right signal light, for

example) disproportionately increases older adults' reaction time compared to that of younger adults (Cerella, Poon, & Williams, 1980; Welford, 1977a, 1977b).

Older adults' movement time, too, shows a very slight slowing (Singleton, 1955), but they maintain the speed of planned, repetitive movements such as tapping (Fieandt, Huhtala, Kullberg, & Saari, 1956). Because almost all behaviors mediated by the central nervous system slow down as an adult ages, central factors are assumed to be largely responsible for slower information processing speed (Birren, 1964). Recognize, though, that the schemata of older adults can be particularly complete and refined for skills with which the adult has had a lifetime of experience. This experience is particularly helpful when accuracy is more important than speed.

---

*When older adults are not pressed to perform as quickly as possible, they demonstrate very accurate performance on well-practiced tasks.*

---

Several studies also document less dramatic slowing in older adults who maintain active lifestyles. When Spirduso (1975) tested both active and inactive older men for simple reaction time, she found the active men were not much slower than younger men. The inactive older men were significantly slower than younger men. All of the older men had slower choice reaction times, but the gap between the younger men and the active older men was smaller than that between the younger men and the inactive older men. The same is true for older women (Rikli & Busch, 1986; Spirduso, 1980).

Because the nature of slowing in older adults implicates CNS functioning, maintaining an active lifestyle must have some effect on central processes. Two possibilities exist. Perhaps exercise enhances the production or functioning of neurotransmitters within the brain (Spirduso, Gilliam, & Wilcox, 1984).

Neurotransmitters carry neural signals between neurons. Or exercise might increase oxygenation of the tissues, and oxygen plays a role in CNS energy metabolism (Birren, Woods, & Williams, 1980; Shephard & Kavanaugh, 1978). In either case, exercisers would maintain better cognitive and motor functioning than nonexercisers.

Dustman et al. (1989) found this to be the case. They placed sedentary 55- to 70-year-olds on a 4-month aerobic exercise program and compared them to both strength-and-flexibility exercisers and nonexercisers on a battery of cognitive and motor tests. Among the tests were a culturally unbiased IQ test and a reaction-time test. Both exercise groups improved, but the aerobic exercisers improved significantly more (see Figure 8.2).

---

Exercise, especially aerobic, is associated with improved information processing for both cognitive and motor tasks in older adults.

---

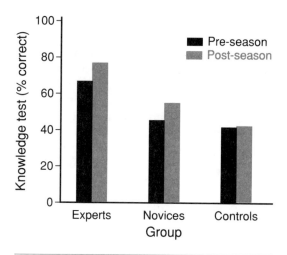

**Figure 8.2** The standard scores (averaged over a battery of eight cognitive and motor tests) for three groups of older adults: aerobic exercisers, strength and flexibility (control) exercisers, and nonexercisers. The exercise programs lasted 4 months. The *p* values indicate that the exercisers improved significantly but the control group did not.
(Reprinted by permission from Dustman et al., 1989.)

## Differing Viewpoints

In chapter 1 we acknowledged that no theoretical perspective is perfect. We should be aware that the information processing perspective has shortcomings, although we appreciate the age-related differences that researchers using this perspective have identified.

Information processing is based on the assumption that humans operate like machines. Although this analogy allows us to study many of the perceptual-cognitive processes, it still includes the idea that an intelligent executive is part of the machine. Movement scientists sometimes call this executive a "little man" or *homunculus* inside the brain, or even a "ghost in the machine" (Kelso, 1982; Koestler & Smythies, 1969). So, some explain the human brain in part by saying it contains something like a human. We could go on and on, explaining each little man with another little man, creating a problem called infinite regress.

Information processing also hypothesizes that all the information an individual needs to move in a skilled way is stored in the brain. To execute complex movements, the brain issues a large number of specific commands to the muscles. In this perspective, these extensive directions are compared to computer programs with subroutines for some of the common, well-learned basic movements. The problem with this notion is that, considering how often we must adapt our movements to different and changing environmental conditions, skilled performers can make an almost infinite number of unique movements. Though our brains have a large capacity, that capacity certainly is not infinite. It logically has limitations.

Recently, the dynamic systems perspective has become more popular because it offers alternative explanations for these weaker aspects of the information processing perspective. Rather than emphasizing the performer alone, dynamic systems emphasize the interaction of the performer, the environment, and the task. Movement is thought to emerge from this interaction, with some aspects of movement being self-organized. The brain, then, does not have to direct every aspect of a movement in detail. The size, shape, and structure of the human body gives its movement typical forms, but the system is flexible enough to meet the varied environmental conditions that an individual encounters.

Dynamicists have not yet dealt with all aspects of human behavior from their perspective. So again, there is no one "correct" perspective on how movement occurs or develops. It will help you, though, to think of the perceptual-cognitive processes as one of the body's many systems that come together when skills are performed. Throughout the life span, the status of this system can influence movement. A child who cannot attend to the relevant environmental conditions cannot perform optimally. An older adult whose cognitive processes have slowed cannot perform as well as a young adult when a task demands optimal speed. A performer of any age is limited by a lack of knowledge of the sport being performed. The perceptual-cognitive processes are an important aspect of movement.

## REVIEW 8.2

We can study age-related differences in each of the perceptual-cognitive processes. As a result of age group comparisons, we know that many of the perceptual-cognitive processes develop over the course of childhood. Among them are attention and selective filtering, the formation of response schemata, and neuromuscular control. The speed of information processing also increases during childhood, which in turn contributes to improved motor performance.

At the opposite end of the life span, older adults demonstrate limitations in information processing. Attentional factors and speed of processing influence declining performance, perhaps reflecting changes in the signal-to-noise ratio within the central nervous system. Repetitive, self-paced tasks and accuracy tasks are not affected as much as tasks requiring a series of rapid movements.

An important aspect of motor performance is an individual's ability to relate present conditions for performance to memories of past experiences. We will discuss this aspect of information processing next.

## MEMORY

From the information processing perspective, memory influences children's improved performance in both motor skills and cognitive skills. When a young batter hits a pitched ball, a large influx of perceptual information combines with memories of previous experiences before the batter can make a response.

Evidence suggests that children do not use their memory systems as effectively as adults, and this could account for some of the performance differences between children and adults. Memory might play a role, too, in performance differences between young adults and older adults. Differences in effective use of the memory system could be due to the available mental capacity, the strategies of memory use, or perhaps a combination of both. Members of the Piagetian school of thought proposed that mental capacity increases with age (Pascual-Leone, 1970; Case, 1972a, 1972b, 1974), but other developmentalists favor the view that processing strategies are deficient in, or unavailable to, children. Both groups present supporting evidence, but current research leans toward the idea that strategies of memory use best explain motor performance differences between age groups (Chi, 1976; Thomas, 1980). These strategies, or control processes, refer to how an individual handles information and include the development and use of remembering strategies; rehearsal strategies; and labeling, grouping, and coding information to be remembered.

Let us examine the evidence supporting the assertion that *control processing strategies* rather than *memory capacity* are the key to memory development. We will also discuss the development of memory strategies and their persistence throughout adulthood.

---

**CONCEPT 8.3**

Children use their memory systems more effectively as they mature, whereas older adults can experience memory deficits.

---

## Models of Memory

Before we discuss the development of memory, it is valuable that you recognize some of the models of memory that explain how adults recall and recognize information. Movement scientists have suggested many such models, but most fall into one of two categories—multistore models or levels of processing models. Neither type of model was originally proposed to explain the development of memory in children, but they provide the context and terminology for much of the developmental research. A basic knowledge of these two frameworks will therefore help you understand the developmental work on memory.

The multistore models of memory have in common the notion of three memory-storage components:

1. The *sensory store*
2. The *short-term store*
3. The *long-term store*

The first holds sensory information for a brief time, perhaps only a second. The short-term store holds information for a matter of seconds but is limited in its capacity for information. The capacity of the long-term store is thought to be unlimited. Of course, the amount of information in long-term store depends on how many experiences you have had, so children would have less information in long-term store than adults would. Once information is placed in long-term store, it can remain there for life, although a person can have difficulty retrieving it from memory storage. An individual uses control processes or strategies to move information through the three storage components.

In the levels of processing models, remembering is related to the depth to which the information is processed. In other words, the more completely a person learns information, the better he remembers it. If a person originally processed the information in a superficial or shallow manner, he will not remember it well. The control processes are critical to this model in that use of these processes moves information to a deeper level of memory. However, both of the memory frameworks, multistore and levels of processing models, consider control processes to be important aspects of memory.

## Memory Capacity

Although researchers have established the importance of control processes to memory, we should consider whether the capacity of the mental space increases as a person ages either instead of or in addition to better usage of the control processes. Chi (1976) examined this point in a review of research studies that analyzed the capacity of children's short-term store. She found several studies that examined what is termed the *recency effect* (see Figure 8.3). In these studies subjects were presented lists of information to remember. On such a task people tend to remember more items from the end of the list (the more recent information)

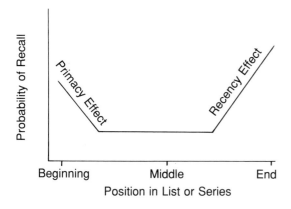

Figure 8.3    The "forgetting curve." Note that the probability of recall is highest for the beginning and the end of a list.

than from the middle. Although children make more errors than adults, the shape of the "forgetting curve" is relatively stable across age groups. Therefore, children evidently do not run out of short-term memory space when they get to the end of the list—that is, their memory capacity is not limited. If it were, children would make many more errors at the end of the list than adults do, which is not the case. Chi also found no evidence that children lose the information in short-term store faster than adults. Thus, research on the topic does not strongly support the view that children have more limited short-term storage capacity than adults do.

## Memory Control Processes

Now consider the various *control processes*, or memory strategies, and their development. These processes facilitate the movement of information into memory, so they can help you remember more effectively.

### Rehearsal

One of the most important control processes is *rehearsal*, in which the individual rehearses the information to be remembered in a serial fashion and continually attends to it in the short-term memory store (Chi, 1976). This process is similar to repeating a phone number, but it need not be overt. Rehearsal is under an individual's control, and it takes time. This strategy is not widely used by children under 5 years old (Chi, 1976; Daehler, Horowitz, Wynns, & Flavell, 1969). Educators can instruct children ages 4 and 5 to use verbal rehearsal in motor performance, such as saying "jump" when they jump, to better remember a sequence of motor tasks. However, this verbal rehearsal fails to help children this young, because they do not realize the rehearsal is a strategy for recalling the task (Weiss, 1983).

After age 5, children begin to use rehearsal strategies, and the strategies become more sophisticated, at least through age 11 (Ornstein & Naus, 1978). You can see this improvement in part by observing the pause time between the items the individual is learning. Young children do not pause to rehearse between items, in contrast to adolescents and adults. Chi (1976) proposes that children learn to rehearse in three stages. They first assemble the rehearsal process, then learn when to execute the process, and finally learn to execute it correctly.

Teaching children a rehearsal strategy in addition to the skill itself will enhance their skill acquisition (Thomas, Thomas, & Gallagher, 1981).

### Labeling

The control process termed naming or *labeling* refers to the attachment of a verbal label to a stimulus. It is likely that children remember less than adults because of a deficient naming process. Very young children might label information to be remembered, but they fail to use the labels to help themselves remember. Instructing children to use labels improves their recall, although it is important that the label be meaningful.

## Grouping

Another memory strategy is *grouping* or chunking, wherein the individual places information to be remembered into subgroups. Adults demonstrate grouping, but young children do not (Belmont & Butterfield, 1971). Yet when children over 7 are taught to use adult grouping strategies, their performance improves (Harris & Burke, 1972; Liberty & Ornstein, 1973; McCarver, 1972). Gallagher and Thomas (1980a) also demonstrated that presenting arm movements in an organized order helped children 7 and older recall the movements.

## Recoding

Another process that young children do not use is *recoding*. This involves searching the short-term store for two or more items that can be combined, based on some similarity, and then reentering the new code into the long-term store as a single item. For example, a tennis player encounters many balls with backspin during a practice session. The player then combines the knowledge gained from these occurrences and recodes them as information about balls with backspin.

## Knowledge Bases

At any age, memory for a particular topic improves as you acquire more knowledge about that topic (Chi, 1981). Children undoubtedly have a smaller base of knowledge than adults because they have had fewer experiences. Perhaps children have poorer memories compared to adults partly because they do not know as much as adults about as many topics. In fact, children who become experts on a particular topic can outperform adults in that area. Chi (1978) observed child experts in chess recall

significantly more chess positions than adult novices in chess. Why would performance be related to size of the knowledge base? There are at least three reasons:

1. Increased knowledge reduces the need to hold a great deal of information in the short-term store (Chase & Simon, 1973).
2. Increased knowledge allows more effective use of the control processes (Ornstein & Naus, 1984, cited in Thomas, French, Thomas, & Gallagher, 1988).
3. Increased knowledge reduces the amount of conscious attention needed to perform some tasks (Leavitt, 1979).

So to play sports well, children need not only to practice their physical skills, they need knowledge of sports as well.

## Types of Knowledge

Before considering the development of knowledge about sport, we must identify the types of knowledge and the differences between experts and novices. Chi (1981) has defined three types of knowledge:

1. *Declarative knowledge*, which is knowing factual information
2. *Procedural knowledge*, which is knowing how to do something and doing it in accordance with specific rules
3. *Strategic knowledge*, which is knowing general rules or strategies that apply to many topics

Declarative and procedural knowledge are specific to a certain topic; strategic knowledge can be generalized. For example, an athlete who understands how to execute a give and go (pass to a teammate, then advance toward the goal or basket for a return pass) in basketball can execute a give and go in hockey or soccer, provided she has the physical skills to do so. Experts have more declarative and procedural knowledge than novices (Chi, 1978; Chi &

Koeske, 1983; Chiesi, Spilich, & Voss, 1979; Spilich, Vesonder, Chiesi, & Voss, 1979). Experts independently organize the information they know in a similar way (Chiesi et al., 1979; Murphy & Wright, 1984)—that is, experts structure information differently than novices. By organizing their information in a methodical structure, such as a hierarchy, experts facilitate their memory recall of information.

Thomas and his colleagues (Thomas et al., 1988, adapted from Berliner, 1986) identified other, sport-specific ways in which experts and novices differ. Those pertinent to our discussion are as follows:

- Experts make more inferences about objects and events. In sport, this helps experts to predict upcoming events and anticipate the most likely occurrences.

- Experts analyze problems at a more advanced level. For example, expert athletes probably think of offensive plays as concepts rather than lists of individual players' movements.

- Experts quickly recognize patterns. For example, expert sport participants quickly recognize defensive configurations.

- Experts preplan their responses for specific situations. Softball infielders, for example, do this before the batter hits, when they identify the base to which they will throw, considering the runners on base and the number of outs.

- Experts tend to organize knowledge in relation to the goal of the game. For example, an expert basketball player thinks of offensive strategies in terms of those that successfully attack a zone defense versus those that attack a player-to-player defense, not as a long list of individual offenses.

- Experts spend much time learning about their topics. Sport expertise, in particular, requires hours of practice and experience, especially if a player wants to develop procedural, how-to knowledge.

Keep in mind that expertise is specific. For sport and dance, this means that individuals become experts in specific sports (tennis, basketball, etc.) or dance forms (modern, ballroom, etc.). In addition, expert performers in sport and dance have a high level of physical skill. Both skill and the knowledge of how to use skills in specific situations are necessary for success (Thomas et al., 1988).

## Development of a Knowledge Base

Let us consider how individuals, especially children, develop a knowledge base in a particular sport. They must acquire declarative knowledge first, to provide a foundation for procedural knowledge (Chi, 1981). Young children often lack declarative knowledge of a sport. They typically are novices who must learn game rules, goals, and strategies before they can exhibit procedural knowledge and make appropriate decisions as to which action to perform. Strategic knowledge is the last to develop. It requires experience with many different types of tasks, enabling children to generalize across topics.

French and Thomas (1987) conducted one of the first studies of knowledge development in sport with children. They proposed that children need both declarative knowledge of basketball and basketball skills to make appropriate decisions while playing basketball. Coaches classified the 8- to 12-year-old boys in a youth basketball program based on their skills, knowledge of the game, and ability to make good judgments in a game. The best third of the group was designated the expert group and the bottom third the novice group. The boys in these two groups then were tested on their basketball knowledge and skills. In individual interviews, they were asked to give the appropriate action for each of five basketball game situations described to them. The researchers also observed the players during games and graded their decisions as appropriate or inappropriate. The experts scored much better than the novices on both the knowledge and skill tests. More importantly, the experts chose the appropriate action in game situations more often than novices. During their situation interviews, experts were more likely to give answers dependent on the action of the opponents and gave more alternatives, indicating better memory of basketball knowledge.

French and Thomas observed some of the 8- to 10-year-old boys from their first study over the course of a season, along with a group of boys who did not play basketball. By the end of the season, both expert and novice players were making better decisions about actions and scored better on the knowledge test (see Figure 8.4). The control group made no significant progress. Interestingly, none of the children improved in physical skill over the season, either on skill tests or in game play. This initial study, then, indicates that basketball knowledge is related to children's skill performance and that children might acquire knowledge faster than they improve their physical skills.

Teachers and coaches would benefit from continued study of knowledge development in

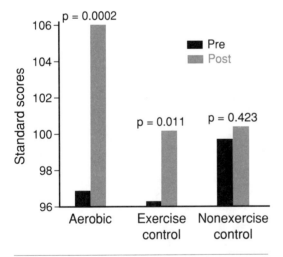

**Figure 8.4** Both expert and novice boys scored better on a postseason basketball knowledge test than on a preseason test. A control group did not improve.
(Drawn from data from French & Thomas, 1987.)

sport. It might well be that educators could improve children's skill acquisition in sport and dance by using appropriately timed instruction of and emphasis on rules, formations, strategies, and goals. Increased knowledge enhances memory.

Gender differences in sport performance might be attributable in part to differences between boys' and girls' knowledge of sport. Society makes it easier for boys to acquire sport knowledge by targeting sport-related merchandise to them—board and electronic games, books, collector cards, and so on. Girls' use of these items is viewed as less appropriate to their gender role, and as a result a performance gap between boys and girls might persist. Also, children who practice more probably acquire more knowledge, so unequal opportunities to participate might widen the performance gap between boys and at least some girls (Thomas et al., 1988).

## Speed of Memory Functions

In addition to the differences in the control processes themselves, there is a difference in the speed with which young children and adults perform memory functions. Children take longer than adults to process information to be remembered. As children get older, they eventually can process either the same amount of information faster or more information in the same amount of time. Because speed is so important in many skills, memory processing speed influences motor performance.

Age-related differences in memory processing speed are apparent when we look at two aspects of processing, encoding and use of *knowledge of results* (KR). For example, Chi (1977a, 1977b) found that speed of encoding is slower in children than in adults. The 5-year-olds she studied required more than twice as much time to identify pictures of classmates, implying that the adults encoded information to be remembered twice as fast as children. This

## Assessing Cognitive Decision Making

In their study of knowledge development in sport, French and Thomas (1987) needed to assess the decisions that young basketball players actually made during games. The written knowledge test and interview yielded useful information, but it was not certain that the players who gave good answers to questions away from the court would make good decisions in a fast-moving, demanding game situation.

To assess decision making in games, French and Thomas designed an observational instrument based on a typical offensive sequence in basketball: When a player catches the ball, he or she must decide to hold the ball, pass, dribble, or shoot. They identified all the decisions a player could make, then categorized them as appropriate or inappropriate.

French and Thomas videotaped youth basketball games. A trained basketball expert watched each player in each game for one quarter of playing time and coded each decision the player made when he received a pass. A second expert watched independently and coded some of the players to assure that an expert observer would code each decision the same way at least 90% of the time. The

observer gave a player a score of 1 for an appropriate decision and a score of 0 for an inappropriate decision. For example, a player received 1 point for passing to an open teammate but 0 for passing to a closely guarded teammate. In this way the researchers could measure the players' decision making in actual games.

Observational instruments are an excellent means of measuring behavior. Performers can be observed in real situations rather than in artificial laboratory conditions. Note, though, that French and Thomas had to develop a coding system that included all of the decisions a player could make. They then had to locate experts and train them to use the assessment instrument. Two experts independently coded some of the trials so the experimenters could cross-check those trials and assure themselves that the coding system was reliable. Finally, the observers coded from videotape so that they could stop the tape to record their judgments, thereby not missing any action. This is obviously a tedious procedure, but it provides an interesting and accurate measure of decision-making behaviors in sport.

---

permitted more time for further processing of the information in the adults' short-term store.

Studies of how children use information about the results of their performance—KR—provide more evidence of slower processing speeds in children. The precision of information given verbally to a performer when he completes a motor task is also important in processing speed; for example, you could say to a batter, "You missed," "You swung ahead of it," "You missed by 2 cm," or "You missed by 2.4 cm." When the time between KR and

the performer's next attempt at the task is held constant, adults typically perform better with more precise KR (unless the information is so precise as to be meaningless). However, this is not true with young children. Thomas, Mitchell, and Solomon (1979) gave both 2nd- and 4th-graders either no KR, general KR (you were short or long), or precise KR (how far short or long) after they performed trials of an arm positioning task. As you can see in Figure 8.5, the precision of KR was associated with reduced positioning error only in the older chil-

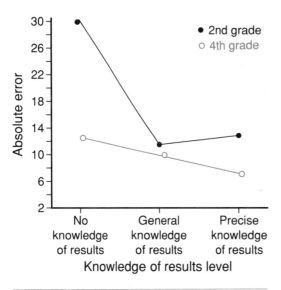

Figure 8.5   The interaction of grade level (age) and precision of knowledge of results for retention. (Reprinted by permission from Thomas, Mitchell, & Solomon, 1979.)

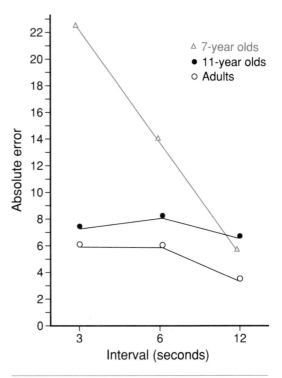

Figure 8.6   The interaction of age level and post-knowledge of results interval during performance of a ballistic movement. (Reprinted by permission from Gallagher & Thomas, 1980.)

dren. The younger children performed more poorly when given precise KR.

Presumably, the more precise the information, the greater the information load that the performer must process during this fixed time. The younger children could not process the increased information load of the precise KR in the time allotted, although it is possible that the precise KR was too complex for them. To clarify this issue, in a follow-up study Gallagher and Thomas (1980b) systematically varied the time following KR (see Figure 8.6). Children at age 7 performed far worse than 11-year-olds or adults when the time span was 3 sec. Their performances improved with 6 sec, but they did as well as the older groups only when they were given 12 sec to process the KR.

Children move information through their memory systems at a slower rate than adults, and this can affect their performance on tasks when speed is important.

## Changes in Memory in Older Adults

Older adults are generally able to recall less information than younger adults (Craik, 1977). There are two plausible explanations for this memory deficit. On one hand, the loss of neurons in the brain that occurs with aging could involve a change in the brain's structure. The other possibility is a change in the functioning of the memory processes. For example, the control processes may not be as efficient in older adults as in younger adults, or perhaps the speed of processing slows in old age. Because some research supports each explanation, we must consider both. It has even been suggested that a structural change is responsible for memory deficits in some older adults, while a functional change is responsible in others (Arenberg, 1980).

Some aspects of memory are affected as adults age, but others do not change. Smith (1980), for example, found little evidence that a storage deficit is involved in poorer memory. The memory span, or the number of information items that a person can hold in short-term store, remains constant at least until the 60s. However, older adults do not remember as well items that exceed the memory span (Welford, 1980a).

Processing deficits that involve encoding items into memory are characteristic of old age. A person's spontaneous organization of material to be remembered is particularly affected. Younger adults regularly organize material in anticipation of recalling the information, whereas older adults do so less often. Older adults may also be deficient in retrieving the information they have encoded into memory, but this is difficult to assess. When older adults fail to recall information, it may be either that they did not encode the information properly or that they encoded it but cannot retrieve it (Smith, 1980).

Persons who study memory using the levels of processing models alternately propose that memory deficits result because older adults' processing is shallower (more superficial), not because of encoding or retrieval deficits (Craik & Simon, 1980). Some evidence indicates that memory loss is due to the slowing of mental functions. Older adults employ the same control processes as younger adults but simply carry them out at a slower rate. For example, older adults rehearse more slowly than younger adults (Salthouse, 1980). The several plausible explanations of memory loss in older adults will be a research frontier for some time to come as investigators attempt to find the best answers.

Some feel that older adults who exercise regularly can better maintain memory functions. You'll recall that oxygen plays an important role in central nervous system energy metabolism. The increased oxygenation that accompanies aerobic exercise in particular could have a positive effect on cognitive functions in general and memory specifically. Abourezk (1989) examined short-term memory efficiency in 50- to 70-year-old men. Half were inactive, and half ran an average of 25 miles a week during the preceding 5 years. The men performed a dichotic listening task in which they listened to numbers spoken simultaneously into both ears through headphones. They had to remember, then say, the number(s) spoken into one or both ears. The active and inactive men performed equally well on simple tasks such as recalling the number spoken into one ear while ignoring the other. But the active men were much better at recalling the number spoken into the second ear, indicating that they could better retain that information in short-term memory.

In another study, geriatric mental patients ages 59 to 89 improved on the Wechsler Memory Scale test after a 12-week walking, calisthenics, and rhythm exercise program (Powell, 1974). Therefore, older adults who maintain their aerobic fitness may be able to forestall declines in memory.

Knowledge bases in older adults have not been widely studied. We can speculate, though, that older adults with expertise in a sport have an advantage in performance. Superior knowledge might offset a loss of physical skill or speed. Also, older adults learning new sports can expect to improve as they acquire knowledge of the sport.

## REVIEW 8.3

Memory plays a role in the performance of motor skills, because the performer matches information associated with skill performance to the memories of previous experiences on similar tasks. For skills involving a speedy response to events in the environment, the memory process must operate efficiently to allow a response within the imposed time. Therefore, memory deficits at any age can limit performance and are exhibited by both the young and the old.

Evidence shows that the control processes that move information through the memory system are not as efficient at either end of the life span. The ability to rehearse, label, organize, and recode information to be remembered generally advances in late childhood. An individual can improve use of the control processes by acquiring knowledge about the activity, including both factual and procedural information. Older adults have more difficulty getting information into memory as well as retrieving it from memory storage, but structural changes in the brain could influence their memory loss.

Regular aerobic exercise may reduce or even eliminate declines in memory function. The speed with which information is processed into memory, too, might be involved in the performance of both children and older adults. Depending on the source of the memory deficit, though, educators may be able to help performers of any age to remember information. To do this, a teacher should allow sufficient time for rehearsal or suggest strategies to organize the information and movements to be remembered.

## SUMMARY

Information processing models hypothesize the perceptual-cognitive steps in human brain function as if they were the calculation steps carried out by computers. Such models facilitate the identification of age-related differences in the perceptual-cognitive processes. We know that children do not attend as well as adults, have fewer and simpler response schemata, cannot handle as much feedback, and are less refined in their neuromuscular control. Children process information more slowly than adults and cannot remember as much. They have less knowledge than adults in general, but can acquire a great deal of knowledge on topics that interest them. Children can be taught to use the control processes, or memory strategies, to improve their memory systems.

Older adults, particularly those who lead sedentary lifestyles, process information more slowly than young adults. This puts them at a disadvantage on tasks that require optimum speed. Older adults also experience memory deficits that seem to relate to use of the control processes rather than a lack of storage space.

At any age, ineffective or slow information processing or a lack of knowledge can limit a person's performance. Many sports demand quick decision making. The inability to make a decision quickly enough or the lack of sufficient knowledge with which to make a sound decision can limit performance as much as a lack of skill or a lack of fitness. The perceptual-cognitive system is just as important to movement as the other body systems.

## Key Terms

channel
choice delay
choice reaction time
control processes
declarative knowledge
encode (encoding)
external feedback
grouping
internal feedback
labeling
long-term (memory) store
memory capacity
procedural knowledge
recency effect
recoding
rehearsal
schema
sensory register
sensory store
short-term (memory) store
simple reaction time
strategic knowledge

subroutines
knowledge of results (KR)

## Discussion Questions

1. What is an information processing model?
2. How do children differ from adults in regard to these steps of information processing: attention, use of schemata, feedback, neuromuscular control, speed of processing?
3. How do older adults differ from younger adults in information processing? What might explain these differences?
4. How do the information processing and dynamic systems perspectives differ in regard to the brain's role in controlling movement?
5. Describe the following control processes and how children differ from adults in their use: rehearsal, labeling, grouping, and recoding.
6. Describe four sport-specific ways that novices and experts differ in regard to their knowledge of a sport.
7. How does maintaining an active lifestyle appear to affect information processing and memory in older adults?

## Suggested Readings

Chi, M. (1976). Short-term memory limitations in children: Capacity or processing deficits? *Memory and Cognition, 4*, 559-572.

Kelso, J.A.S. (Ed.) (1982). *Human motor behavior: An introduction.* Hillsdale, NJ: Erlbaum.

Poon, L.W., Fozard, J.L., Cermak, L.S., Arenberg, D., & Thompson, L.W. (Eds.) (1980). *New directions in memory and aging.* Hillsdale, NJ: Erlbaum.

Rothstein, A.L. (1977). Information processing in children's skill acquisition. In R.W. Christina & D.M. Landers (Eds.), *Psychology of motor behavior and sport—1976* (pp. 218-227). Champaign, IL: Human Kinetics.

Thomas, J.R., French, K.E., & Humphries, C.A. (1986). Knowledge development and sport skill performance: Directions for motor behavior research. *Journal of Sport Psychology, 8*, 259-272.

Welford, A.T. (1980). Motor skill and aging. In C.H. Nadeau, W.R. Halliwell, K.M. Newell, & G.C. Roberts (Eds.), *Psychology of motor behavior and sport—1979* (pp. 253-268). Champaign, IL: Human Kinetics.

Wickens, C.D. (1974). Temporal limits of human information processing: A developmental study. *Psychological Bulletin, 81*, 739-755.

# Chapter 9

# Psychosocial and Cultural Influences in Motor Development

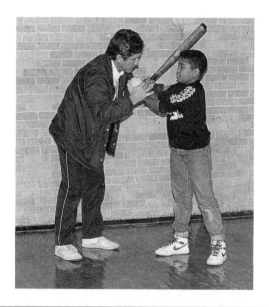

## CHAPTER CONCEPTS

**9.1**
Children and adults are socialized into physically active lifestyles.

**9.2**
Self-esteem influences sport participation and skill mastery and becomes more accurate as a person ages.

**9.3**
Racial and ethnic differences in motor development are related to the environmental variables affecting group members.

303

Social learning is one of the most potent environmental factors in development. Children learn certain behaviors by observing others, who serve as models, and by internalizing those behaviors (Bandura, 1969; Bandura & Walters, 1963). Models, especially those significant to the child (called significant others), can encourage or discourage behaviors by either engaging in them or not, or by how they label them. For example, telling a young boy that only girls cry influences him to believe it is inappropriate for him to cry. Learners need not reproduce behaviors outwardly or receive direct encouragement from models to internalize the behaviors, although encouragement strengthens the chances that the learner will reproduce the behaviors.

The toys and furnishings provided to children are also a part of the socialization process, because they stimulate particular kinds of play. The neighborhoods and geographic regions where children live offer opportunities for certain activities but not others. Thus, beginning at a very young age, children are socialized for participation as functioning members of society, both broadly and for specific social roles, including their gender role (Loy, McPherson, & Kenyon, 1978). This process of social learning, however, extends throughout life as other people and situations influence individuals.

*Socialization* involves many types of behavior, including social skills, physical skills, traits, values, knowledge, attitudes, norms, and dispositions. Socialization is critical for motor development, because motor experiences are vital to the full development of motor skills. Children who are socialized into motor experiences are more likely to learn motor skills. Increased proficiency in skill performance is enjoyable and rewarding in itself and in turn promotes continued participation. On the other hand, children who are not exposed to motor experiences are less likely to master motor skills. With only limited practice, children are more likely to fail and lose interest in physical activities (Greendorfer, 1983). When individuals expect failure at motor skills, this expectation becomes a limitation to their skill performance.

For example, consider a family in which the parents are physically active. They exercise regularly and join recreational sport leagues. Their children see them in these settings. When the parents go to the tennis courts just a few blocks from their home, the children accompany them and get a turn to play tennis. The parents may buy tennis rackets for the children and teach them some basic tennis skills. It would be of little surprise to find that these children become active sport participants when they reach adolescence and adulthood.

# SOCIALIZATION INTO SPORT

An individual's early sport and physical activity socialization is a key factor in both motor development and the likelihood of later participation in physical activities. People and situations continue to influence individuals in their choice of activities throughout life. Peers, for example, influence which recreational activities, active or sedentary, a person undertakes and, over a period of time, whether that person adopts an active or inactive lifestyle. Certainly, the socialization process and the individuals who are influential in the process deserve attention as major environmental influences on motor development.

Three major elements of the socialization process lead an individual to learn his or her societal role:

1.  Socializing agents (i.e., significant others)
2.  Social situations
3.  Personal attributes (Kenyon & McPherson, 1973; see Figure 9.1)

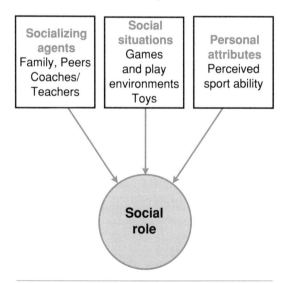

**Figure 9.1** The three major elements of the socialization process that lead to the learning of a societal role for participation in physical activity. (Based on Kenyon & McPherson, 1973.)

Developmentalists are interested in which, if any, element is the most important in the sport socialization process. (We use the word *sport* here, in a broad sense, to include all types of physical activity.) Among the important *socializing agents* are family members, peers, teachers, and coaches. Likewise, developmentalists want to know if one group of agents is more influential than the others. Let's review each of the socialization elements to see if some are indeed more important than others.

---

### CONCEPT 9.1
Children and adults are socialized into physically active lifestyles.

---

## Socializing Agents

Socializing agents are the people who are most likely to play a role in a person's socialization process—family members, peers, teachers, and coaches. We will look at how each of these groups might influence participation in sport and exercise. Before we examine the roles of specific agents in the sport socialization process, we will discuss how boys and girls are socialized into sport differently, especially into stereotypical gender-related behaviors.

### Stereotypical Behavior

Parents and other significant socializing agents can encourage children toward different types of behavior. Societies commonly socialize boys and girls into different societal roles. This practice is often termed *sex typing*, *gender role stereotyping*, or *gender typing*. Traditionally, Western societies carry gender typing through to sport involvement. Sports are considered appropriate, even important, activities for boys, but not always for girls. Therefore, adults often permit and encourage vigorous, outgoing play for toddler boys, whereas girls are discouraged from or even punished for running, climbing, venturing away from parents, and so on (DiPietro, 1981; Eaton & Enns, 1986; Eaton & Keats, 1982; Fagot & Leinbach, 1983; Lewis, 1972; Liss, 1983; Lloyd & Smith, 1985). Society reinforces constrained, sedentary types of play for girls, and thus many girls *self-select* away from vigorous play (Greendorfer, 1983), leaving a comparatively small number of girls as active participants in vigorous, skilled play.

With such limited involvement and practice, many girls never develop their motor skills to their full potential. Even those girls who do participate may feel that all-out effort and skilled performance are inappropriate to their gender role. This in turn could affect a girl's or woman's motivation for participating, for training, or for striving for high achievement standards that rival those of boys and men. Thus, this pervasive societal influence on boys' and girls' sport participation is believed to be a factor in measurements of skill and fitness that compare the sexes. Despite a growing awareness during the 1970s and 1980s that these societal roles potentially limit girls' opportunities to enjoy the many benefits of sport participation, research studies conducted in the mid-1980s confirm that parents still tend to interact differently with sons and daughters in play environments (Power, 1985; Power & Parke, 1983, 1986; see Williams, Goodman, & Green, 1985, on tomboys). For example, parents tend to direct their girls' play but allow boys more opportunities for independent, exploratory play (Power, 1985).

The roles various agents play in the socialization of children, then, can vary with the sex of the child. In addition, the sex of the agent serving as a model for behavior may differentially influence the child's internalization of the behavior.

---

*In any discussion of the socialization process, you must keep in mind the sex of the socializing agent as well as that of the individual.*

---

## Family Members

A person's family is a major influence in the sport socialization process (Kelly, 1974; Snyder & Spreitzer, 1973), just as it is in the socialization of children into other pursuits, such as music (Snyder & Spreitzer, 1978). This is partly because the family's influence begins so early in a child's life. Family members expose their infant to certain experiences and attitudes. They reinforce the behaviors they deem appropriate through their gestures, praise, and rewards and punish inappropriate behaviors. The process is systematic, but at times it is so subtle that family members may hardly realize what and how they communicate to the infant.

### Parents

Older children, adolescents, and adults who participate in sport reflect in part their parents' interest and encouragement during their early years. Parents can encourage children to engage in active play that involves motor skills, or they can support sedentary play. As children become physically active, parents can encourage or discourage games and, eventually, specific sports. Little doubt exists that socialization into sport begins in childhood; about 75% of eventual sport participants become involved in sport by age 8 (Greendorfer, 1976; Snyder & Spreitzer, 1976), and the best predictor of adult sport involvement is participation during childhood and adolescence (Greendorfer, 1979; Loy et al., 1978; Snyder & Spreitzer, 1976).

Individual family members might play differential roles in the sport socialization process. Snyder and Spreitzer (1973) proposed that a child's same-sex parent is most influential in the extent of that child's sport involvement, and McPherson (1978) suggested specifically that mothers serve as sport role models for their daughters. Some researchers believe that fathers are stricter in their reinforcement of gender-appropriate behavior (Lewko & Greendorfer, 1988). Greendorfer and Lewko (1978b) identified fathers as a major influence in the sport involvement of both boys and girls, whereas mothers did not appear to be a factor in sport socialization. In contrast, Lewko and Ewing (1980) found that boys between the ages of 9 and 11 who were highly involved in sports were influenced by their fathers and that highly involved girls were influenced by their mothers. A difference between boys and girls, however, was that to become involved, girls seemed to need a higher level of encouragement than boys did from their families, and they needed it from many members of the family (see Table 9.1). A similar pattern was found in Japanese children (Ebihara, Ikeda, & Myiashita, 1983). That girls needed a higher level of encouragement from more of their significant others probably reflects society's traditional attitude that sports are more appropriate for boys than for girls.

## Siblings

Some investigators feel that siblings are also important agents in the sport socialization process because they form an infant's first play group. Brothers, for example, are often considered important to girls' sport involvement (Weiss & Knoppers, 1982), although sisters can influence girls' participation, too (Lewko & Ewing, 1980). On the other hand, some chil-

dren and teens report that older siblings were not important in their sport involvement (Greendorfer & Lewko, 1978b; Patriksson, 1981). It is possible that for most children, siblings merely reinforce the sport socialization pattern established by parents rather than act as a major socializing force (Lewko & Greendorfer, 1988).

## Patterns of Influence

It is obvious that various investigators reached different conclusions about the influence of family members on sport socialization. Greendorfer and Lewko (1978a) attempted to clarify these various conclusions by questioning children from a broad range of social backgrounds. They found some differences in the pattern of significant influences. The agent who exerted the most influence in sport socialization varied somewhat among children according to sex, social background, race, and geographic location. For example, fathers were influential in socializing Caucasian American boys into sport, but not African-American boys (Greendorfer & Ewing, 1981).

Perhaps we should focus our attention on the relative influence of each family member both within particular groups of children and for individual children. For example, the pattern

Table 9.1   Family Members' Influence on Sport Involvement

| | Sport involvement level | | | | | | | |
| | Males | | | | Females | | | |
| | Low | | High | | Low | | High | |
| Family member | M | SD | M | SD | M | SD | M | SD |
|---|---|---|---|---|---|---|---|---|
| Father | 15.13 | 4.63 | 18.46 | 4.34 | 14.92 | 3.53 | 18.53 | 4.06 |
| Mother | 12.66 | 3.25 | 14.48 | 3.66 | 13.62 | 3.59 | 17.74 | 3.67 |
| Brother | 13.32 | 6.98 | 15.61 | 7.14 | 14.14 | 5.71 | 16.24 | 7.26 |
| Sister | 11.32 | 5.18 | 11.21 | 5.29 | 11.89 | 5.22 | 14.60 | 6.77 |

Note. Mean scores (M) and standard deviations (SD) from a questionnaire are given in the table; higher means reflect stronger influence.
Adapted by permission from Lewko & Ewing, 1980.

of socializing influences for girls is more variable regardless of social background. One explanation for the inconsistent pattern of girls' sport involvement is the lack of a specific family member to take responsibility for socializing a girl into sport. In comparison, fathers feel responsible for initiating their sons' interest in sport. Think, too, of a boy highly involved in sport who did not have a father present in the home. His mother or an older brother may have made a special effort to involve him in sport. Despite the minor inconsistencies in pattern of influence among various groups of children, family members, especially parents, are clearly important agents in the sport socialization process.

## Peers

A child's peers have the potential to reinforce the sport socialization process begun in the family (Greendorfer & Lewko, 1978b). If a peer group tends to participate in active play or sports, individual members are drawn to such activities. If the group prefers passive activities, individual members tend to follow that lead. Adult athletes typically report that peer groups or friends influenced the extent of their sport participation when they were in school, although the strength of this influence varies among sports. The first peer group a child encounters is typically a play group. Children become involved in such groups when they are about 3 to 4 years old and continue in them during their early school years.

Boys and girls from several countries, including the United States, Japan, and Canada, report that peers influenced their childhood sport participation (Ebihara et al., 1983; Greendorfer & Ewing, 1981; Greendorfer & Lewko, 1978b; Yamaguchi, 1984). During preadolescence, children enter more formalized peer groups, such as cliques or gangs. These peers continue to be influential during adolescence (Brown, 1985; Butcher, 1983, 1985; Higginson, 1985; Patriksson, 1981; Schellenberger,

1981; Smith, 1979; Yamaguchi, 1984). In fact, among the women she questioned, Greendorfer (1976) found that the peer group was the only socializing agent that influenced sport involvement throughout all phases of the life cycle studied: childhood, adolescence, and young adulthood. Other socializing agents were important at some ages but not at others. For example, the family, so important to young children, probably is less influential to adolescents.

Peers often provide a stronger influence for participation in team sports than for participation in individual sports during childhood and adolescence (Kenyon & McPherson, 1973). Children's and adolescents' supportive peer groups are usually made up of others the same sex as the participant. For adults, especially women and particularly after marriage, spouses and friends of the opposite sex become more influential in either encouraging or discouraging involvement in certain activities (Loy et al., 1978). As individuals leave school and enter new social environments as members of the work force, they often leave their peer groups. If a peer group had been sport-oriented, a reduction in sport involvement might follow. New peer groups at the workplace, on the other hand, could stimulate sport involvement; the individual may join a team in a recreational sport league or perhaps participate in a company-sponsored exercise and recreation program (Loy et al., 1978).

It is likely that the typical middle-aged adult, even one who was involved in sport as a young adult, reduces sport involvement. This trend might be due in part to a lack of programs aimed specifically at middle-aged and older adults. The emphasis on fitness that began in the late 1970s has led to a greater availability of exercise and recreation programs for members of these age groups. Additionally, adult participation in sport and exercise programs has become acceptable and even desirable in Western societies. With specific programs now available, peer groups might once again influence older adults' recreational involvement. Once involved, adults keep participating to be a part of the peer group.

Despite the strong influence of peer groups on sport participation throughout life, it is still not clear that membership in a sport-oriented peer group always precedes participation—that is, that a person is drawn to an activity because of a desire to associate with peers. Possibly individuals first select groups that fit their interests, including an interest in sports (Loy et al., 1978). Although it is not clear which comes first, the interest in sports and the desire to be a part of a peer group make it likely that an individual will continue to participate and to select membership in active groups. Peers apparently play just as important a role in sport socialization as the family plays (Lewko & Greendorfer, 1988).

## Coaches and Teachers

Coaches and teachers are also socializing agents who influence an individual's sport involvement (Greendorfer & Lewko, 1978b). Male athletes consistently report that coaches and teachers influenced both their participation and their selection of sports, particularly when they were adolescents and young adults (Ebihara et al., 1983; Kenyon & McPherson, 1973). Female athletes report that teachers and coaches influenced them during childhood (Greendorfer & Ewing, 1981; Weiss & Knoppers, 1982) and adolescence (Greendorfer, 1976, 1977). In contrast, Yamaguchi (1984) found that schoolteachers and coaches were not influential. Participants rarely name teachers and coaches as the most influential agents in their sport involvement. Perhaps the role of teachers and coaches is to strengthen the sport socialization processes begun earlier by family and friends.

Nevertheless, teachers and coaches should not overlook their potential to influence their students' sport involvement. They can introduce children and adolescents to exciting new activities and stimulate them to learn the skills and attitudes associated with sport. Conversely, teachers and coaches also must recognize the potential they have to turn their students away from sport and physical activity. Bad experiences in school can have lifelong consequences for a person's overall lifestyle (Snyder & Spreitzer, 1983). Such negative experiences are known as *aversive socialization*; this can occur when teachers or coaches embarrass children in front of their peers, overemphasize performance criteria at the expense of learning and enjoyment, and plan class activities that result in overwhelming failure rather than success. Children who experience aversive socialization naturally avoid physical activities and fail to learn skills well; consequently, any attempts they make to participate frustrate and discourage them.

---

Though teachers and coaches can take pride in students who achieve success in sport and dance, they can also strive to make physical activities enjoyable for all their students.

---

## Social Situations

The situations in which children spend their formative years are a part of the socialization process. We will discuss how play environments, activities, and the toys children use can influence their later activities.

### Play Environments and Games

An adequate environment for play, such as a backyard or playground, can provide the social situation and environment a child needs to begin sport involvement. Play spaces probably influence sport selection as well. A child who lacks an adequate play space has a diminished opportunity to get involved in activity and practice skills, which thus discourages participation in sports. Children who grow up in urban areas where playing fields are limited are typically exposed to sports that require little space and equipment, such as basketball. Colder climates provide children an opportunity to learn to ice skate; warmer climates encourage swimming. Some play environments could influence boys and girls to participate in gender-typed activities. A boy might be labeled a sissy for jumping rope or a girl a tomboy for playing basketball. Western society has traditionally considered certain types of games to be appropriate for boys but not for girls, and vice versa. This labeling is particularly apparent as children enter adolescence.

The pressure to participate in gender role–appropriate games has implications for children's opportunities to practice skills. Traditional boys' games are typically complex and involve strategy. They encourage work toward specific goals and promote negotiation to settle disputes over rules. Traditional girls' games, on the other hand, are typically noncompetitive, and rather than encouraging interdependence among group members, they involve waiting for turns to perform simple repetitive tasks, such as jumping rope or playing hopscotch. Such games rarely give girls opportunities to increase game complexity or to develop increasingly more difficult skills. In fact, the games often end because the participants lose interest, not because they achieve a goal (Greendorfer, 1983).

---

Though sex typing through games has diminished in recent years, educators should keep in mind that a play environment that channels boys and girls into sex-typed games perpetuates a situation in which boys can develop their skills but girls cannot.

---

## Play With Toys

Children's toys are another facet of the socialization process. Toys can encourage children to be active or inactive and can stimulate them to model sport figures. For example, a hockey stick encourages a child to run or skate, dodge obstacles, and develop an accurate shot; a board game encourages sedentary play. Obviously, each kind of toy has its advantages, but certainly some toys facilitate children's socialization into sport more than others.

Toys are also a means by which gender typing can occur in the socialization process. For example, toys marketed to boys tend to be complex and encourage more vigorous activity than those marketed to girls. The typical girls' toy promotes quiet indoor play, such as playing house (Greendorfer, 1983; Liss, 1983). Gender typing through toys is well entrenched in society. Manufacturers often use gender-typed strategies to advertise their products. For example, commercials or packaging for racing-car sets and action-oriented video games feature boys, and toy kitchen sets picture girls (see Figure 9.2a and b). Children as well as their parents are influenced by these marketing ploys.

Parents also enjoy giving their children the same kinds of toys they played with as children, thus tending to perpetuate traditional gender typing. For example, a father might buy a Lincoln Log building set for his son, remembering the hours he spent with one as a child, despite more modern, complex toys on the market. Moreover, parents can promote gender typing by negatively reinforcing play with toys they judge to be gender-inappropriate (Fagot, 1978), such as telling boys they should not play with dolls. Such gender typing through toys is slow to change, and recent surveys find little evidence of change (Eisenberg, Wolchick, Hernandez, & Pasternack, 1985; Lloyd & Smith, 1985).

In recent years, our society has become more aware of the many ways children are sex typed and the implications of this process. Yet little evidence shows any substantial change away from sex typing (Huston, 1984; Kaiser & Phinney, 1983; Langlois & Downs, 1980; Schwartz & Markham, 1985). Teachers must

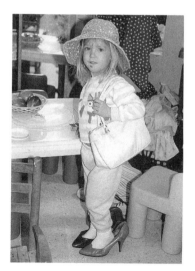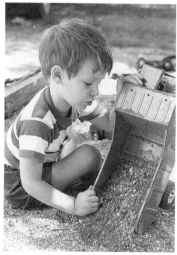

**Figure 9.2** Children are often led to stereotypical, gender-typed play by the toys marketed and given to them.

realize they influence this aspect of socialization (Fagot, 1984). They can reinforce early sex typing by continuing to label certain activities as more important or appropriate for one sex than for the other, choosing different activities for boys and girls, and holding different expectations for boys' and girls' achievements. Or they can make every attempt possible to eliminate such distinctions and allow individuals to explore their full potentials. Again, the evidence shows that teachers still behave differently toward the play of boys compared to that of girls (Fagot, 1984; Oettingen, 1985; Smith, 1985). It is likely that such day-to-day decisions and expectations accumulate over time to produce differences in boys' and girls' motor development by channeling their practice opportunities (Brundage, 1983; Greendorfer & Brundage, 1984).

## Personal Attributes

Socializing agents and situations interact with an individual's personal attributes to influence sport involvement. Certainly, perceived ability is one attribute important to your choice of

activity (Kukla, 1978). You are not likely to continually choose an activity if you expect to achieve little success. On the other hand, you would probably persist in an activity, such as a sport, if you perceived your ability as high, even in the face of limited real success. We will discuss the development of these perceptions and expectations in more detail later in this chapter. The information provided to boys and girls, upon which they base their perceptions, can depend on their gender. Let us now examine how the socialization process can lead to different perceptions of physical ability in boys and girls.

## Perceived Sport Ability in Boys and Girls

Lewko and Ewing (1980) questioned children about their *perceived ability* and level of involvement in sport. Interestingly, boys as a group perceived their ability as high regardless of their level of sport involvement. This may reflect the boys' tendency to respond in accordance with a male stereotype. In contrast, only girls involved in sport perceived their ability as high; girls uninvolved perceived their ability as low. These findings suggest that the sport socialization process can deliver two very different messages to young boys and girls.

Boys are expected to be capable of sport participation. For most boys this is an advantage in that they enter sports with positive expectations. Of course, boys with low expectations and subsequent failures in sport are left feeling inadequate and often withdraw from sport and exercise. The message many girls get through the sport socialization process is that they are incapable of highly skilled performance. Even though the message is invalid, they approach skills expecting to fail. To compound these negative expectations, girls frequently have limited motor experiences and practice opportunities; therefore, they have a greater propensity to fail. When this happens, many girls lose their interest in physical activities (Greendorfer, 1983).

Even those girls who develop good skills can have lingering doubts about their potential or the appropriateness of their sport involvement. Although this scenario need not be true, it is important for educators to realize that many girls come to believe they have limited potential for skilled performance, and failure only tends to reinforce this belief. Boys who have low levels of skill can feel they are not living up to their gender role, particularly if their fathers and coaches pressure them. This can contribute to a poor self-image that affects many behaviors.

## Adult Socialization

As a result of childhood and adolescent socialization, individuals form identities based on social roles with certain social expectations. These expectations are the basis of new social learning in adulthood. Changes in identity are a function of new adult roles, such as those associated with a career or being a parent (Brim, 1966). Whereas children are socialized into cultural values transmitted by parents and the school system, adults learn behaviors

attached to specific roles (Inkeles, 1969). Individuals also anticipate the roles they will occupy in future years. For example, a young executive might learn to play golf because all his superiors play golf with their clients. He comes to associate that activity with successful business and believes it might help him get a promotion. So children play-act roles they might adopt as adults, young adults anticipate achieving a certain economic standard of living by middle age, middle-aged adults anticipate leisure activities in retirement, and so on. People often form these anticipated roles by conforming to the age-linked behaviors society holds as appropriate for a particular age group. Acting outside the accepted social roles often invites negative reactions from others and brings about discord within the individual.

Following the typical pattern of social behavior in Western societies, adults decrease their involvement in active sports such that older adults are often considered sedentary or even feeble. Older adults often anticipate that their roles include cessation of vigorous activity. Recently, attitudes have shifted to favor exercise and activity throughout life. This change has probably been stimulated by medical research, but undoubtedly it involves a redefinition of the appropriate age-linked behaviors related to sport and exercise. Therefore, in recent years society has come to accept middle-aged and older adults wearing exercise clothes and running shoes. Activity groups for older adults have emerged, and special sport-related functions for older adults, such as the Senior Olympics, are popular.

---

Whereas older adults might previously have been socialized into sedentary lifestyles, recent attitude shifts have allowed for their socialization into active lifestyles.

---

New activity-oriented peer groups are an important aspect of this emerging active lifestyle. Older adults might join exercise and recreational groups as much for the social benefits as for the physical benefits. They establish new friendships and peer groups. These activity-oriented friends encourage continued involvement in the activity program. As a result, exercise and activity become normal characteristics of the lifestyle.

Although older adults who are active and exercise have gained acceptance in recent years, some older adults remain uncomfortable adopting this role. The extent of an individual's sport socialization during youth likely affects his or her participation throughout life. Peer groups and the availability of sport situations undoubtedly influence adult sport involvement, but they often do so against the backdrop of early sport socialization. Therefore, those socialized into roles characterized by sedentary lifestyles probably persist in these lifestyles, even when exercise and activity become critical to their overall health. The older adult who was very active as a younger person finds it easier to become active, even if years of inactivity have intervened, than someone who was not active during youth. This emphasizes the importance to lifelong health of socializing both males and females into active lifestyles, if not sport, when they are young.

## REVIEW 9.1

Young people learn social behaviors by observing and internalizing the behaviors of their significant others, who serve as models. Further, reinforcement from these significant people contributes to the likelihood that young people will adopt certain behaviors. Involvement in sport is one of the behaviors affected by this process. Family members—especially parents, peer groups, teachers, and coaches—can successfully encourage a child to participate in sports. Appropriate environmental spaces and objects can also help a child develop skills and participate in sports, although gender typing through games and toys can limit the skills that girls achieve.

The strong influence of social factors on motor development raises questions when we compare males and females on skill achievements. Are differences primarily biological? Or might social factors be so pervasive as to limit the achievements of girls and women more than any relevant biological factors? These questions are difficult to answer because most female athletes are still products of a socialization process that tends to be different for girls than for boys.

In the past, the socially acceptable role for middle-aged and older adults did not include participation in exercise and vigorous activity, but recently a new model has emerged for adults. In this new role, exercise and physical activity are integral to the lifestyle. Exercise and recreation programs for middle-aged and older adults foster the formation of new, activity-oriented peer groups that in turn encourage continued involvement.

We mentioned that a person's perception of his or her physical abilities can affect expectations of success and failure. This in turn influences whether an individual will seek opportunities to participate in physical activities or choose to avoid them. Let us learn more about the development of self-judgments of ability.

## SELF-ESTEEM

Each of you evaluates yourself as a person in general and in more specific areas, such as physical ability, physical appearance, academic ability, and social skills. We have many names for such self-judgments, including self-esteem, self-concept, self-image, self-worth, and self-confidence. In this discussion we will use the term *self-esteem*. Self-esteem is your personal judgment of your own capability, significance, success, and worthiness, and you convey it to others in words and in actions (Coopersmith, 1967, p. 5). Whether your self-evaluations are accurate is not as important to your self-esteem as your belief that they are accurate (Weiss, 1993). Others can identify your level of self-esteem through what you say to others as well as your nonverbal behaviors in joining or avoiding certain activities. For example, someone with a high self-esteem for physical skills is likely to join a recreational sport team, whereas someone with a low self-esteem for physical activity is likely to avoid it. This is one of the reasons that self-esteem is so important. It influences one's motivation to join and sustain particular activities.

Self-esteem is not just a general sense. It is specific to *domains* or situations. For example, a teenage boy may evaluate himself as high in the physical and social domains but low in the academic domain. Within each domain, individuals may differentiate their abilities at even more specific levels (Fox & Corbin, 1989). Academic ability may be perceived in terms of ability in mathematics, writing, foreign languages, and so on. Here, we will focus on self-evaluations in the physical domain and the specific levels related to physical skills.

Professionals interested in motivating people to be active must understand self-esteem and the factors that influence people's judgments of their capabilities. Those working with children should know how self-esteem develops. Those working with people of any age should be aware of the criteria people use as a basis for their evaluations and whether these criteria change as individuals grow older.

---

**CONCEPT 9.2**

Self-esteem influences sport participation and skill mastery and becomes more accurate as a person ages.

---

## Development of Self-Esteem

Children's self-esteem is greatly influenced by verbal and nonverbal communications from others who are significant to them, including parents, siblings, friends, teachers, and coaches (see Figure 9.3). Verbal comments such as "Good" or "Why can't you do better?" are sources of information, as are facial expressions and gestures (Weiss, 1993). Children are likely to compare themselves to other children, too, and the results of this evaluation influence self-esteem. These appraisals and comparisons, though, do not have an equal influence throughout life. Let's examine how the pattern of influence changes.

## Social Interactions

Children as young as age 5 can compare themselves to others (Scanlan, 1988), but under the age of 10 they depend more on parental appraisals and the outcomes of contests than on comparisons (Horn & Hasbrook, 1986, 1987; Horn & Weiss, 1991). Young children, too, are not as accurate as teenagers in their evaluations of their physical competence. The level of intrinsic motivation and the extent to which children believe they control their lives influ-

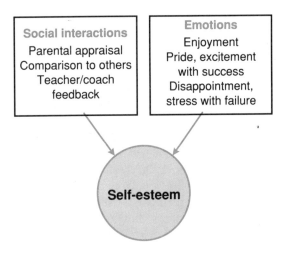

**Figure 9.3**  Social interactions and emotions influence the development of self-esteem for physical performance. Interactions are both verbal and nonverbal.

ence the accuracy of children's physical ability perceptions. Children older than 10 come to rely on comparisons to and appraisals given by their peers.

Feedback and appraisal from teachers and coaches contribute to the development of self-esteem in the physical domain (Smoll & Smith, 1989). For example, male athletes 10 to 15 years old show higher self-esteem when they play for coaches who give frequent encouragement and corrective feedback, especially if the athletes begin with somewhat low self-esteem (Smith, Smoll, & Curtis, 1979). Teenage girls, too, are influenced by coaches' appraisals and self-perceptions of improvement, but the pattern of coaches' influence is interesting: In a study by Horn (1985), self-esteem did not increase when girls received reinforcement from coaches after successful performances. Instead, an increase in perceived competence was associated with criticism. Apparently the coaches' positive comments were general and did not relate specifically to the girls' performance, whereas the criticisms were associated with a skill error and often included a suggestion for improvement. So teachers and coaches cannot expect global praise to automatically raise a child's self-esteem. Feedback should relate to performance (Horn, 1986, 1987).

## Emotions

The development of self-esteem is also related to emotions associated with participation. The pride and excitement associated with success or the disappointment and stress associated with failure influence a person's self-esteem and motivation to sustain participation (Weiss, 1993). Enjoyments leads to higher levels of self-esteem and motivation to participate. In turn, perceptions of high ability and mastery, low parental pressure, and greater parent/coach satisfaction lead to enjoyment in preadolescents and young adolescents (Brustad, 1988; Scanlan & Lewthwaite, 1986; Scanlan, Stein, & Ravizza, 1988).

## Influence of Self-Esteem on Motivation

Self-esteem can influence behavior because people tend to act in ways that confirm their beliefs of themselves; that is, people tend to be *self-consistent*. These beliefs often are evident in the reasons they give for their successes and failures. These reasons are called *causal attributions*. We can expect people of any age with high self-esteem to make attributions that are

1. internal, believing that their behavior influences outcome;
2. stable, believing that the factors influencing outcome are consistent from situation to situation; and
3. controllable, believing that they personally control the factors influencing outcome.

For example, competitors with high self-esteem attribute their successes to talent (internal), think they can win again (stable), and believe they were responsible for their successes, not merely lucky (controllable). They view their failures as temporary and meet them with renewed effort and continued practice to improve skills.

In contrast, people with low self-esteem attribute failure to factors that are

1. external, believing they could not change such outcomes;
2. unstable, believing outcome is a product of fluctuating influences such as good and bad luck; and
3. uncontrollable, believing that nothing they do could result in a different outcome.

Competitors with low self-esteem often attribute losing to a lack of ability and winning to luck or a task so easy that anybody could win.

Examining causal attributions can help us understand adult behavior, but few researchers have studied the causal attributions of children in sport. Such information is interesting because children are in the process of developing self-esteem. We have seen that children use different factors in judging themselves as they develop. So we must be concerned with the accuracy of their self-estimates and the roles adults play in helping children make appropriate attributions.

---

Children who perceive their physical abilities as low are not likely to persist in physical activities and realize the associated health and psychosocial benefits (Weiss, 1993). They will not be motivated to participate.

---

## Children's Attributions

The little information available on age-related changes in children's attributions indicates that children 7 to 9 years old attribute outcomes to effort and luck more than older children and teens (Bird & Williams, 1980). These factors are both unstable. The children in this study reacted to stories the researchers provided rather than actual outcomes they experienced, however, and a more recent study failed to find age differences in attributions following actual participation (Weiss, McAuley, Ebbeck, & Wiese, 1990). Because young children might not be able to distinguish between ability and effort very well, more information is needed on age differences.

Differences do exist in the attributions made by children who differ in their perceived physical competence (Weiss et al., 1990). As expected, children with high physical self-esteem give internal, stable, and controllable reasons for their successes. Their attributions for success are more stable and their future expectations for success higher than those of children with low physical self-esteem. As we mentioned previously, children vary in the accuracy of their physical estimates (Weiss & Horn, 1990). Girls

who underestimate their physical abilities typically choose less challenging skills and attribute outcomes to external factors, unlike those who estimate their physical abilities accurately or overestimate them. Boys who underestimate their physical abilities report little understanding of what is responsible for their successes or failures. Children with low perceptions of their physical abilities who also tend to underestimate their abilities probably make inaccurate attributions about the outcomes of their efforts. Their behavior is characterized by

- an unwillingness to try challenging tasks,
- a lack of effort to do well, and
- avoidance of participation.

Parents, teachers, and coaches can help children, especially those with low self-esteem, make appropriate attributions. Adults can help children with low self-esteem retrain their attributions (Horn, 1987; see Figure 9.4). Rather than letting children attribute failure to lack of ability and success to luck, adults can emphasize

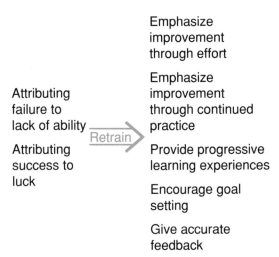

Attributing failure to lack of ability

Attributing success to luck

Retrain

Emphasize improvement through effort

Emphasize improvement through continued practice

Provide progressive learning experiences

Encourage goal setting

Give accurate feedback

**Figure 9.4** Adults must help children who have low self-esteem for physical performance improve their self-esteem. Retraining can change causal attributions.
(Based on Horn, 1987.)

## Measuring Self-Esteem in Children

It is easier to imagine how developmentalists measure running and jumping, or strength and flexibility, than self-esteem in children. Susan Harter (1985) of the University of Denver uses a question format ("Some kids . . . BUT Other kids . . .") to measure children's self-perceptions. For example, one pair of statements is "Some kids feel that they are better than others their age at sports BUT Other kids don't feel they can play as well." Next to each statement are two boxes, one labeled *really true for me* and one labeled *sort of true for me*. Children check one of the boxes, indicating which kids they perceive as being like themselves and to what extent.

Harter's Self-Perception Profile for Children contains 36 different statements for five specific domains (scholastic competence, athletic competence, social acceptance, physical appearance, and behavioral conduct) and a global score for self-worth. This profile is appropriate for children age 8 through early adolescence. For children under 8, Harter and Pike (1984) designed a pictorial scale. Instead of two statements, two pictures are presented: One shows a competent or accepted child; the other shows a child unaccepted or unable to do the pictured task. Children say whether they are a lot or a little like the child in the picture. Hence, the scale is made more concrete for young children and can be given to children who cannot read or understand written statements. The pictorial scale assesses four domains: cognitive competence, physical competence, peer acceptance, and maternal acceptance. Scales available for adolescents and adults typically cover many more domains.

improvement through effort and continued practice. They also can encourage children to set goals and can provide accurate feedback about the children's progress. Children who come to think their situations are hopeless (have learned helplessness) need challenges that are accurately matched to their abilities and in which difficulty is increased in steps much smaller than those presented to other children. Children with high self-esteem for physical competence probably possess high levels of intrinsic motivation to participate in physical activities. If children with low self-esteem are ever to enjoy physical activities and ultimately realize the benefits of participation, adults must make special efforts to improve their self-esteem (Weiss, 1993).

### Adults' Attributes

Self-esteem also influences the motivation of adults. Just as with children, adults tend to be-

have according to their beliefs about themselves. Recall that children obtain the information on which they base their self-judgments largely from their significant others and their own comparisons. Adults obtain information from four sources (Bandura, 1986):

1. Actual experiences (previous accomplishments or failures)
2. Vicarious experiences (observing a model)
3. Verbal persuasion from others
4. Their physiological state

An individual's actual experiences are particularly influential, and changing physiological status is a reality for most older adults. For example, failing eyesight lowers an older adult's confidence for participating in racket sports. In contrast, verbal persuasion is a much weaker influence. The models available to older adults vary considerably. Some older adults have opportunities to see others like themselves participating in a wide range of activities; others do not, especially on a personal basis rather than in a magazine or on television. Given these influences, it is obvious that a person's self-esteem can increase or decrease throughout life.

A few investigators have related adults' physical self-esteem and their motivation to maintain or improve their fitness. Ewart, Stewart, Gillilan, and Kelemen (1986) involved men with coronary artery disease, ages 35 to 70, in either a walk/jog plus circuit weight training program or a walk/jog plus volleyball program for 10 weeks. They measured self-esteem before and after the program as well as arm and leg strength and treadmill running performance.

The researchers found that those with higher pretraining self-esteem improved more in arm strength than those with lower self-esteem, even when accounting for beginning strength level, type of training, and frequency of participation. Self-esteem did improve with training, but only when participants received information indicating their performance was improving. For example, the weight training group improved their self-esteem for lifting weights but not for jogging, even though they improved on both tests in a postprogram assessment. They could monitor their improvements in weight training during the program, but their jogging distance remained constant, so they had no indication they were improving. Hogan and Santomier (1984) also observed an increase in self-esteem for swimming in older adults after a 5-week swimming class. So older adults' self-esteem can influence how much improvement they realize in a program, but participation can raise self-esteem when participants have information about their actual improvements.

## Motivation

The motivation to participate in activities of a certain type involves many factors. One aspect of motivation is the set of factors that lead people to initiate or join an activity. Another aspect is the set of factors that encourage people to persist in an activity and to exert effort to improve. Still another aspect concerns those factors that lead people to end their involvement. In Concept 9.1, we considered those factors that encourage children's initial sport involvement, or the sport socialization process. Let us turn now to those factors that keep children involved in sport or lead them to drop out. We also will consider how the factors that motivate people to participate in physical activities change over the life span.

## Persistence

Researchers have focused quite a bit of attention on the reasons children and teens continue to participate in sport (see Weiss, 1993). In general, the reasons include the following:

1. A desire to be competent by improving skills or attaining goals
2. A desire to affiliate with or make new friends
3. A desire to be part of a team
4. A desire to undertake competition and be successful
5. A desire to have fun
6. A desire to increase fitness

Most individuals will cite several of these reasons for participating rather than one or two. Harter (1978, 1981a) proposed a competence motivation theory to explain this: Children are motivated to demonstrate their competency, and therefore they will seek out mastery attempts, opportunities to learn and demonstrate skills. Those who perceive they are competent and believe they control situations have more intrinsic motivation to participate than others.

Membership in subgroups also can influence a person's motivation to persist in sport. Examples of subgroups are age groups, starters versus bench warmers, elite athletes versus recreational participants, and so on. Consider age groups. Brodkin and Weiss (1990) studied varying age groups of competitive swimmers: ages 6 to 9, 10 to 14, 15 to 22, 23 to 39, 40 to 59, and 60 to 74. They found that children cited wanting to compete, liking the coaches, and pleasing family and friends as reasons to participate. The 15- to 22-year-olds gave social status reasons, as the young children did to an extent, and fitness motives were important to the young and middle-aged adults. Children and older adults did not consider fitness as important. Young children and older adults named fun as the most important reason to participate.

Another investigation of children involved in swimming found that children younger than 11 were motivated to participate by external factors: encouragement from family and friends, liking the coaches, social status, and activities that they enjoyed (Gould, Feltz, & Weiss, 1985). Teenagers in this study cited more internal factors: competence, fitness, and the excitement of swimming. So different age groups have different reasons for participating, but more research is needed on other activities and with participants of varying skill levels (Weiss, 1993).

## Dropping Out

Withdrawal from sport programs is a very real aspect of youth involvement in physical activity. Changing from one type of activity to another might be part of developing or might reflect a person's changing interests or desire to try something new, but withdrawing from activity has serious repercussions for health at any point in life. It is often difficult for surveys and research studies to distinguish between participants who switch activities and those who withdraw from activities altogether. In addition, dropouts do not always quit by choice. Injuries or high monetary costs might force some to withdraw. The reasons participants give for quitting deserve our attention.

Some young dropouts cite very negative experiences as reasons for withdrawing from sport, including the following:

- Dislike for the coach
- Lack of playing time
- Too much pressure
- Too much time required
- Overemphasis on winning
- Lack of fun
- Lack of progress
- Lack of success (McPherson, Marteniuk, Tihanyi, & Clark, 1980; Orlick, 1973, 1974)

Such negative reactions come from a small number of dropouts (Feltz & Petlichkoff, 1983; Gould, Feltz, Horn, & Weiss, 1982; Klint & Weiss, 1986; Sapp & Haubenstricker, 1978). The majority of dropouts withdraw to pursue other interests, try different sport activities, or participate at lower intensity levels. Teens often report dropping out to take jobs. Many plan to reenter their sport later. So, much of the attrition from youth sports reflects shifting interests and involvement levels rather than negative experiences. Professionals, though, should be concerned about negative experiences, because they can be detrimental to a person's psychological development and can lead to a lifelong avoidance of healthful activities.

## Adult Activity Levels

As mentioned in earlier chapters, the amount and intensity level of physical activity decreases as adults grow older, especially among women (Boothby, Tungatt, & Townsend, 1981; Curtis & White, 1984; McPherson, 1983; Rudman, 1986). This withdrawal from and reduction in physical activity is not due to changes in physiological health alone (Spreitzer & Snyder, 1983). Psychosocial factors influence adults' activity levels (McPherson, 1986). These factors include the following:

- stereotypes of appropriate activity levels,
- limited access to facilities and programs,
- childhood experiences,
- concerns over personal limitations on exercise,
- a lack of role models,
- a lack of knowledge about appropriate exercise programs, and
- beliefs that exercise is harmful or ineffective in preventing disease (see Duda & Tappe, 1989a).

Yet indications exist that adults, especially older ones, are becoming more interested in health and the influence of physical activity on health status (Howze, DiGilio, Bennett, & Smith, 1986; Maloney, Fallon, & Wittenberg, 1984; Prohaska, Leventhal, Leventhal, & Keller, 1985).

Duda and Tappe (1988, 1989a, 1989b) proposed that adult exercise participation reflects three interrelated factors:

1. Personal incentives, such as a desire to demonstrate mastery, to compete, to be with others, to receive recognition, to maintain health, to cope with stress, and to improve physical fitness
2. A sense of self, particularly in regard to one's self-esteem for physical activity
3. Perceived options, or the opportunities a person has in a given situation, such as transportation to various sites where adult programs are offered (see Figure 9.5)

Personal incentive values and self-esteem can change throughout life. For example, the desire to compete can decrease and the desire to be with others can increase as an adult ages. Older adults also can come to perceive that their physical abilities have declined over time. Duda and Tappe surveyed 144 adults in three age groups (25 to 39, 40 to 60, and 61+ years) who were participating in an exercise program. Personal incentives differed among the age

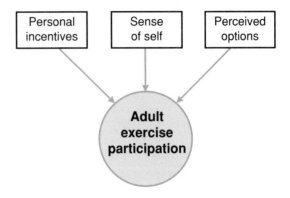

**Figure 9.5**   Three interrelated factors can influence the level of adults' exercise participation. (Based on Duda & Tappe, 1989a, and Maehr, 1984.)

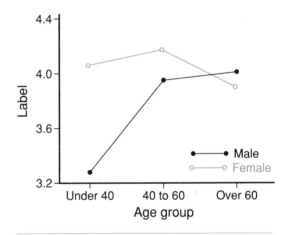

**Figure 9.6**   Personal incentives to exercise differ among adult age groups and between the genders. Group averages on the coping with stress category of the Personal Incentives for Exercise Questionnaire (a 5-point Likert-type scale) are plotted here.
(Reprinted by permission from Duda & Tappe, 1989.)

groups and between men and women (see Figure 9.6). Middle-aged and older adults placed more value on the health benefits of exercise than did young adults. For example, Figure 9.6 shows the extent to which men and women in each age group valued the stress-reducing benefits of exercise. Young adult men put little emphasis on this exercise benefit, as shown by their low average on the Personal Incentives for Exercise Questionnaire, a 5-point Likert-type scale. Men also, more so than women, valued competitive activities. Exercise leaders, then, might help older adults stick to their exercise programs by emphasizing social interaction, health benefits, and stress reduction (Duda & Tappe, 1989b).

Among these older adults there were no age group differences in self-esteem, but differences did exist between men and women. The women had lower physical self-esteem and less feeling of control over their health status than the men had. These beliefs are typically associated with less involvement, but fortunately the women felt they had more social support for their involvement than the men, and they continued to participate.

Exercise leaders who adopt strategies targeted at those adults who might have low physical self-esteem can improve participants' self-esteem and exercise involvement (Duda & Tappe, 1989b). Another group of adults might not have the same characteristic incentives and perceptions as those Duda and Tappe surveyed. Yet exercise leaders can encourage older adults to persist in their exercise programs by being aware of the incentives and perceptions of their particular groups. They then can emphasize the aspects and benefits of exercise that are most important to those participants.

## REVIEW 9.2

It is clear that a person's self-esteem in a particular domain influences behavior. People with higher physical self-esteem are more likely to seek out physical activities, to maintain their participation levels, and to exert the effort needed to improve than those with lower physical self-esteem. Parents and educators can help children develop strong self-esteem for physical activities. They can make sure that children experience success in physical endeavors and

can give children information about their progress.

Likewise, exercise leaders working with adults can provide feedback about their progress. Leaders can emphasize and provide those factors important to the particular adults in their programs. For example, they could emphasize the social dimension by pairing up participants or planning occasional social events. It is important for professionals to be aware of psychosocial influences. Very often they can structure these influences to increase the motivation and enjoyment of people of any age and help them realize the benefits of sport and exercise.

We have seen that social values and norms influence a person's sport participation and lifestyle. Certainly these values and norms differ among various cultures and ethnic groups. So, too, do standards of living, including diet. Next we will discuss what effects these and other factors might have on the motor development of various ethnic and cultural groups.

## RACIAL AND ETHNIC DIFFERENCES

Throughout our discussions we have emphasized the influence of environmental factors on motor development. For example, motor development can lag if nutrition is poor, if disease is prevalent, if environmental pollutants abound, or if physical growth is subsequently slowed, but it can be maximized if a child receives good nutrition and health care and numerous opportunities for skill practice. Educational programs can stimulate thought and creativity to maximize a child's cognitive development. The activities that family members demonstrate and the behaviors reinforced by persons important to the child can either encourage or discourage an individual's involvement in physical activities.

Child-rearing practices can lend themselves to stimulation of active play and skill development or can limit these opportunities. Economic status can influence the amount of play space and the number and type of toys available, which in turn can affect the child's opportunities to attempt and practice skills. These are just some of the environmental factors that can vary for a developing individual.

Many of these environmental factors are similar for whole groups of people—races, cultures, or ethnic groups. Could this lead to differences between such groups in the pattern or tempo of motor development? Identifying any such differences would have at least two benefits. First, if such differences exist, norms for a particular group can be established, and teachers can consider these norms when working with members of the group. Second, if researchers can identify the environmental conditions that vary between groups, then they can identify the effects of those environmental factors on the acceleration or retardation of motor development. The focus of our discussion is whether differences actually exist in motor performance between racial, ethnic, and cultural groups and which environmental factors could influence or account for these differences.

---

**CONCEPT 9.3**

Racial and ethnic differences in motor development are related to the environmental variables affecting group members.

---

## African-American and Caucasian Children

The two ethnic groups in the United States whose motor performance is tested most often are Caucasians of European ancestry and African-Americans. Sometimes, investigators have noted performance differences between the groups, although at other times and on some tests, they have detected no differences.

### Infancy and Early Childhood

Most of the performance differences found in research studies come between birth and 2 years of age and consist of temporal differences in the emergence of the motor milestones. The sequence of motor development is remarkably stable across these two groups (Malina, 1973). The timing differences are usually in favor of African-American children. For example, Bayley (1965) observed that African-American infants were ahead of Caucasian infants in mean score on the Bayley Scale of Infant Development at every month of age from 1 month to 14 months (see Table 9.2). This advantage existed on most of the 60 test items, so one type of skill was not responsible for the difference in the scale scores.

A study of African-American and Caucasian infants in the 1980s generally confirmed Bayley's observations. Capute and colleagues (1985) observed infants from 2 weeks until 2 years of age for selected milestone skills. All of the infants surpassed a minimum score on the Bayley mental and motor scales and were judged clinically normal at 2 years of age to make a fair comparison more likely. African-American children reached the motor milestones slightly earlier than Caucasian children, with a greater difference between the girls than between the boys. Socioeconomic status also was recorded. African-American infants were underrepresented in the upper socioeconomic group, the group associated with slower motor development. Therefore, it is difficult to assess racial differences independently of socioeconomic and environmental factors. Despite a few studies that failed to find significant differences between African-American and Caucasian infants (see Malina, 1973, for a summary), we can expect African-American infants on the

**Table 9.2   Performance on the Bayley Infant Scale of Motor Development for Babies by Race**

| Age (mos) | Caucasian babies | | | African-American babies | | |
| --- | --- | --- | --- | --- | --- | --- |
| | N | M | SD | N | M | SD |
| 1 | 41 | 6.34 | 2.03 | 41 | 6.39 | 2.98 |
| 2 | 45 | 9.31 | 2.20 | 37 | 9.89 | 2.22 |
| 3 | 42 | 12.12 | 2.57 | 41 | 13.39 | 2.82 |
| 4 | 47 | 14.57 | 3.20 | 31 | 16.29 | 2.92 |
| 5 | 41 | 18.83 | 3.32 | 40 | 21.25 | 3.46 |
| 6 | 44 | 25.73 | 4.40 | 42 | 25.76 | 4.78 |
| 7 | 47 | 28.47 | 4.88 | 41 | 30.46 | 4.64 |
| 8 | 61 | 34.41 | 5.27 | 51 | 35.67 | 5.02 |
| 9 | 54 | 37.13 | 4.06 | 44 | 38.95 | 4.17 |
| 10 | 53 | 40.11 | 3.62 | 40 | 41.32 | 3.93 |
| 11 | 43 | 42.84 | 3.06 | 26 | 44.00 | 2.97 |
| 12 | 49 | 44.22 | 3.16 | 43 | 45.88 | 4.42 |
| 13 | 44 | 46.45 | 6.49 | 36 | 47.08 | 3.27 |
| 14 | 48 | 48.33 | 3.01 | 38 | 48.68 | 4.03 |

*Note.* Mean scores (*M*) and standard deviations (*SD*) on the Bayley Infant Scale of Motor Development are given. Reprinted by permission from Bayley, 1965.

average to reach the motor milestones at a younger age than Caucasian infants.

Less information on ethnic-group differences in motor development is available for children between 2 and 6 years old. Further, the results of the studies of these age groups tend to be inconclusive. For example, Sessoms (1942) found African-American 3- and 4-year-olds to be ahead of Caucasian children in fine-motor tasks, but Rhodes (1937) found no fine-motor differences in a sample of preschoolers. More recently, Sandler, Van Campen, Ratner, Stafford, and Weismar (1970) compared the performance of lower class, urban African-American children at 4 to 6 years to the Denver Developmental Screening Test norms that were established primarily on Caucasian children. The African-American children compared favorably with or scored slightly ahead of the norms on gross-motor skill items and some fine-motor items. On fine-motor items involving cognitive operations, however, the

African-American children fell below the norms.

---

No clear racial trends emerge from studies of motor development in preschool children.

---

## Childhood

Comparisons of school-aged African-American and Caucasian children tend to be based on quantitative, or product-oriented, measures, including measures of functional muscle strength. Many of these comparisons also documented higher performance levels for African-American children and adolescents than for their Caucasian counterparts. For example, African-American children scored better than Caucasians on the following:

• Running dashes (boys and girls) (Hutinger, 1959; Malina, 1969; Malina and Roche,

1983; Milne et al., 1976) and agility runs (DiNucci & Shows, 1977; see Figure 9.7)
- A throw for distance (girls) (Temple, 1952)
- The standing long jump (boys and girls) (Malina & Roche, 1983; Temple, 1952)
- The vertical jump/jump and reach (boys and girls) (Jones, Buis, & Harris, 1986; Martin, 1966; Martino, 1966; Temple, 1952)

On the other hand, some studies reported little difference between African-American and Caucasian children on motor skills such as these:

- Softball throw for distance (Malina, 1969)

- Pull-ups, push-ups, or ball put (Walker, 1938)
- Sit-ups, flexed-arm hang, soccer wall volley, agility run, and 600-yd walk/run (Jones et al., 1986)

On occasion, differences in favor of Caucasian children were found, such as on these tasks:

- The broad jump and the dash (Walker, 1938)
- The vertical jump (girls) (DiNucci & Shows, 1977)
- The standing long jump (girls) for these age groups: ages 6 to 9 (Malina & Roche, 1983), kindergarten and 2nd grade (Milne et al., 1976), and age 8 (Temple, 1952)

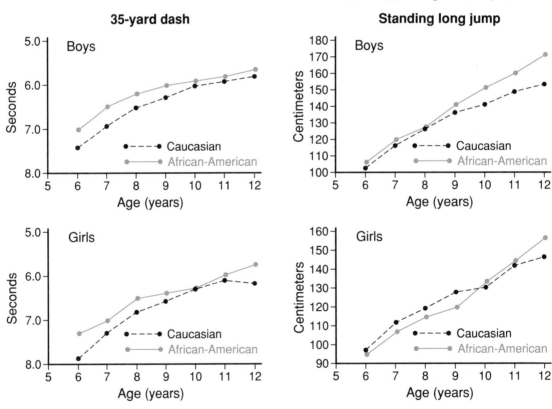

**Figure 9.7** Running dash and standing long jump performance of African-American and Caucasian boys and girls in a mixed-longitudinal study by Malina and Roche (1983).

(Reprinted by permission from Malina & Bouchard, 1991.)

- An eye-hand coordination task (Jones et al., 1986)

Our effort to find trends in these results is frustrated by repeated measures that show one group ahead at one testing but the other group ahead at the next (Malina, 1969). The findings are just as variable on measures of functional muscle strength (see Malina, 1973, for a summary). In attempting to summarize these studies, we can only conclude that performance differences between African-American and Caucasian children of school age tend to vary, with few overall trends.

## Factors Contributing to Differences

Any motor performance differences between African-American and Caucasian children could relate to genetic factors, environmental factors, or a combination of both. Let us consider the possibility of each type of factor.

### Genetic Factors

Consider whether genetic factors might explain any motor performance differences between African-Americans and Caucasians. We know that the skeletal growth of African-American infants is ahead of that of Caucasian infants (Malina, 1969), suggesting a faster maturation rate in African-Americans. Racial differences in body proportions (Martorell et al., 1988) and composition also have implications for performance. Recent studies have detected slight physiological differences between African-Americans and Caucasians. On the average, African-Americans have approximately 9% more Type II muscle fibers in the vastus lateralis thigh muscle than Caucasians, but lower performance on a maximal leg extension task after the first 45 s (Ama et al., 1986; Ama, Lagasse, Bouchard, & Simoneau, 1990). Much more research is needed on physiological differences.

The difficulty with attributing all motor development differences to genetic factors is that some studies found no developmental differences between African-Americans and Caucasians (Knobloch & Pasamanick, 1958).

---

If innate racial characteristics are operating alone, observed group differences in development should be consistent. If transient environmental variables influence the differences, different studies might produce variable results, as is the case.

---

For this reason, we emphasize environmental factors in the explanation of racial and ethnic differences in motor development.

### Environmental Factors

Environmental factors often vary between ethnic groups. We will now focus on three of these factors:

1. Economic conditions
2. Child-rearing practices
3. Socialization into sport

**Economic Conditions.** Many of the environmental conditions that could influence motor development are related to economic factors. For example, poor nutrition often results when families lack enough money to buy adequate amounts of nutritious foods. A higher incidence of infectious disease can accompany poor nutrition, poor living conditions, and lack of access to quality medical care. A shortage of toys and sport equipment can limit the practice opportunities available to children.

In the United States, more African-Americans than Caucasians are in the lower socioeconomic levels. Due to this and the pervasive effects that poverty can have on a person's life, it is clear that motor performance differences between the two races may, in many cases, ultimately be traced to economic factors. Therefore, it is vital that you remember that motor development differences may actually reflect economic rather than true racial differences.

***Child-Rearing Practices.*** Developmentalists believe that child-rearing practices influence motor performance. Because racial groups fall disproportionately into different socioeconomic classes, differences in child-rearing practices between these classes might contribute to motor performance differences between the racial groups.

In 1953, Williams and Scott found that families from the lower socioeconomic class typically permitted infants to explore their environments and manipulate objects more freely than families from higher socioeconomic levels. This would facilitate motor development. In contrast, infants in upper-class families were often placed in playpens or more restricted environments. Today some children in upper-class families are similarly restricted. For example, they are not allowed to climb on the good furniture, turn the dials on the home entertainment center, or play with the computer. Such constraints restrict a child's learning and practicing experiences and may slow motor development. Although such practices are probably not followed so rigidly by today's socioeconomic classes, these findings do remind us that child-rearing practices can influence motor development.

Another practice common today in families where both parents work is placing children in day-care facilities. The quality of care in these facilities varies widely, and if young children spend much time there, day-care centers can have a major influence on their motor development. For example, one center might have more caretakers than another and thus supervise the children more closely, perhaps unknowingly restricting their exploration of the environment. Others may be understaffed and utilize playpens more in an effort to ease the staff's work load. Still others might offer programs specifically designed to encourage chil-

dren to explore and experience their environments.

Sometimes, but not always, these characteristics of day-care centers depend on their budgets, which may in turn reflect how much parents pay. In such cases, a child's day-care experience could be related to the family's socioeconomic status.

***Socialization Into Sport.*** Some research indicates that socialization into sport differs between races. With regard to sport, Greendorfer and Ewing (1981) found that Caucasian children were primarily influenced by specific socializing agents, whereas African-American children were more influenced by social structure or contextual factors such as values and opportunities. Therefore, African-American children receive more diffuse influences than Caucasians do. African-American athletes successful in professional sports serve as role models for young African-American children because media coverage of these athletes keeps them highly visible. African-Americans successful in other areas rarely enjoy similar visibility, resulting in a lack of role models outside of the sports arena. Caucasian children have numerous role models available in a far wider range of careers, so their interests could easily shift to other areas.

Success in sport skills, then, takes on relatively more importance for African-American youths, especially boys, than it does for Caucasian youths. Again, by examining socioeconomic factors, we find some explanations for this. Sport might be one of the few leisure activities accessible to impoverished people because some sports require limited equipment and expense. In contrast, middle- and upper-class families have access to, and the resources to afford, numerous entertainment options. Lower income families may also see sport as a chance for fame and fortune and subsequently encourage their children's sport involvement (see Snyder & Spreitzer, 1983, pp. 146-153, for a review). Sports participation can provide these children opportunities to move ahead, to perhaps earn college scholarships and ultimately participate at the professional level.

Differences in the sport socialization process among racial and ethnic groups seem to indicate that in general African-American families emphasize sport participation more heavily than Caucasian, Asian-American, or Hispanic-American families. Such an emphasis could result in an earlier introduction to sport participation and more practice time for African-Americans. This could enhance motor development.

## Unanswered Issues

Although environmental factors seem to have more influence than genetic factors on motor development differences between African-Americans and Caucasians, many questions remain unexplored. We still do not clearly understand the role of socioeconomic status in motor development, in part because socioeconomic status is so intertwined with almost every aspect of a person's life. Some child-rearing practices in lower socioeconomic classes favor motor development; however, children in higher socioeconomic levels are often advanced in development as a result of better nutrition, prenatal care, and health care.

Certainly child-rearing practices and living conditions have changed since much of the initial research in these areas was conducted; consequently, comparing research studies conducted on different cohorts is questionable. More recent research is simply not available. Environmental conditions involved in racial differences might change from generation to generation, yielding variable results. As a further complication, an environmental factor in one case can offset differences due to genetic factors or other environmental factors, masking the true nature of group differences. Yet in another case, that same factor might not be strong enough to offset the others.

## Other Ethnic Groups

Mexican-Americans, other Hispanic-Americans, and Asian-Americans are sometimes included in studies of ethnic differences in motor development. Unfortunately, data on these groups are limited, and the results are even more variable than those comparing African-American and Caucasian children.

For example, Thompson and Dove (1942) and Thompson (1944) found that Spanish- and Mexican-American boys in their early teens outperformed Caucasian boys on a battery of six quantitative motor tasks (baseball throw, base running, chinning, 60-yd dash, jump and reach, and shot put). However, Miller (1968) reported the opposite results for 13- to 15-year-old boys taking the California Physical Performance Test. Obviously, the same environmental factors that may be responsible for differences noted between African-Americans and Caucasians can affect Hispanic and Asian groups as well. Both of these latter groups also tend to be smaller in physical size and stature than Caucasians, possibly accounting for some performance differences and further limiting our ability to generalize from the scant number of research studies conducted to date. It is presently impossible to identify any differential trends in the motor development of these ethnic groups.

## REVIEW 9.3

Most of the available information on racial and ethnic differences in motor development compares African-Americans and Caucasians. African-Americans typically reach motor milestones before Caucasians in the early months of life, though not all studies have found differences for this time span. But in later years it is difficult to identify trends in group differences. These results suggest that a variety of environmental factors might be operating. In a practical sense, an educator must assess on an individual basis the environmental factors influencing a single child. Knowing what factors are likely to influence a member of an ethnic group is valuable as an initial guideline if the knowledge is accepted as a generalization instead of an absolute, but further individual assessment allows for a more accurate prescription of motor activities and experiences.

## SUMMARY

We are social beings. The interactions children have with the significant others in their lives, the situations in which they live, and the feedback they receive about their activities and talents all influence their feelings about engaging in sport and exercise activities. If these feelings are negative, psychosocial factors can limit their motor performance as much as any physical deficiency or disability. If these feelings are positive, the door is open for them to enjoy activities and the feeling of mastery that accompanies achievement.

When we compare the motor performance of various racial and ethnic groups, it is difficult to identify significant trends. This indicates that environmental factors are probably more influential than genetic factors in motor performance, especially when we observe average rather than elite performers. So economic conditions, child-rearing practices, and the socialization process vary among ethnic groups and influence the extent to which individuals participate in sport and exercise, their choices of activities, and the activities in which they excel. Understanding these patterns of influence helps professionals work with individuals.

## Key Terms

aversive socialization
causal attributions
gender typing
perceived ability
self-consistent
self-esteem
sex typing
socialization
socializing agents

## Discussion Questions

1. Who are the socializing agents most likely to influence children's socialization into sport?
2. How might gender role stereotyping result in fewer women participating in sport and exercise activities?
3. How might physical education teachers turn some children away from sport and exercise participation?
4. Describe how toys are part of the socialization process.
5. How does perceived ability influence children's involvement in sport and exercise? Adults' involvement?
6. What is self-esteem? Is it general or specific? How is it developed?
7. People tend to attribute their successes and failures to various causes. What are the differences in the causal attributions made by those with high self-esteem and those with low self-esteem? To what do children tend to attribute the outcome of their performance?
8. How does perceived competence change children's causal attributions?
9. What factors are associated with children's persisting in sport activities? With dropping out?

10. Describe any differences in motor development that exist between African-American and Caucasian children. What environmental differences might play a role in ethnic differences in motor performance? How?

## Suggested Readings

Greendorfer, S. (1983). Shaping the female athlete: The impact of the family. In M.A. Boutilier & L. Sangiovanni, *The sporting woman* (pp. 135-156). Champaign, IL: Human Kinetics.

Kenyon, G.S., & McPherson, B.D. (1973). Becoming involved in physical activity and sport: A process of socialization. In G.L. Rarick (Ed.), *Physical activity: Human growth and development* (pp. 303-332). New York: Academic Press.

Malina, R.M. (1973). Ethnic and cultural factors in the development of motor abilities and strength in American children. In G.L. Rarick (Ed.), *Physical activity: Human growth and development* (pp. 333-363). New York: Academic Press.

Ostrow, A.C. (Ed.) (1989). *Aging and motor behavior*. Indianapolis: Benchmark.

Smoll, F.L., Magill, R.A., & Ash, M.J. (Eds.) (1988). *Children in sport* (3rd ed.). Champaign, IL: Human Kinetics.

# Epilogue: Every Person Is Unique

People interested in observing and teaching motor skills naturally want information about the average performances and capabilities of different age groups. Averages provide reference points against which individuals may be compared and a general idea of what to expect from members of a group. However, the study of developmental processes and the factors influencing them repeatedly demonstrates the uniqueness of individuals. Though physical growth and maturation proceed in a consistent pattern dictated by genetic makeup, a variety of environmental factors act throughout the life span to alter motor development patterns and tempos. Various experiences, including those that are perceptual, cognitive, and social, all have an impact. Differences among individuals are further manifested in the ways they progress qualitatively from unskilled to skilled performances. Thus, regardless of age, individual motor development is a reflection of genetically inherited attributes coupled with impinging environmental influences.

The challenge confronting motor developmentalists, teachers, coaches, and parents is to tailor goals and expectations to individual capabilities and characteristics. Optimal motor skill development is likely related to the degree that practice opportunities and insightful instruction are matched to individual capability and potential. Although it is both complex and time-consuming to individualize motor development goals and instruction in most institutional settings, findings from motor development research at various stages of the life span point in this direction. Continued research and observation of motor development will undoubtedly yield a better understanding of developmental processes, but our task remains to find ways of using our knowledge to foster optimal motor development in every individual.

# Glossary

**acceleration curve** — A plot of the rate of change in velocity over time. In the study of physical growth, the velocity of growth in height, weight, or some anthropometric measure is often plotted to highlight landmarks or important periods of growth. An acceleration curve is a representation of the second derivative of the function represented by the distance curve, the extent of change plotted over time.

**accommodation** — 1. Action of the ciliary muscle to change the curvature of the eye's lens to view objects of varying distance. 2. Adaptation to constant sensory stimulation by a raising of the absolute threshold level—that is, the minimal level of strength necessary for detection of a stimulus.

**aerobic capacity** — Total energy available to meet the demands of prolonged exercise, met by oxidative breakdown of food stores.

**aerobic power** — Highest amount of oxygen the body can consume during work for the aerobic production of adenosine triphosphate (ATP), which stores energy in the body.

**affordances** — The actions or behaviors provided or permitted an actor by the places, objects, and events in and of an environment. For example, a small rock affords throwing, but a boulder does not. Some hypothesize that the affordance, the behaviors allowed with respect to an environment, is perceived by animals and humans (J.J. Gibson).

**aging** — 1. The normal process of growing old, without regard to chronological age, characterized by a loss of the ability to adapt. 2. Continuing molecular, cellular, and organismic differentiation.

**anaerobic capacity** — Maximal amount of energy that a person's body can create by anaerobic glycolysis, the primary metabolic pathway for short-term, high-intensity exercise.

**anaerobic power** — Maximal rate (amount per unit time) at which the adenosine triphosphate (ATP)-PC system can produce energy.

**anaerobic threshold** — The work load or oxygen consumption level where lactate production by the working muscle exceeds the rate of lactate removal by the liver; at approximately 50% to 80% of $\dot{V}O_2max$; a higher lactate threshold has been associated with better endurance performance. Also called *lactate threshold*.

**anthropometer** — An instrument used to measure the linear breadth or width of a body segment, such as the shoulders or hips. The instrument might have straight arms (blade anthropometer), in which case a fixed arm is positioned, then a movable arm is slid into place; or C-shaped, curved arms (bow caliper), in which case the arms close onto the body segments.

**anthropometry** — The branch of science concerned with comparative measurements of the human body and its parts and proportions, often to establish frequency of occurrence among cultures, races, sexes, age groups, cohorts, etc.

**anticipation time** — The error score on a coincident timing task, in units of time, often carrying an indication of direction—usually negative numbers as early responses and positive numbers as late responses.

**anticipation timing** — The coordination of a movement response to an environmental event that the performer must predict—for example, a baseball batter coordinating the swing of the bat to the arrival of the pitch. See also **coincidence-anticipation**.

**appositional growth** — Growth by addition of new layers upon previously formed layers, prevalent when rigid materials such as bone are involved.

**asymmetrical tonic neck reflex** — An infant's extending the arm and leg on one side of the body in an unconscious reaction to turning the head to that side while lying supine.

**atrophy** — The gradual shrinking or wasting away of muscle tissue from disease or disuse.

**auditory acuity** — A person's sensitivity in detecting the presence of a sound at any given pitch.

**auditory discrimination** — The ability to distinguish two sounds on a characteristic such as pitch, loudness, or speech sound.

**auditory figure-ground** — The ability to hear the auditory stimuli of interest amidst irrelevant background noises and sounds. See also **figure-and-ground perception**.

**auditory localization** — The ability to indicate the location from which a sound originates.

**auditory pattern perception** — The ability to detect the nonrandom relationships among sounds based on one or more of the properties of time, intensity, and frequency.

**auditory-tactile integration** — The matching of an auditory event with its corresponding tactile stimulation—that is, the matching of a sound with the event that also caused tactile stimulation.

**auditory-visual integration** — The matching of an auditory event with its corresponding visual object, source, or event—that is, the matching of a sound with sight of the object/event from which the sound comes.

**aversive socialization** — Social learning through negative experiences resulting in avoidance of such experiences.

**balance** — 1. The ability to maintain or control upright body position. 2. The ability to maintain body equilibrium or steadiness.

**ballistic skills** — Motor tasks in which force is applied to an object, with or without an implement. Ballistic skills are a subdivision of fundamental manipulative skills; they include throwing, striking, volleying, and kicking.

**base of support** — The area of body part(s) in contact with a resistive surface that provides a reaction force to the applied force of the body.

**Bayley Scales of Infant Development** — A norm-referenced test, consisting of three scales, for children between 2 and 30 months of age. The mental scale measures a child's object manipulation and response to visual and auditory stimuli; it consists of 163 test items. The motor scale measures fine- and gross-motor coordination; it consists of 81 items. The behavior scale assesses various factors, such as attention and social behavior, through interview. A modified version for handicapped children is available. Split-half reliabilities, wherein the odd-numbered scores are correlated with the even-numbered scores from a large sample of children, range from .68 to .93.

**biacromial breadth** — The anthropometric measure of skeletal breadth across the shoulders, taken at the outside edges of the right and left acromial processes of the scapulae.

**bicristal breadth** — The anthropometric measure of skeletal breadth across the hips, taken at the outside edges of the iliac crests.

**biiliac breadth** — See **bicristal breadth**

**bimanual** — Pertains to two arms acting or moving at the same time, although not necessarily symmetrically.

**bimanual reaching** — Movement of the two arms toward an object.

**block rotation** — Simultaneous forward movement (lateral rotation) of the upper trunk and pelvis in ballistic skills.

**body awareness** — 1. Recognition, identification, and differentiation of the location, movement, and interrelationships of body parts and joints. 2. A performer's spatial orientation and perceived location of the body in the environment.

**body composition** — In physical growth, the partitioning of body mass into nonfat or lean body mass and fat.

**body dimensions** — The lengths, breadths, and circumferences of various body parts or segments. Often, such measurements are used to monitor an individual's physical growth and maturation.

**body image** — The concept of how one's body appears to others and the nature of its performance.

**body part identification** — The component of body awareness wherein a child can name parts of the body or locate them in response to a label.

**body-scaling** — Adapting objects, distances, and/or tasks according to the overall physical size of an individual or a body component; hence, object size or distance is scaled to an individual's body size when group members vary in body size.

**body sway** — Small, oscillatory movements of the body around a base center during balanced standing, sometimes studied for a period following a disturbance in balance.

**bow caliper** — See **anthropometer**.

**breadth caliper** — See **anthropometer**.

**breech birth** — Birth wherein the infant emerges feet, knees, or buttocks first rather than headfirst.

**Bruininks-Oseretsky Test of Motor Proficiency** — A norm-referenced test battery, for children 4.5 to 14.5 years old, that tests motor proficiency and fine- and gross-motor skills. It can help educators distinguish normal and gross-motor dysfunction populations. The long form has eight subtests and 46 test items; a short form has 14 items. Test-retest reliability is .87 for the long form, .86 for the short.

**cardiac output** — Quantity of blood pumped from the left and right ventricles per unit of time; the product of heart rate and heart stroke volume.

**cardiorespiratory endurance** — The ability to perform physical work for extended periods, dependent on an individual's maximal oxygen consumption and the percentage of maximal oxygen consumption at which he or she can maintain steady-rate exercise.

**catch-up growth** — An increase in growth rate with restoration of favorable environmental conditions after a period of influence by one or more negative factors. The extent of growth restoration depends on the length, timing, and severity of the negative condition.

**causal attributions** — Factors cited as explanations of performance outcome. Also called *causal elements.*

**cephalocaudal development** — The sequential direction of growth and behavioral development that proceeds from head to "tail."

**channel** — In information processing models, the path whereby signals are transmitted from input to output.

**choice delay** — In information processing models, the function wherein the chosen response is waiting to be performed at the appropriate time.

**choice reaction time** — A reaction time measurement requiring the earliest possible response to more than one stimulus, usually with a different response matched to each of the possible stimuli. See also **reaction time** and **simple reaction time**.

**chronological age** — An individual's calendar age, from birth to a specified date.

**chunking** — The control process (memory strategy) in which individual bits of information are organized into units, such as three numbers into a telephone area code.

**co-contraction** — Simultaneous agonistic and antagonistic muscle actions.

**cohort** — A group of individuals with a common characteristic. In motor development, the characteristic is often time of birth, although there is no definitive time span for inclusion.

**coincidence-anticipation task** — A task of watching a moving stimulus and accurately timing a response to coincide with the arrival of the stimulus at a designated target. An example is batting a pitched ball.

**coincident timing** — The skill of making a response at the instant a moving object coincides with a fixed object or target. Also called **coincidence-anticipation task**; *transit reaction*.

**component steps** — Levels within the intra-task sequences of skill development as classified by body area, such as legs or trunk.

**confidence interval** — A range outside of which an event or score is not expected to occur.

**congenital** — Pertains to a trait, condition, or disease present at birth, due either to heredity or to an influence arising during gestation.

**consolidation** — A characteristic of developmental stages indicating that the behaviors of a stage gradually emerge and mix with behaviors of the previous stage, with the latter behaviors being reworked and performance improved.

**constancy scaling** — The tendency for a person to perceive objects and distances as the same size or the actual distance despite their distance from the observer and, therefore, their size on the eye's retina.

**continuous skill** — A motor task with an arbitrary beginning point and an arbitrary end point, often but not necessarily cyclic (antonym: *discrete skill*).

**continuous tracking task** — A task in which a subject, using a stylus, control stick, or sight, stays as close as possible to a continuously moving target, which is often on a pursuit rotor apparatus.

**contralateral** — On the opposite side of the body.

**contrast sensitivity** — The ability to visually resolve spatial structures, varying from fine to coarse, at various levels of contrast.

**control processes** — 1. Functions that facilitate transfer of information within the nervous system. Many of these functions are involved in memory. Some are under direct control of an individual whereas others are automatic. 2. Memory strategies at the disposal of an individual that, when applied, can help an individual remember more effectively.

**coordinative structure** — A class of movements with common active muscle groups (sometimes spanning many joints) constrained to function as a single unit. The collective is part of a hierarchy of organized movement execution to reduce the number of parameters that must be controlled.

**correlation coefficient** — A statistic that expresses the degree of relationship between two variables. Correlation coefficients range from .00 to 1.00, positive or negative. The closer a coefficient is to 1.00, the greater the relationship. A positive correlation indicates the same standing on both variables—that is, high on both, low on both, etc. A negative correlation indicates high standing on one variable but low on the other.

**co-twin method** — Use of one twin as a standard, or control, to which the other is compared after some particular training.

**crawling** — Locomotion with the body in a prone position, trunk on the ground. The feet or knees exert a pushing motion and the arms engage in pulling (often confused with creeping).

**creeping** — Locomotion on hands and knees with the trunk off the ground. Although first attempts can be characterized by movement of one limb at a time, or homolateral movement of the arm and leg (i.e., arm and leg on the same side of the trunk), the developmentally advanced pattern is contralateral (i.e., opposite arm and leg). It is often confused with crawling.

**criterion-referenced scale** — Evaluation of performance based on a behaviorally established standard or level of mastery to meet an educational goal when available norms are not applicable or available; standards are generally based on biomechanical or developmental criteria.

**critical period** — A span of time during which a developing organism is most susceptible to the influence of an event, stimulus, or mitigating factor. For example, early childhood is a critical period for the acquisition of language.

crossing midline — The component of body awareness wherein (a) a task is completed by a body part crossing the body's midline, or (b) movements on each side of the midline are sequenced.

cross-modal functioning — A form of intersensory integration in which information presented in two different sensory modalities—tactile and visual, for instance—is interrelated based on a concept or principle, such as smoothness.

cross-sectional research design — The experimental technique used to imply development by studying groups of varying ages at one time rather than following a single group for a longer time to obtain repeated observations.

declarative knowledge — Factual information.

degrees of freedom — 1. The number of free variables. In movement control, these free variables (muscles, joints) must be regulated to produce intentional or purposeful movement. 2. The number of planes in which motion at a joint is possible. 3. In statistical analysis, the number of observations minus the number of restrictions on these observations, which is equal to the number of independent calculations used to derive a given statistic.

Denver Developmental Screening Test — A norm-referenced test for children from birth to age 6 that screens children for developmental delays. Four areas are assessed: personal-social, fine-motor adaptive, language, and gross-motor. The test includes 105 items, but typically only 20 need to be administered to each child. A short form of 12 items is available.

depth perception — A person's judgment of the distance from self to an object or place in space.

derotative righting — Body righting and neck righting reflexes.

development — The process of continuous change to a state of specialized functional capacity and adaptation to maintain that state. Often confused with growth and maturation.

developmental age — An indicator of physical or psychological maturation based on important physiological landmarks rather than chronological age or growth.

developmental delay — 1. Failure of a developing organism to exhibit a skill or behavior within the chronological age span during which most members of the species exhibit that behavior. 2. Initial exhibition of a skill or behavior at an older age than the age at onset for the majority of a species.

developmental lag — See developmental delay.

developmental sequence — A progression of qualitative changes in behavior or movements that eventually lead to mature behavior or mechanically efficient movement. This progression is assumed to be consistent across normal individuals, and the changes intransitive (fixed in order).

diaphysis — The shaft of a long bone, located between the epiphyses.

dichotic listening task — A task in which one must listen to different sounds or speech in the two ears at the same time.

differential threshold — The smallest difference between stimuli, correctly reported 75% of the time.

differentiated trunk rotation — The preferred movement pattern in a forceful overarm throw and similar skills, in which first the lower trunk unwinds or rotates to the front-facing position, then the upper trunk.

differentiation — Development of a mass of homogeneous cells into specialized tissues.

directional awareness — The understanding of concepts about movement direction, including such concepts as laterality and directionality.

directionality — 1. The ability to identify or project dimensions to the space external to the body. 2. The grasp of spatial concepts about the movements or locations of objects in the environment.

**discrimination tasks** — Tasks based on the ability to decipher variations in sensory stimuli.

**distance curve** — A plot of the extent to which some measurement increases over time. Regarding physical growth, often plots height, weight, circumference, limb length, and so on against advancing age.

**domain** — A sphere of behavior or a field of knowledge.

**dominant genetic disorder** — A disorder that results when an individual inherits one normal gene and one defective gene, the defective gene subsequently dominating the normal gene. Offspring of a carrier have a 50% chance of inheriting the defective gene.

**double-knee lock** — The pattern of walking or running where the knee changes from extension (at foot strike) to flexion (near midstance) to extension again (near toe-off).

**double support phase** — The portion of a cyclic locomotor skill when the two legs support the body's weight, not necessarily evenly, as exhibited by contact with the surface.

**dynamic balance** — Maintenance of equilibrium either on a moving surface or while moving the body through space.

**dynamic environment** — A changing setting.

**dynamic systems theory** —A branch of ecological psychology proposing that the organization of the body's physical and chemical systems restricts behavior to certain limits, although behavior is seen to emerge from the organism, the environment, and the goal of the task. The organism is considered to consist of cooperative systems that may self-organize. These systems develop at different rates such that one or more may dictate the appearance of new behaviors.

**ecological psychology** — A branch of psychology whose proponents argue that individuals (both humans and animals) perceive their environment directly, without the intervention of memories and representations—

in contrast to what information processing proponents argue.

**effect size** — A statistical term that refers to the difference between means divided by the standard deviations, thus providing a standardized contrast or difference in units of standard deviation.

**embryo** — The prenatal human organism from conception until 8 weeks.

**encoding** —The transformation of perceptual information where input is identified into a form that can be stored in the central nervous system (memory).

**epiphyseal (growth) plate** — The area near the ends of long bones between the epiphysis and shaft. This is where new bone cells are deposited, allowing lengthening of the bone.

**epiphysis** — A center for ossification (bone formation) at each end of a long bone.

**equilibration process** —The alternation between periods of stability and instability as an individual moves through developmental stages. The instability is brought about by imbalance between the individual's mental structure and the environment, and the stability is brought about by consolidation, or the mixing of developmental stages for improved performance (Piaget).

**equilibrium** — 1. A balanced or stabilized state. 2. The ability to maintain or control upright body position. 3. In dynamics, the zero length of a springlike element.

**external feedback** —1. Information received as the result of a response or act from an outside source. 2. Feedback obtained through an external sense receptor, usually the eye or ear.

**eye-hand coordination** —The ability to perform hand movements precisely based on visual information.

**feedback** — 1. Any kind of information received as a result of a particular response or act. 2. The afferent neural information produced by sensory receptors as a result of movement (sensory feedback). 3. The means by which input and output are linked to regulate a system.

fetus — The unborn human infant from the end of the 8th week after conception to birth.

fifty percent (50%) phasing — Cyclic movements of two limbs in which one limb passes through corresponding points of its trajectory exactly one-half cycle after the other limb.

figure-and-ground perception — A person's ability to see an object of interest as distinct from the background.

fine-motor skill — The type of skill performed by the small musculature, particularly of the hands and fingers.

flexibility — The range of motion about a joint.

foot strike — Contact of a foot or feet with a surface in a locomotor skill after a period of flight or recovery from a preceding step.

form constancy — A person's ability to recognize a shape or form as the same regardless of its orientation, size, color, or the context in which it is present.

front facing — The moment in throwing when the thrower's shoulders rotate to a position facing (parallel with) the target.

functional strength tests — Evaluations of strength from performance of fundamental motor skills, necessarily confounding strength and motor coordination.

gait pattern — The spatial-temporal (space-time) relationship exhibited by the legs during locomotion.

galloping — The locomotor pattern wherein one foot takes the lead to step forward and the trailing foot closes with a leap-step. The landing of the leap-step is even with the lead foot. The pattern is repeated with the same foot always leading.

gender typing — See sex typing

genetic disposition — A tendency to develop a disease or condition, based on inheritance, if an individual encounters certain environmental conditions. Hence, a genetic disposi-

tion for an allergic condition is manifested only with exposure and sensitization to an allergen.

genotype — The genetic makeup of an individual.

gestation age — The length of time the fetus remains in the uterus, beginning with conception.

gross-motor skill — A motor task either requiring large musculature or moving the body in space.

grouping — The control process (memory strategy) wherein individual bits of information are organized into groups.

growth — Quantitative increase in the size or mass of a living being or any of its parts as a result of an increase in already complete units and the transformation of nonliving nutrients into protoplasm.

hand dominance — A person's consistent preference to use one hand rather than the other.

hand-eye coordination — See eye-hand coordination.

hand preference — A person's choice to use one hand rather than the other for a given task. It may or may not be the dominant hand.

hand shaping — Appropriate, anticipatory positioning of the hand and fingers when reaching to grasp an object.

haptic perception — The component of kinesthetic perception that combines information from the cutaneous receptors and the proprioceptors.

Hawthorne effect — The tendency of participants to perform with more effort when they perceive an event to be new or special.

head circumference — The anthropometric measurement of head size, taken as the minimum circumference obtainable 1 inch above the ears and above the eyebrows. Large deviations from average head circumference for age in infants may indicate a need for medical attention, often because of abnormal brain growth.

**hemispheric dominance** — The concept that one hemisphere of the brain is more important than the other in controlling particular bodily functions and mental processes. For example, some consider the left hemisphere more important than the right due to its role in language.

**hemoglobin** — The iron-protein molecule in the red blood cell that carries oxygen throughout the body; approximately 1.34 ml of oxygen combines with each gram of hemoglobin.

**heredity** — The characteristics parents biologically transmit to offspring at conception.

**hierarchical integration** — The characteristic of developmental stages (Piaget) indicating that subsequent stages incorporate the previous stage and that new structures are formed by transforming or reorganizing the preceding structures.

**high guard** — The arm position in locomotor skills wherein the arms are abducted at the shoulders, the elbows flexed, and the hands held at or above shoulder level; often seen in early development of a locomotor skill.

**homolateral** — On the same side of the body. Also called *ipsilateral*.

**hopping** — The locomotor pattern wherein the body is projected from the floor by one leg and lands on the same leg while either stationary or traversing a distance.

**horizontal decalage** — The developmental lag between an individual's entrance into a developmental stage and the appearance of a behavior that is characteristic of that stage (Piaget). All of the characteristic behaviors do not appear at once.

**humerus lag** — A characteristic of efficient overhand throwing in which the arm follows the trunk in rotating forward. The humerus does not horizontally flex past the trunk before the trunk faces front.

**hyperplasia** — Growth in a tissue or organ through an increase in the number of cells.

**hypertrophy** — Growth in a tissue or organ through an increase in the size of tissue elements, not cell number.

**hypokinetic circulation** — Type of vascular circulation characteristic of children in which cardiac output is relatively low.

**hypoxia** — Insufficient amount of oxygen.

**infantile reflexes** — Involuntary responses to specific stimuli, present prenatally, in infancy, or both but that disappear or are inhibited as the infant matures. Also called **neonatal reflexes**.

**information processing** — Manipulation of information in humans or machines through a number of operations leading to a response or output.

**information processing perspective** — The view that humans and machines manipulate information through a number of operations—including sensory input, perception, the retrieval and storage of information (memory), and response selection—before making a response.

**interception skills** — Fundamental skills wherein control of a moving object is gained by catching, fielding, trapping, or similar means.

**internal feedback** — 1. Information available to a performer, through one or more of the senses, as an inherent consequence of performing a task. 2. Information available to a performer through the proprioceptors, as a consequence of performing a task.

**internalize** — To incorporate attitudes or standards of conduct into one's own behaviors.

**intersensory integration** — The ability to match sensory information from multiple sources—for example, visual, auditory, and tactual—simultaneously.

**intransitivity** — The characteristic of developmental stages (Piaget) indicating that the order or sequence of the stages cannot be changed.

**intrasensory discrimination** — The ability to distinguish stimuli within an individual sensory system.

**intratask development** — See **developmental sequence**.

in utero — 1. Within the uterus. 2. Referring to the fetus in the womb.

jumping — The locomotor skill in which the performer takes off on one foot or both feet and after a period of flight lands on both feet simultaneously.

kinesthesis — 1. Information that is derived from a combination of senses—the muscle spindles, Golgi tendon organs, joint receptors, cutaneous receptors, semicircular canals, and hair cells in the utricle and saccule—that gives the performer a sense of limb position and body position in space. 2. Sense of movement.

kinesthetic discrimination — The ability to identify differences in objects—such as size, weight, texture, and shape—through kinesthetic (tactual) exploration or manipulation.

kinesthetic perception — The perceptual system that yields information about limb and body position in space and movement, and about aspects of the external environment with which the body comes in contact. See also kinesthesis.

kinesthetic system — The sensory systems that provide information about position of the limbs and the body in space.

knowledge base — The amount of information a person possesses on a specific topic, consisting of declarative knowledge and possibly procedural and strategic knowledge.

knowledge of results (KR) — Information given to the performer at the conclusion of performance regarding the outcome of a movement response. It is often verbal.

knowledge structure — The manner in which a person organizes information about a topic, typically expressed in hierarchical fashion. Experts on a topic tend to structure information in similar ways.

kwashiorkor — A disease of malnutrition, particularly protein deficiency, characterized by edema, potbelly, change in hair color, anemia, bulky stools, and depigmentation of the skin.

labeling — A rehearsal strategy that helps a person recall a movement by attaching to it a meaningful verbal label.

lag — A delay, slowing, or stoppage in the forward movement of a limb, limb component, or implement held by a limb during execution of a ballistic skill. See also developmental delay.

lateral dominance — The consistent preference for use of one eye, ear, hand, or foot instead of the other, although the preference for different anatomical units is not always on the same side.

laterality — The awareness that one's body has two distinct sides that can move independently; a component of body awareness.

lean body mass — Fat-free body plus essential fat stores; equals body mass minus storage fat.

leaping — The locomotor pattern consisting of an elongated running step. It can be interspersed in a run or performed continuously with an alternating foot pattern.

leg length — The anthropometric measure of the leg's linear size, measured in one of three ways: (a) the distance from the greater trochanter to the lateral malleolus, (b) the distance from the greater trochanter to the bottom of the foot (or floor, if subject stands), or (c) the difference between standing height and sitting height (sometimes termed functional leg length).

limited capacity channel — An hypothesis that the amount of stimulus information a person can handle simultaneously in the central nervous system to produce multiple responses is limited. This limitation is likely due to the person's optimal capacity to process information. Exceeding this capacity often results in cognitive interference between tasks, which slows response time and increases errors.

locomotor reflexes — The group of reflexes so named because the automatic response resembles a voluntary locomotor skill in spatial-temporal pattern, such as the walking reflex.

locomotor skills — The group of skills in

which the performer transports the body through space from one place to another.

**longitudinal research design** — A research technique in which the same individual is observed performing the same task or observed on the same measurement over a long time to determine developmental change.

**long-term memory store** — 1. Recall, recognition, and retrieval of information after a delay of hours, days, or years without rehearsal. 2. Structure within the information processing areas of the brain in which input is selectively and permanently stored. The input may be forgotten or subsequently retrieved through recall or recognition after a delay of hours, days, or years without rehearsal.

**low birth weight** — A birth weight usually below 2,500 g, without regard to length of gestation.

**low guard** — The arm position in locomotor skills wherein the arms hang down at the sides and do not swing in coordination with leg action.

**manipulative skills** — Gross skills involving the hands or feet that impart force to objects or receive force from them, often to gain control of them. Manipulative skills are one type of fundamental motor skill; the other categories are locomotor and nonlocomotor skills. The manipulative skills include, but are not limited to, throwing, catching, kicking, trapping, volleying, dribbling, striking, and fielding.

**marasmus** — Wasting due to prolonged dietary deficiency of calories and protein.

**mark-time pattern** — Locomotion wherein the swing leg touches down alongside the support leg rather than swinging past the support leg to move the body forward. Often seen in young children in their early attempts to ascend or descend stairs.

**maturation** — 1. Qualitative advancement in biological makeup. 2. Cellular, organ, or system advancement in biochemical composition.

**maximal oxygen consumption** — Highest amount of oxygen the body can consume during work for the aerobic production of adenosine triphosphate (ATP), which stores energy in the body.

**maximum exercise test** — A test measuring maximum aerobic capacity by exercising an individual until the oxygen uptake plateaus and does not increase further with an increase in work load.

**meiosis** — A process of cell division that forms gametes and reduces the number of chromosomes by one half.

**memory capacity** — The amount of information that can be held in memory.

**memory span** — The number of items that can be repeated after one presentation.

**menarche** — Time of a female's first menstrual period.

**meta-analysis** — Statistical analysis technique that permits researchers to pool the results of many research studies by expressing differences on a scale independent of the specific measurement used in each study.

**metabolic rate** — Amount of energy expended in a given time.

**middle guard** — The arm position in locomotor skills wherein the hands are held nearly motionless at waist level.

**midsupport** — The point approximately halfway through the support phase in the step of a locomotor skill.

**mitosis** — Cell division wherein the chromosomes split, going to daughter cells each containing the same number of chromosomes as the original cell.

**mixed dominance** — The consistent preference for using one eye, hand, or foot over the other when the preference is for different sides and different parts of the body (e.g., left eye, right hand, left foot).

**mixed longitudinal design** — A research technique combining longitudinal and cross-sectional observations. Some subjects are observed over the full length of the study, whereas others are monitored part of the time or just once.

**modal** — Pertaining to the mode, or the score or behavior that occurs most often in a set of observations. In motor development, modal often refers to the behavior within a developmental sequence that is most frequently observed.

**modal level** — The level within a developmental sequence a subject exhibits most often on the trials composing an observation session.

**modeled behavior** — Imitated action following the observance of a demonstration of that action.

**Moro reflex** — An infant's reflexive response to a sudden noise or jolt, a sneeze, or being dropped a short distance through the air; consists of spinal extension and horizontal arm abduction, then adduction. Also called *startle reflex*.

**morphological age** — An assessment of biological maturation wherein a measurement of an individual's body height, limb length, breadth, or physique is compared to the average measurement for a given chronological age.

**morphologic growth** — Growth in terms of body structure, proportions, and physique.

**motor behavior** — The movement responses made by an organism.

**motor control** — The subdisciplinary area of study concerned with the mechanisms, both voluntary and reflexive, that control human movement.

**motor development** — The subdisciplinary area of study concerned with change and stability in motor behavior from conception to death.

**motor learning** — 1. A relatively permanent improvement in skill resulting from practice and inferred from performance. 2. The subdisciplinary area of study concerned with the acquisition of skills as a result of practice and the manner in which skills are taught (instructional strategies) and executed.

**motor milestones** — A set of fundamental skills a person acquires during infancy in a relatively fixed order that varies among individuals. So named because they are often landmarks (key points) in motor development.

**motor pattern** — A combination of limb and trunk movements organized in a particular temporal-spatial (time and space) arrangement.

**motor program** — An abstraction of one or more movements scientists believe to be previously learned and stored in the central nervous system. In traditional views, a person selects and initiates the movement without regard to sensory feedback, with corrections based on sensory feedback only after at least one reaction time has elapsed. Other views incorporate sensory feedback correction of movement execution, but not movement selection.

**motor scale** — See **Bayley Scales of Infant Development**

**motor unit** — Smallest controllable muscular unit consisting of a single motor neuron and the muscle fibers it innervates.

**movement awareness** — Knowledge of the extent of movement that takes place at one or more body joints, and that a person often demonstrates by reproducing some movement as accurately as possible.

**movement generator** — The functional stage in an information processing model wherein, once the decision mechanism loads one or motor programs into the generator, the individual organizes and initiates the program, selecting the appropriate musculature to achieve the movement goal.

**movement pattern generator** — See **pattern generator**

**movement process** — The spatial-temporal pattern of a movement.

**movement product** — The outcome of a movement, typically gauged quantitatively.

**neonatal reflexes** — See **infantile reflexes**

**neonate** — A newborn infant.

**neural noise** — Random activity in the nervous system that interferes with the individual's perception of external stimuli.

**norm-referenced scale** — Evaluation consisting of standardized tasks administered under conditions that are similar to, and comparisons based on variables that are consistent with, the assessed group.

**ontogenesis** — The progressing life history of an individual.

**ontogenetic** — 1. Refers to the development of an individual. 2. Refers to behavioral changes resulting from learning.

**opening up** — Body movements in throwing and striking skills wherein body parts are moving in the opposite direction simultaneously (e.g., contralateral leg forward, arm and shoulder back) to ultimately produce force in the direction of object projection. (If observed from the side, the performer appears to "stretch out.")

**open kinetic chain** — Sequence of movements that permit transfer of momentum from one body part to another, typically from more massive body parts to less massive body parts, to maximize the performance of ballistic skills.

**opposition** — The movement pattern wherein the arm and the leg on opposite sides of the body swing forward and back in unison, with the remaining arm and leg swinging in the opposite direction.

**optic array** — The reverberating flux of light waves resulting from the characteristic way each surface in the environment reflects light according to its color, texture, and angle of inclination. This flux of light waves provides the viewer the stimulus for visual perception.

**optic flow** — A change in the pattern of optical texture as the viewer moves forward or back in a stable environment.

**Osgood-Schlatter disease** — Condition affecting the area below the knee in which osteochondrosis or separation of the tibial tubercle occurs at the epiphyseal junction.

**ossification** — The formation of bone or a bony substance.

**out-toeing** — A characteristic of walking and running wherein the feet are planted with the toes pointed to the front and side, oblique to the line of progression. Sometimes the feet are also swung forward after toe-off at an oblique (outward) angle.

**palmar grasp reflex** — An infant's reflexive contraction of the finger flexor muscles in response to a tickling of the palm.

**parachute** — To extend the arms to the front and side in anticipation of losing balance when landing from a jump.

**pattern generator** — The oscillator mechanism in the central nervous system that provides muscular synergies to the various motor units involved in a movement. Also called *central pattern generator*.

**patterning** — A proposed method of treating children with developmental delays wherein they repeatedly perform active and passive movements similar to patterns for crawling, creeping, and walking.

**pattern perception** — The ability to detect nonrandom relationships among stimuli.

**pattern recognition** — The ability to perceive a relationship among stimuli such that a person visually perceives certain lines as a shape or auditorily perceives certain spoken sounds as a word.

**peak oxygen uptake** — See **maximal oxygen consumption**.

**peak velocity** — A point during growth when the rate of growth is the greatest.

**perceived ability** — One's subjective assessment of one's own skills, on which is based one's stable, internal explanation (causal attribution) for one's performance outcomes.

**perception** — The multistage process of knowing objects and events through the senses.

**perception-action perspective** — A proposal that properties of perception and action each are rationalized by the other; that is, perception is manifested in action, and actions are constrained by perceptions.

perceptual anticipation — The acquisition or matching of a moving target along a predictable path at a predictable rate, requiring a prediction of target position at the end of the response movement.

perceptual constancy — A person's ability to recognize objects or distances as stable and consistent even when their dimensions vary at the sensory receptor. For example, a person perceives a chair to be stable in size if he or she views it at a distance, yielding a small image on the retina, then views it nearby, yielding a large image on the retina.

perceptual filter — A functional operation during information processing wherein certain input is screened out while other information is identified and passed on for processing (e.g., storage, decision making, rehearsal), the distinction in humans being influenced by past experience.

perceptual-motor skills — 1. Pertains particularly to motor skills in which perception plays a large role, with perceptual discrimination often dictating the appropriate response. 2. Pertains to the motor skills children acquire.

perceptual size constancy — See perceptual constancy.

perturbation — 1. A disturbance to a movement that is not anticipated by the performer. 2. A disturbance in balance, induced in experimental settings to measure subsequent postural sway, or the latency and pattern of a movement in response to the disturbance.

phase — 1. A step in a developmental sequence based on a qualitative change in behavior. The term is sometimes used when the sequential change is not known to meet the criteria of a stage of behavior. 2. A portion of the life cycle that is temporary but characterized by typical behavior. 3. In cyclic motion, the factor on which two or more cyclic motions can be compared for identical period, frequency, and starting time.

phylogenesis — The progressing life history of a species.

phylogenetic — 1. Refers to the development of a race or species. 2. Refers to behavioral changes that occur automatically as an individual matures.

physical fitness — Physiological state of well-being that provides a degree of protection against disease.

physique — The physical structure of the body; body build.

pincer grasp — A hand grasp that employs opposition of the thumb with a finger to obtain a small object.

plasticity — 1. Adaptability and flexibility. 2. In growth, the ability of cells or tissue to take on a new function in the event of injury or damage to other cells.

postural reactions — The group of reflexes whose automatic responses change the body's orientation or posture. Also called gravity reflexes.

postural sway — See body sway.

power — The amount of work done per unit of time. Mean power is the average over some time period. Peak power is the highest value attained.

power grip — A hand grasp in which a person holds a handle against the palm so that he or she may generate power in using the implement.

precision grip — A hand grasp in which a person holds the object near the ends of the fingers so that it may be shifted or manipulated.

prehension — The grasping of an object, usually with the hand.

preparatory crouch — The position a person takes before takeoff in a jump wherein the hips, knees, ankles, and trunk are flexed so that they can extend more fully in the takeoff.

prereaching — Arm movements toward objects of interest that newborn infants make before they are capable of reaching for and grasping them.

**pressure epiphysis** — In growing children, the growth plate located at the ends of long bones, especially those that bear weight (hence the term *pressure*).

**primacy-recency effect** — The principle that the initial and ending portions of a series of items or movements are remembered better than those in the middle.

**primitive reflexes** — The class of reflexes that appear prenatally or early after birth; these are often necessary for early survival. They are typically mediated by the lower brain centers.

**procedural knowledge** — Information about how to do something in accordance with applicable rules.

**progressive overload** — Training wherein resistance, intensity, distance, repetitions, and so on are gradually increased as performance improves.

**proprioception** — Sensory information about (a) position of the body and its parts, (b) extent and force of movement, (c) muscular tension, and (d) physical pressure, all arising from the vestibular apparatus, Golgi tendon organs, muscle spindles, and/or joint receptors.

**proprioceptive system** — The sensory modality including the muscle spindle receptors, the Golgi tendon organs, the joint receptors, and the vestibular apparatus.

**proprioceptors** — The set of sensory receptors that includes the muscle spindle receptors, the Golgi tendon organs, the joint receptors, and the vestibular apparatus.

**proximodistal trend** — The tendency for development in structure or function to advance first in the trunk, then in the near limbs, in the far limbs, and finally in the hands and the feet.

**qualitative change** — Variation of movement in terms of the spatial-temporal movement patterns; the movement process rather than its outcome.

**quantitative change** — Variation of movement in numerical terms reflecting the movement's outcome.

**rate controller** — The elements or systems that change the slowest in maturation or the fastest in aging, thus controlling the rate of change when other elements or systems would permit the behavior.

**rate limiter** — The elements or systems that mature slowly, thereby delaying the appearance of a skill during development, even though other elements or systems are advanced.

**reaction time** — The interval between onset of a stimulus, presented to one or more of the sensory modalities, and initiation of a response to that signal. See **choice reaction time** and **simple reaction time**.

**recapitulation theory** — The viewpoint that an individual organism passes through stages that approximate the development of the species to which that individual belongs.

**recency effect** — See **primacy-recency effect**.

**reception skills** — Gross skills, such as catching, trapping, and fielding, in which an individual receives force from some object.

**receptor anticipation** — Acquisition or matching of a target moving along a displayed path, requiring the performer to predict the duration of the response movement.

**recessive genetic disorder** — A disorder resulting from inheritance of a defective gene from both parents who were both unaffected. Approximately one in four offspring of parents carrying (but not displaying) the gene are affected.

**reciprocity** — 1. An aspect of social learning theory in which the interaction between individual and environment consists of internalizing a model's behavior and attempting to match this internalization in progressive approximations. 2. A child's belief that punishment of misbehavior should logically follow from the misbehavior (Piaget).

**recoding** — A control process (memory strategy) wherein two or more items in short-term memory are combined based on some similarity, then encoded in long-term memory as one item.

**recumbent length** — The anthropometric measure of body length taken while the subject is lying in a standard (specified) body position. Typically used to measure the height of children younger than 2 years old.

**reflex** — Involuntary response of the central nervous system to a specific stimulus.

**regression** — 1. In motor development, the appearance of a movement pattern or technique that the individual has previously outgrown or suppressed but that is evident as he or she attempts to learn a new skill. 2. A return to an earlier level of learning. 3. In conditioning, reappearance of a previously extinguished conditioned response after punishment.

**rehearsal** — A control process (memory strategy) in which the individual repeats information or movement or accumulates experience.

**reliable score** — Outcome of a test that yields consistent scores upon repeated measurements of the same group.

**retinal disparity** — Difference in the images the two eyes receive as a result of their distinct locations; a cue in depth perception.

**reversion** — See **regression**.

**righting reflexes** — Reflexes that bring the body to its normal position in space when any force tending to put it into a false position stimulates any one of a variety of sensory receptors in the labyrinth, eyes, muscles, or skin.

**right-left discrimination** — The ability to label the lateral dimensions of the body as right or left.

**rooting reflex** — An infant's involuntary turning of the head to the side in reaction to touching the cheek on that side with a smooth object.

**rotational velocity** — The time ,rate of change of angular position.

**running** — The locomotor pattern in which weight is transferred from one leg to the other. There is a period of flight between toe-off of the rear leg and touchdown of the forward leg.

**saccule** — A small membranous pouch in the vestibule of the inner ear that responds to movement of the head in a straight line in relation to the force of gravity.

**schema** — 1. A set of rules, formed by abstracting information from related movement experiences, that includes the underlying movement principle for this class of responses. 2. A unit of thought that grows and differentiates with the experiences of childhood (Piaget).

**secondary sex characteristics** — Aspects of form or structure appropriate to males or females, often used to assess biological maturity in adolescents.

**secular trend** — Change in a landmark of physical growth or development, such as menarche, over successive generations, usually by influence of environmental factors.

**selective attention** — The ability to focus on specific stimuli or features, ignoring other (presumably irrelevant) concurrent stimuli.

**selective filter** — See **perceptual filter**.

**self-adjusting system** — See **self-organizing system**.

**self-consistent** — Behaving with a high degree of interrelationship; reliable behavior.

**self-efficacy** — Capability to make a certain response that produces a successful outcome; a situation-specific factor that can influence a person's choice of activities, amount of effort expended, and how long a person will persist in the face of obstacles and aversive experiences. 2. Situation-specific form of self-confidence; the belief that one is competent and can do whatever is necessary in a specific situation; may fluctuate from time to time. Also called *efficacy*, *efficacy expectations*.

**self-esteem** — Feelings of competence or self-worth.

**self-organizing system** — A system that can establish relationships among its elements without a detailed higher order command. In dynamic models of human interlimb coordination, muscle collectives acting as limit cycle oscillators can entrain to act as a single unit by mutual synchronization, not higher order control.

self-select — Process whereby individuals anticipate outcomes and act consistent with anticipated favorable outcomes. For example, a short individual might want to play basketball but, in anticipation of not being selected for a basketball team, instead tries out for the tennis team.

sensation — Stimulation of one or more sensory receptors and subsequent transmission of nerve impulses along afferent pathways to the brain.

sensitive period — A span of time during which a developing organism is particularly susceptible to the influence of an event, stimulus, or mitigating factor. Sometimes used as a more accurate term for critical period.

sensoriperceptual development — Refinement of the sensory processes and perception based on sensory information such that more and more complex sensory information can be detected and evaluated.

sensory integration — The ability to match or combine sensory information from multiple sources simultaneously, either within or between modalities. Also see intersensory integration.

sensory register — See sensory store.

sensory store — The functional memory location where a physiological representation of information is held for a brief time, usually 2 to 3 s for vision and up to 15 s for other modalities.

sequential research design — See mixed longitudinal design.

sex-linked disorder — A disorder involving genes carried on the sex chromosomes (X and Y chromosomes). Also called sex-linked recessive disorder. See also recessive genetic disorder.

sex typing — Labeling an activity as appropriate or inappropriate for individuals of a given sex—for instance, labeling a sport as masculine or feminine.

sexual age — An assessment of biological maturity based on primary and secondary sex characteristics.

shape discrimination — The ability to match or differentiate between shapes or forms.

shape identification — The ability to name various shapes and forms.

short-term memory store — The component of memory with a relatively short duration (thought to be less than 60 s) and limited capacity (thought to be seven items or chunks of information, plus or minus two).

sigmoid curve — The name given the plot of typical whole-body growth measures because of its S appearance, resulting from rapid gain in infancy and early life, steady gain in middle childhood, rapid gain during adolescence, and then a slowing in late adolescence until the cessation of growth.

simple reaction time — The interval between the onset of a single stimulus and the initiation of a single response to that signal.

single knee-lock — A characteristic of immature walking in infants consisting of one knee extension action during the entire support phase following foot strike with a partially flexed knee. In the mature double knee-lock, the knee is extended at foot strike, then flexes as body weight transfers over the foot, then extends again.

sitting height — The anthropometric measure of trunk plus head and neck length, recorded from the sitting surface to the vertex of the skull when the body is in a standard sitting position (i.e., when the head is in the horizontal plane).

size constancy — The recognition that an object maintains its size even if its distance from the observer varies and the size of the retinal image therefore changes.

skeletal age — An assessment of biological age based on the extent of change in the developing skeleton in selected body areas.

skill — 1. A learned movement task. 2. A qualitative indicator of performance denoting proficient execution. 3. Use of the optimal value in the control and coordination of movement such that the movement is proficient and efficient.

skipping — The locomotor pattern in which each leg executes a walking step and a hop before weight is transferred to the other leg. The step is temporally longer than the hop, resulting in an uneven rhythm.

sliding — The locomotor pattern in which one foot steps sideways, then the other foot closes with a leap-step; a type of sideways galloping.

small-for-age infant — A neonate born after a full prenatal term who is markedly below the population average birth weight; typically under 2,500 g.

socialization — The process whereby developing individuals learn age- and gender-appropriate social roles over a period of years.

socializing agent — A person, significant to a developing individual, who influences that individual's behaviors, choices, attitudes, values, or dispositions.

somatosensory — 1. Refers to the sensory receptors located throughout the body and yielding body sensations. 2. Refers to the skin receptors and proprioceptors.

somatotype — In physical growth, a physique assessment conducted to study the sex differences and age-related changes in physique during childhood and adolescence.

sound localization — See auditory localization.

Southern California Sensory Integration Tests — Norm-referenced tests, including the Ayres Space Test, Southern California Motor Accuracy Test, Southern California Kinesthetic and Tactile Perception Test, and the Southern California Visual Perception Test, to detect dysfunctions in sensory integration and determine their nature. There are 17 subtests for children 4 to 8 years old. The Motor Accuracy Test has internal

consistency reliabilities ranging between .67 and .94 for various age groups, but the other tests generally have low stability coefficients, below .40.

spatial awareness — An appreciation of the arrangement of objects, symbols, or the body in space and the ability to make judgments about space, such as the required amount of space needed for a given object.

spatial compatibility — Harmonious relationship in space between a signal or stimulus and the response. For example, requiring an individual to respond to a row of lights by pressing a button immediately under the lamp that is lit is spatially compatible, whereas requiring the respondent to press the button two spaces to the right of the lamp that is lit is not compatible.

spatial orientation — A person's ability to appreciate the orientation or position of objects as they are located in space or as a two-dimensional drawing.

spatial relationships — The ability to recognize associations between two or more objects as they are located in space.

spatial-temporal integration — The ability to match sensory information of a spatial (defined in three-dimensional space) nature to that of a temporal (time) nature.

spinal pattern generator — Oscillator mechanism in the interneurons of the spinal cord that provide muscular synergies or collectives to the various motor units involved in certain basic movements, such as the step in locomotor movement.

S-shaped — 1. Pertains to the plot of performance index over units of practice that depicts initially slow improvement, then rapid improvement, followed by decreasing gains. 2. In growth, pertaining to a plot of a growth measure over age depicting rapid growth in infancy, then decreasing gains until a rapid increase (adolescent growth spurt), then a leveling off to adult size.

stability — 1. Balance or a state of body equilibrium. 2. Pertains to skills executed in a static, balanced position, as opposed to loco-motion.

stadiometer — A calibrated device to measure stature. Consists of a base, a rule at a perfect right angle to the base, and an adjustable piece attached to the rule at a perfect right angle. This piece contacts the vertex of the skull and simultaneously indicates the stature measurement on the rule.

stage — 1. A level in a predictable sequence of change, such that each step in the sequence is qualitatively different, intransitive, universal for individuals, and hierarchical. A period of flux occurs as an individual moves to a new stage, with new behaviors appearing gradually until they consolidate into a period of stability (Piaget). 2. Atheoretically, a level of difficulty, phase, step, point, type, pattern, time, or mood, usually in regard to a developmental behavior or a shift in a learning process.

static balance — The ability to maintain equilibrium in a stationary position or pose.

stature — The anthropometric measure of standing height, from the floor to the vertex of the skull, taken when the subject is in an erect posture without shoes.

step — A qualitative change in the movement or behavior comprising a developmental sequence, often used if the change does not meet the criteria for a stage.

step cycle — The step of a locomotor pattern from a designated point to a return to that point after movement through a complete pattern.

strategic knowledge — Information regarding general rules or strategies that can apply to many topics.

strength — Ability of a muscle or muscle group to exert force against a resistance.

stride length — Horizontal distance covered along the line of progression during one stride of a locomotor skill.

striking — Fundamental motor skills in which an object is hit, with or without an implement.

stroke volume — Amount of blood pumped from a ventricle in each cardiac cycle; increases with an increase in exercise intensity up to approximately 50% to 60% of an individual's maximal oxygen consumption, and then levels off; maximum stroke volume increases with training and is a factor related to the increase in maximum oxygen transport that accompanies the training response.

structural wholeness — The characteristic of developmental stages indicating an organic interconnection among a stage's processes such that a person approaches related tasks in the same way (Piaget).

submaximal exercise test — An evaluation of exercise performance that is terminated at a predetermined heart rate such that peak oxygen uptake can be estimated or predicted.

subroutine — A group of neural motor commands an individual uses to execute a component of a movement that, combined with other subroutine commands, comprises a motor program.

subthreshold — A level of stimulation or information below that needed to identify the stimulus.

sucking reflex — An infant's sucking motion as an involuntary response to a touch above or below the lips.

support leg — The leg in a locomotor skill that is in contact with the ground, and therefore holding the weight of the body, while the other leg is recovering to take the next step; the leg from touchdown to takeoff.

support phase — The portion of locomotor travel between periods of flight when one or both legs contact the ground, therefore holding the body weight.

swing leg — 1. The leg in a locomotor skill that is recovering, usually from an extension to propel the body to a position where body weight can again be supported—the leg from takeoff to touchdown. 2. In hopping, the nonsupport, nonhopping leg.

swing phase — The portion of a step when

a leg is recovering from an extension to propel the body to a position where it can again support body weight; the time from takeoff to touchdown of a limb.

tactile localization — The ability to identify the exact spot on the skin that has been touched.

tactile perception — The perceptual system that yields information about stimuli in contact with the skin, arising mostly from cutaneous receptors.

takeoff — The moment in a locomotor skill when the support limb(s) leave the ground to project the body into flight.

takeoff leg — The last leg to leave the ground in a locomotor skill to project the body into flight.

task analysis — Identification of all the characteristics of a task, including those pertinent in the environment, that can vary without changing the task components and objectives. Examples include speed, weight and size of implements used, and projection trajectory.

teratogen — A drug or agent that causes abnormal development in a fetus upon exposure.

Test of Gross Motor Development — A criterion-referenced assessment for children 3 to 10 years old that includes 12 locomotor and object control skills. Split-half reliability is .85 for locomotor skills and .78 for object control skills.

test-retest reliability — Measure of the extent to which an evaluation yields consistent scores upon repeated measurement of the same group.

threshold value — The minimal level of stimulation or information required to identify a stimulus.

toe-off — The moment in a locomotor skill when the toes of the support leg(s) leave the ground.

touchdown — The landing of a limb during a locomotor skill after a period of flight or recovery from a preceding step.

traction epiphysis — A growth area in the part of a bone where a muscle tendon attaches.

trailing leg — In locomotor skills such as galloping and sliding, the leg that closes the step initiated by the opposite, leading leg.

trapping — A reception skill wherein a person gains control of an oncoming ball by absorbing its force with the legs, head, or trunk, but not the arms or hands.

universal sequence — The characteristic of developmental stages indicating that individuals advance through the stages in the same order (Piaget).

utricle — A membranous pouch in the vestibule of the inner ear that responds to movement of the head in a straight line in relation to the force of gravity.

velocity curve — A plot of the rate of change; a representation of the first derivative of the function represented by the distance curve. See also acceleration curve.

vestibular apparatus — Structures of the inner ear, including the vestibule (containing the utricle and saccule) and semicircular canals, that give rise to position and balance sense.

vestibular system — The aspect of proprioception arising from stimulation of the semicircular canals and otolith organs (vestibule) in the inner ear and giving information about head position in space and sudden changes in direction of body movement.

visual acuity — 1. Sharpness of vision. 2. The ability of the visual system to resolve detail.

visual-kinesthetic integration — The matching of a visual event with its corresponding kinesthetic stimulation.

visually directed reaching — Voluntary arm movement toward an object in the visual field.

visually elicited reaching — Voluntary arm movement toward an object that is stimulated by sight of the object but does not require sight for the movement's completion.

**visually guided reaching** — Voluntary arm movement toward an object in the visual field in which the individual adjusts the hand in anticipation of the target; reaching to pick up a pencil, for example.

**visual-tactile integration** — The matching of a visual event with its corresponding tactile stimulation.

**vital capacity** — Maximal volume of air forcefully expired after a maximal inspiration.

**walking** — The locomotor pattern of alternate-limb stepping. In humans, at least one foot is in contact with the support surface at all times, and the trunk is upright.

**walking reflex** — Movement of an infant's legs in a walking pattern in involuntary response to being held upright, then being lowered toward a flat surface.

**weight-transfer skills** — Fundamental skills characterized by the support of body weight on various body parts successively.

**whole-and-part perception** — The ability to discriminate parts of a picture or an object from the whole, yet integrate the parts into the whole, perceiving them simultaneously.

**whole-part perception** — See **whole-and-part perception**.

**winging** — An arm action sometimes seen in inefficient jumping and leaping. Consists of shoulder retraction and backward arm extension, often with elbows bent while the body is being projected forward.

**working capacity** — The greatest exercise load that a person can tolerate before reaching exhaustion.

Adapted from Anshel, M.H., Freedson, P., Hamill, J., Haywood, K., Horvat, M., & Plowman, S.A. (1991). *Dictionary of the sport and exercise sciences*. Champaign, IL: Human Kinetics. Adapted by permission.

# References

Abourezk, T. (1989). The effects of regular aerobic exercise on short-term memory efficiency in the older adult. In A.C. Ostrow (Ed.), *Aging and motor behavior* (pp. 105-113). Indianapolis: Benchmark.

Adams, F.H. (1973). Factors affecting the working capacity of children and adolescents. In G.L. Rarick (Ed.), *Physical activity: Human growth and development* (pp. 80-96). New York: Academic Press.

Adams, G.M., & DeVries, H.A. (1973). Physiological effects of an exercise training regimen upon women aged 52 to 79. *Journal of Gerontology*, **28**, 50-55.

Adams, J.E. (1965). Injury to the throwing arm. *California Medicine*, **102**, 127-132.

Adrian, M.J. (1980). Biomechanics and aging. In J.M. Cooper & B. Haven (Eds.), *Proceedings of the Biomechanics Symposium* (pp. 132-141). Indianapolis: Indiana State Board of Health.

Adrian, M.J. (1981). Flexibility in the aging adult. In E.L. Smith & R.C. Serfass (Eds.), *Exercise and aging: The scientific basis* (pp. 45-57). Hillside, NJ: Enslow.

Adrian, M.J. (1982, April). *Maintaining movement capabilities in advanced years*. Paper presented at the annual convention of the American Alliance for Health, Physical Education, Recreation and Dance, Houston, TX.

Alexander, M.J., Ready, A.E., & Fougere-Mailey, G. (1985). The fitness level of females in various age groups. *Canadian Journal of Health, Physical Education, and Recreation*, **51**, 8-12.

Allon, N. (1973). The stigma of overweight in everyday life. In G.A. Bray (Ed.), *Obesity in perspective* (pp. 83-102) (Fogarty Report No. 017-053-00046-9). Washington, DC: U.S. Government Printing Office.

Ama, P.F.M., Lagasse, P., Bouchard, C., & Simoneau, J.A. (1990). Anaerobic performances in Black and White subjects. *Medicine and Science in Sports and Exercise*, **22**, 508-511.

Ama, P.F.M., Simoneau, J.A., Boulay, M.R., Seresse, O., Theriault, G., & Bouchard, C. (1986). Skeletal muscle characteristics in sedentary Black and Caucasian males. *Journal of Applied Physiology*, **61**, 1758-1761.

American Alliance for Health, Physical Education, Recreation and Dance. (1976). *Youth Fitness Test manual, revised*. Reston, VA: Author.

American Alliance for Health, Physical Education, Recreation and Dance. (1988). *Physical best*. Reston, VA: Author.

American Health and Fitness Foundation. (1986). *Fit youth today*. Austin, TX: Author.

Ames, L.B. (1937). The sequential patterning of prone progression in the human infant. *Genetic Psychology Monographs*, **19**, 409-460.

Aniansson, A., & Gustafsson, E. (1981). Physical training in elderly men with special reference to quadriceps muscle strength and morphology. *Clinical Physiology*, **1**, 87-98.

Aniansson, A., Hedberg, M., Henning, G.B., & Grimby, G. (1986). Muscle morphology, enzymatic activity and muscle strength in elderly men: A follow-up study. *Muscle Nerve*, **9**, 585-591.

Arenberg, D. (1980). Comments on the processes that account for memory declines with age. In L.W. Poon, J.L. Fozard, L.S. Cermak, D. Arenberg, & L.W. Thompson (Eds.), *New directions in memory and aging*. Hillsdale, NJ: Erlbaum.

Arnheim, D.D., & Sinclair, W.A. (1979). *The clumsy child: A program of motor therapy*. St. Louis: Mosby.

Aronson, E., & Rosenbloom, S. (1971). Space perception in early infancy: Perception within a common auditory visual space. *Science*, **172**, 1161-1163.

Asano, K., Ogawa, S., & Furuta, Y. (1978). Aerobic work capacity in middle and old-aged runners. In F. Landry & W.A.R. Orban (Eds.), *Exercise physiology: Proceedings of the International Congress of Physical Activity Sciences* (Vol. 4). Quebec: Symposia Specialists.

Asmussen, E. (1973). Growth in muscular strength and power. In G.L. Rarick (Ed.), *Physical activity: Human growth and development* (pp. 60-79). New York: Academic Press.

Asmussen, E., & Heebøll-Nielsen, K. (1955). A dimensional analysis of physical performance and growth in boys. *Journal of Applied Physiology*, **7**, 593-603.

Asmussen, E., & Heebøll-Nielsen, K. (1956). Physical performance and growth in children: Influence of sex, age, and intelligence. *Journal of Applied Physiology*, **8**, 371-380.

Åstrand, P. (1976). The child in sport and physical activity-physiology. In J.G. Albinson & G.M. Andrew (Eds.), *Child in sport and physical activity* (pp. 19-33). Baltimore: University Park Press.

Åstrand, P.O., & Rodahl, K. (1986). *Textbook of work physiology*. New York: McGraw Hill.

Atkinson, J., & Braddick, O. (1981). Acuity, contrast sensitivity, and accommodation in infancy. In R. Aslin, J. Alberts, & M. Peterson (Eds.), *Development of perception* (pp. 245-277). New York: Academic Press.

Auerbach, C., & Sperling, P. (1974). A common auditory-visual space: Evidence for its reality. *Perception and Psychophysics*, **16**, 129-135.

Ayres, A.J. (1965). Patterns of perceptual-motor dysfunction in children: A factor analytic study. *Perceptual and Motor Skills*, **20**, 335-368.

Ayres, A.J. (1966). *Southern California sensory-motor integration tests*. Los Angeles: Western Psychological Corporation.

Ayres, A.J. (1969). *Southern California perceptual-motor tests*. Los Angeles: Western Psychological Services.

Ayres, A.J. (1972). *Southern California sensory-motor integration tests manual*. Los Angeles: Western Psychological Services.

Bachman, J.C. (1961). Motor learning and performance as related to age and sex in two measures of balance coordination. *Research Quarterly*, **32**, 123-137.

Bailer, I., Doll, L., & Winsberg, B.G. (1973). *Modified Lincoln-Oseretsky Motor Development Scale*. New York: New York State Department of Mental Hygiene.

Bailey, D.A. (1976). The growing child and the need for physical activity. In J.G. Albinson & G.M. Andrew (Eds.), *Child in sport and physical activity* (pp. 81-93). Baltimore: University Park Press.

Bailey, D.A., Malina, R.M., & Rasmussen, R.L. (1978). The influence of exercise, physical activity, and athletic performance on the dynamics of human growth. In F. Falkner & J.M. Tanner (Eds.), *Human growth* (Vol. 2, pp. 475-505). New York: Plenum.

Baldwin, B.T. (1920). *The physical growth of children from birth to maturity*. Iowa City: University of Iowa.

Baldwin, K.M. (1984). Muscle development: Neonatal to adult. In R.L. Terjung (Ed.), *Exercise and sport science reviews* (Vol. 12, pp.1-19). Lexington, MA: Collamore.

Bandura, A. (1969). Social learning theory of identificatory process. In D. Goslin (Ed.), *Handbook of socialization theory and research* (pp. 213-262). Chicago: Rand McNally.

Bandura, A. (1977). *Social learning theory*. Englewood Cliffs, NJ: Prentice-Hall.

Bandura, A. (1986). *Social foundations of thought and action: A social cognitive theory*. Englewood Cliffs, NJ: Prentice-Hall.

Bandura, A., & Walters, R.H. (1963). *Social learning and personality development*. New York: Holt, Rinehart, and Winston.

Banks, M., Aslin, R., & Letson, R. (1975). Sensitive period for the development of human binocular vision. *Science*, **190**, 675-677.

Bard, C., Fleury, M., Carriere, L., & Bellec, J. (1981). Components of the coincidence-anticipation behavior of children aged 6 to 11 years. *Perceptual and Motor Skills*, **52**, 547-556.

Bard, C., Fleury, M., & Gagnon, M. (1990). Coincidence-anticipation timing: An age-related perspective. In C. Bard, M. Fleury, & L. Hay (Eds.), *Development of eye-hand coordination across the life span* (pp. 283-305). Columbia, SC: University of South Carolina Press.

Bar-Or, O. (1983). *Pediatric sports medicine for the practitioner*. New York: Springer-Verlag.

Bar-Or, O. (1988). Exercise performance of the sick child. In R.M. Malina (Ed.), *Youth athletes: Biological, psychological, and education perspectives* (pp. 99-117). Champaign, IL: Human Kinetics.

Bar-Or, O. (1989). Temperature regulation during exercise in children and adolescents. In C.V. Gisolfi & D.R. Lamb (Eds.), *Perspectives in exercise science and sports medicine. Vol. 2: Youth, exercise and sport* (pp. 369-400). Indianapolis: Benchmark.

Bar-Or, O., Shephard, R.J., & Allen, C.L. (1971). Cardiac output of 10- to 13-year-old boys and girls during submaximal exercise. *Journal of Applied Physiology*, **30**, 219-223.

Bar-Or, O., & Zwiren, I.D. (1973). Physiological effects of increased frequency of physical education classes and of endurance conditioning on 9- to 10-year-old girls and boys. In O. Bar-Or (Ed.), *Pediatric work physiology, 4th International Symposium* (pp. 183-198). Natanya, Israel: Wingate Institute.

Barrett, K.R. (1979). Observation for teaching and coaching. *Journal of Physical Education and Recreation*, **50**, 23-25.

Barsch, R.H. (1965). *Achieving perceptual-motor efficiency*. Seattle: Special Child Publications.

Bayley, N. (1935). The development of motor abilities during the first three years. *Society for Research in Child Development Monograph*, **1**, 1.

Bayley, N. (1965). Comparisons of mental and motor test scores for ages 1–15 months by sex, birth order, race, geographical location and education of parents. *Child Development*, **36**, 379-411.

Bayley, N. (1969). *Manual for the Bayley scales of infant development*. New York: The Psychological Corporation.

Beck, M. (1966). *The path of the center of gravity during running in boys grades one to six*. Unpublished doctoral dissertation, University of Wisconsin, Madison.

Belisle, J.J. (1963). Accuracy, reliability and refractoriness in a coincidence-anticipation task. *Research Quarterly*, **34**, 271-281.

Belmont, J.M., & Butterfield, E.C. (1971). What the development of short-term memory is. *Human Development*, **14**, 236-248.

Benson, J.B. (1985). *The development of crawling in infancy*. Paper presented to the International Society for the Study of Behavioral Development, Tours, France.

Benson, J.B. (1987, April). *New lessons on how infants learn to crawl*. Paper presented at the biannual meeting of the Society for Research in Child Development, Baltimore.

Benson, J.B. (1990). The significance and development of crawling in human infancy. In J.E. Clark & J.H. Humphrey (Eds.), *Advances in motor development research* (Vol. 3, pp. 91-142). New York: AMS Press.

Bergstrom, B. (1973). Morphology of the vestibular nerve. II. The number of myelinated vestibular nerve fibers in man at various ages. *Acta Otolaryngology*, **76**, 173-179.

Berliner, D.C. (1986). In pursuit of the expert pedagogue. *Educational Researcher*, **15**, 5-13.

Bertenthal, B.I., & Bai, D.L. (1989). Infants' sensitivity to optical flow for controlling posture. *Developmental Psychology*, **25**, 936-945.

Bertenthal, B.I., & Campos, J.J. (1987). New directions in the study of early experience. *Child Development*, **58**, 560-567.

Bertenthal, B., Campos, J., & Barrett, K. (1984). Self-produced locomotion: An organizer of emotional, cognitive and social development in infancy. In R. Emde & R. Harmon (Eds.), *Continuities and discontinuities in development* (pp. 175-210). New York: Plenum.

Beunen, G., & Malina, R.M. (1988). Growth and physical performance relative to the timing of the adolescent spurt. *Exercise and Sport Sciences Reviews*, **16**, 503-540.

Beunen, G., Malina, R.M., Van't Hof, M.A., Simons, J., Ostyn, M., Renson, R., & Van Gerven, D. (1988). *Adolescent growth and motor performance: A longitudinal analysis of Belgian boys*. Champaign, IL: Human Kinetics.

Birch, L.L. (1976). Age trends in children's time-sharing performance. *Journal of Experimental Child Psychology*, **22**, 331-345.

Bird, A.M., & Williams, J.M. (1980). A developmental-attributional analysis of sex-role stereotypes for sport performance. *Developmental Psychology*, **16**, 319-322.

Birren, J.E. (1964). The psychology of aging in relation to development. In J.E. Birren (Ed.), *Relations of development and aging* (pp. 99-120). Springfield, IL: Charles C Thomas.

Birren, J.E., Woods, A.M., & Williams, M.V. (1980). Behavioral slowing with age: Causes, organization, and consequences. In L.W. Pool (Ed.), *Aging in the 1980s*. Washington, DC: American Psychological Association.

Boileau, R.A., Lohman, T.G., Slaughter, M.H., Ball, T.E., Going, S.B., & Hendrix, M.K. (1984). Hydration of the fat-free body in children during maturation. *Human Biology*, **56**, 651-666.

Boileau, R.A., Lohman, T.G., Slaughter, M.H., Horswill, C.A., & Stillman, R.J. (1988). Problems associated with determining body composition in maturing youngsters. In E.W. Brown & C.F. Branta (Eds.), *Competitive sports for children and youth* (pp. 3-16). Champaign, IL: Human Kinetics.

Boone, P.C., & Azen, S.P. (1979). Normal range of motion of joints in male subjects. *Journal of Bone and Joint Surgery*, **61A**, 756-759.

Boothby, J., Tungatt, M., & Townsend, A. (1981). Ceasing participation in sports activity: Reported reasons and their implications. *Journal of Leisure Research*, **13**, 1-14.

Botuck, S., & Turkewitz, G. (1990). Intersensory functioning: Auditory-visual pattern equivalence in younger and older children. *Developmental Psychology*, **26**, 115-120.

Bouchard, C., Perusse, L., LeBlanc, C., Tremblay, A., & Theriault, G. (1988). Inheritance of the amount and distribution of human body fat. *International Journal of Obesity*, **12**, 205-215.

Bovend'eerdt, J.H.F., Bermink, M.J.E., van Hijfte, T., Ritmeester, J.W., Kemper, H.C.G., & Verschuur, R. (1980). *De MOPER fitness test: Onderzoeksverslag.* Haarlem: De Vrieseborch.

Bower, T.G.R. (1972). Object perception in infants. *Perception*, **1**, 15-30.

Bower, T.G.R. (1977). *A primer of infant development.* San Francisco: W.H. Freeman.

Bower, T.G.R., Broughton, J.M., & Moore, M.K. (1970a). The co-ordination of visual and tactual input in infants. *Perception and Psychophysics*, **8**, 51-53.

Bower, T.G.R., Broughton, J.M., & Moore, M.K. (1970b). Demonstration of intention in the reaching behavior of neonate humans. *Nature*, **228** (5272), 679-681.

Bower, T.G.R., Broughton, J.M., & Moore, M.K. (1970c). Infant responses to approaching objects: An indicator of response to distal variables. *Perception and Psychophysics*, **9**, 193-196.

Bowlby, J. (1978). Evidence on effects of deprivation. In J.P. Scott (Ed.), *Critical periods.* Stroudsburg, PA: Dowden, Hutchinson, & Ross.

Boyd, E. (1929). The experimental error inherent in measuring the growing human body. *American Journal of Physical Anthropology*, **13**, 389-432.

Braddick, O., & Atkinson, J. (1979). Accommodation and acuity in the human infant. In R.D. Freeman (Ed.), *Developmental neurobiology of vision.* New York: Plenum.

Brandfonbrener, M., Landowne, M., & Shock, N.W. (1955). Changes in cardiac output with age. *Circulation*, **12**, 557-566.

Brandt, I. (1978). Growth dynamics of low-birth-weight infants with emphasis on the perinatal period. In F. Falkner & J.M. Tanner (Eds.), *Human growth: Vol. 2. Postnatal growth.* New York: Plenum.

Branta, C., Haubenstricker, J., & Seefeldt, V. (1984). Age changes in motor skill during childhood and adolescence. In R.L. Terjung (Ed.), *Exercise and sport science reviews* (Vol. 12, pp. 467-520). Lexington, MA: Collamore.

Brewer, V., Meyer, B.M., Keele, M.S., Upton, S.J., & Hagan, R.D. (1983). Role of exercise in prevention of involutional bone loss. *Medicine and Science in Sports and Exercise*, **15**, 445-449.

Brim, O.G. (1966). Socialization through the life cycle. In O.G. Brim & S. Wheeler (Eds.), *Socialization after childhood: Two essays* (pp. 1-49). New York: Wiley.

Brodkin, P., & Weiss, M.R. (1990). Developmental differences in motivation for participating in competitive swimming. *Journal of Sport & Exercise Psychology*, **12**, 248-263.

Brown, B.A. (1985). Factors influencing the process of withdrawal by female adolescents from the role of competitive age group swimmers. *Sociology of Sport Journal*, **2**, 111-129.

Brown, C.H., Harrower, J.R., & Deeter, M.F. (1972). The effects of cross-country running on pre-adolescent girls. *Medicine and Science in Sports*, **4**, 1-5.

Brown, K.W., & Gottfried, A.W. (1986). Cross-modal transfer of shape in early infancy: Is there reliable evidence? In L.P. Lipsitt & C. Rovee-Collier (Eds.), *Advances in infancy research* (Vol. 4, pp. 163-170). Norwood, NJ: Ablex.

Brozek, J. (1952). Changes of body composition in man during maturity and their nutritional implications. *Federation Proceedings*, **11**, 784-793.

Bruininks, R.H. (1978). *Bruininks-Oseretsky test of motor proficiency.* Circle Pines, MN: American Guidance Service.

Brundage, C.L. (1983). *Parent/child play behaviors as they relate to children's later socialization into sport.* Unpublished master's thesis, University of Illinois, Urbana.

Bruner, J.S. (1970). The growth and structure of skill. In K.J. Connolly (Ed.), *Mechanisms of motor skill development* (pp. 63-94). London: Academic Press.

Brustad, R.J. (1988). Affective outcomes in competitive youth sport: The influence of intrapersonal and socialization factors. *Journal of Sport & Exercise Psychology*, **10**, 307-321.

Bull, D., Eilers, R., & Oller, K. (1984). Infants' discrimination of intensity variation in multisyllabic stimuli. *Journal of the Acoustical Society of America*, **76**, 13-17.

Bullen, B.A., Reed, R.B., & Mayer, J. (1964). Physical activity of obese and nonobese adolescent girls appraised by motion picture sampling. *American Journal of Clinical Nutrition*, **14**, 211-223.

Burke, W.E., Tuttle, W.W., Thompson, C.W., Janney, C.D., & Weber, R.J. (1953). The relation of grip strength and grip-strength endurance to age. *Journal of Applied Physiology*, **5**, 628-630.

Burnett, C.N., & Johnson, E.W. (1971). Development of gait in childhood, Part II. *Developmental Medicine and Child Neurology*, **13**, 207-215.

Buros, O.K. (Ed.) (1972). *The seventh mental*

*measurement yearbook*. Highland Park, NJ: Gryphon.

Bushnell, E.W. (1982). The ontogeny of intermodal relations: Visions and touch in infancy. In R. Walk & H. Pick (Eds.), *Intersensory perception and sensory integration* (pp. 5-36). New York: Plenum.

Bushnell, E.W. (1985). The decline of visually guided reaching during infancy. *Infant Behavior and Development*, **8**, 139-155.

Bushnell, E.W. (1986). The basis of infant visual-tactual functioning—amodal dimension or multi-modal compounds? In L.P. Lipsitt & C. Rovee-Collier (Eds.), *Advances in infancy research* (Vol. 4, pp. 183-194). Norwood, NJ: Ablex.

Butcher, J. (1983). Socialization of adolescent girls into physical activity. *Adolescence*, **18**, 753-766.

Butcher, J. (1985). Longitudinal analysis of adolescent girls' participation in physical activity. *Sociology of Sport Journal*, **2**, 130-143.

Butterworth, G., & Hicks, L. (1977). Visual proprioception and postural stability in infancy. A developmental study. *Perception*, **6**, 255-262.

Campbell, W.R., & Pohndorf, R.H. (1961). Physical fitness of British and United States children. In L.A. Larson (Ed.), *Health and fitness in the modern world* (pp. 8-16). Chicago: Athletic Institute.

Capute, A.J., Shapiro, B.K., Palmer, F.B., Ross, A., & Wachtel, R.C. (1985). Normal gross motor development: The influences of race, sex, and socioeconomic status. *Developmental Medicine and Child Neurology*, **27**, 635-643.

Carron, A.V., & Bailey, D.A. (1974). Strength development in boys from 10 through 16 years. *Monographs of the Society for Research in Child Development*, **39**.

Carson, L.M., & Wiegand, R.L. (1979). Motor schema formation and retention in young children: A test of Schmidt's schema theory. *Journal of Motor Behavior*, **11**, 247-252.

Case, R. (1972a). Learning and development: A neo-Piagetian interpretation. *Human Development*, **15**, 339-358.

Case, R. (1972b). Validation of a neo-Piagetian mental capacity construct. *Journal of Experimental Child Psychology*, **14**, 287-302.

Case, R. (1974). Structures and strictures: Some functional limitations on the course of cognitive growth. *Cognitive Psychology*, **6**, 544-573.

Cerella, J., Poon, L.W., & Williams, D.M. (1980). Age and the complexity hypothesis. In L.W. Poon (Ed.), *Aging in the 1980s* (pp. 332-340). Washington, DC: American Psychological Association.

Cerney, L. (1970). The results of an evaluation of skeletal age in boys 11-15 years old with different regime of physical activity. In J. Kral & V. Novotny (Eds.), *Physical fitness and its laboratory assessment* (pp. 56-59). Prague: Charles University.

Cerny, F.J., & Armitage, L.M. (1989). Exercise and cystic fibrosis: A review. *Pediatric Exercise Science*, **1**, 116-126.

Chapman, E.A., DeVries, H.A., & Swezey, R. (1972). Joint stiffness: The effects of exercise on young and old men. *Journal of Gerontology*, **27**, 218-221.

Chase, W.G., & Simon, H.A. (1973). Perception in chess. *Cognitive Psychology*, **4**, 55-81.

Chi, M. (1976). Short-term memory limitations in children: Capacity or processing deficits? *Memory and Cognition*, **4**, 559-572.

Chi, M. (1977a). Age differences in memory span. *Journal of Experimental Child Psychology*, **23**, 266-281.

Chi, M. (1977b). Age differences in the speed of processing: A critique. *Developmental Psychology*, **13**, 543-544.

Chi, M.T.H. (1978). Knowledge structures and memory development. In R.S. Siegler (Ed.), *Children's thinking: What develops?* (pp. 73-105). Hillsdale, NJ: Erlbaum.

Chi, M.T.H. (1981). Knowledge development and memory performance. In M.P. Friedman, J.P. Das, & N. O'Connor (Eds.), *Intelligence and learning* (pp. 221-229). New York: Plenum.

Chi, M.T.H., & Koeske, R.D. (1983). Network representation of a child's dinosaur knowledge. *Development Psychology*, **19**, 29-39.

Chiesi, H.L., Spilich, G.J., & Voss, J.F. (1979). Acquisition of domain related information in relation to high and low domain knowledge. *Journal of Verbal Learning and Verbal Behavior*, **18**, 257-273.

Chrysler Fund–Amateur Athletic Union (1987). *Physical fitness program*. Bloomington, IN: Author.

Clark, J.E. (1982). Developmental differences in response processing. *Journal of Motor Behavior*, **14**, 247-254.

Clark, J.E., & Philips, S. (1985). A developmental sequence of the standing long jump. In J. Clark & J. Humphrey (Eds.), *Motor development: Current selected research* (Vol. 1, pp. 73-85). Princeton, NJ: Princeton Books.

Clark, J.E., Phillips, S.J., & Petersen, R. (1989). Developmental stability in jumping. *Developmental Psychology*, **25**, 929-935.

Clark, J.E., & Whitall, J. (1989a). What is motor development? The lessons of history. *Quest*, **41**, 183-202.

Clark, J.E., & Whitall, J. (1989b). Changing patterns of locomotion: From walking to skipping. In M.H. Woollacott & A. Shumway-Cook (Eds.), *Development of posture and gait across the life span* (pp. 128-151). Columbia, SC: University of South Carolina Press.

Clark, J.E., Whitall, J., & Phillips, S.J. (1988). Human interlimb coordination: The first 6 months of independent walking. *Developmental Psychobiology*, **21**, 445-456.

Clarke, H.H. (Ed.) (1975). Joint and body range of movement. *Physical Fitness Research Digest*, **5**, 16-18.

Clouse, F. (1959). *A kinematic analysis of the development of the running pattern of preschool boys*. Unpublished doctoral dissertation, University of Wisconsin, Madison.

Cobb, K., Goodwin, R., & Saelens, E. (1966). Spontaneous hand positions of newborn infants. *Journal of Genetic Psychology*, **108**, 225-237.

Colling-Saltin, A.S. (1980). Skeletal muscle development in the human fetus and during childhood. In K. Berg & B.O. Eriksson (Eds.), *International Congress on Pediatric Work Physiology: Children and exercise IX* (pp. 193-207). Baltimore: University Park Press.

Collins, J.K. (1976). Distance perception as a function of age. *Australian Journal of Psychology*, **28**, 109-113.

Conel, J.L. (1939). *The postnatal development of the human cerebral cortex*. Cambridge, MA: Harvard Press.

Connolly, K.J. (Ed.) (1970). *Mechanisms of motor skill development*. New York: Academic Press.

Connolly, K.J., & Elliott, J.M. (1972). The evolution and ontogency of hand function. In N. Burton-Jones (Ed.), *Ethological studies of child behavior* (pp. 329-383). Cambridge, England: Cambridge University Press.

Coopersmith, S. (1967). *The antecedents of self-esteem*. San Francisco: Freeman. (Reprinted in 1981 by Consulting Psychologists Press, Palo Alto, CA)

Corbetta, D., & Mounoud, P. (1990). Early development of grasping and manipulation. In C. Bard, M. Fleury, & L. Hay (Eds.), *Development of eye-hand coordination across the life span* (pp. 188-216). Columbia, SC: University of South Carolina Press.

Corso, J.F. (1977). Auditory perception and communication. In J.E. Birren & K.W. Schaie (Eds.), *Handbook of the psychology of aging* (pp. 535-553). New York: Van Nostrand Reinhold.

Craik, F.I.M. (1977). Age differences in human memory. In J.E. Birren & K.W. Schaie (Eds.), *Handbook of the psychology of aging* (pp. 384-420). New York: Van Nostrand Reinhold.

Craik, F.I.M., & Simon, E. (1980). Age differences in memory: The roles of attention and depth of processing. In L.W. Poon, J.L. Fozard, L.S. Cermak, D. Arenberg, & L.W. Thompson (Eds.), *New directions in memory and aging* (pp. 95-112). Hillsdale, NJ: Erlbaum.

Craik, R. (1989). Changes in locomotion in the aging adult. In M.H. Woollacott & A. Shumway-Cook (Eds.), *Development of posture and gait across the life span* (pp. 176-201). Columbia, SC: University of South Carolina Press.

Cratty, B.J. (1979). *Perceptual and motor development in infants and children* (2nd ed.). Englewood Cliffs, NJ: Prentice-Hall.

Crossman, E.R.F.W., & Szafran, J. (1956). Changes with age in the speed of information intake and discrimination. *Experientia* (Suppl.), **4**, 128-135.

Crouchman, M. (1986). The effects of babywalkers on early locomotor development. *Developmental Medicine and Child Neurology*, **28**, 757-761.

Cureton, K.J., Collins, M.A., Hill, D.W., & McElhannon, F.M. (1988). Muscle hypertrophy in men and women. *Medicine and Science in Sports and Exercise*, **20**, 338-344.

Curtis, J.E., & White, P.G. (1984). Age and sport participation: Decline in participation with age or increased specialization with age? In N. Theberge & P. Donnelly (Eds.), *Sport and the sociological imagination* (pp. 273-293). Fort Worth, TX: Texas Christian University Press.

DaCosta, M.I. (1946). The Oseretsky tests (E.J. Fosa, Trans.). *Training School Bulletin*, **43**, 1-13, 27-38, 50-59, 62-74.

Daehler, M.W., Horowitz, A.B., Wynns, F.C., & Flavell, J.H. (1969). Verbal and non-verbal rehearsal in children's recall. *Child Development*, **40**, 443-452.

Davies, C.T.M. (1972). The oxygen transporting system in relation to age. *Clinical Science*, **42**, 1-13.

de Garay, A.L., Levine, L., & Carter, J.E.L. (1974). *Genetic and anthropological studies of Olympic athletes*. New York: Academic Press.

Dehn, M.M., & Bruce, R.A. (1972). Longitudinal variations in maximum oxygen intake with age and activity. *Journal of Applied Physiology*, **33**, 805-807.

Dekaban, A. (1970). *Neurology of early childhood*. Baltimore: Williams and Wilkins.

Delacato, C.H. (1959). *Treatment and prevention of reading problems*. Springfield, IL: Charles C Thomas.

Delacato, C.H. (1966). *Neurological organization and reading*. Springfield, IL: Charles C Thomas.

Demany, L., McKenzie, B., & Vurpillot, E. (1977). Rhythmic perception in early infancy. *Nature*, **266**, 718-719.

Dennis, W. (1935). The effect of restricted practice upon the reaching, sitting, and standing of two infants. *Journal of Genetic Psychology*, **47**, 17-32.

Dennis, W. (1938). Infant development under conditions of restricted practice and of minimum social stimulation: A preliminary report. *Journal of Genetic Psychology*, **53**, 149-158.

Dennis, W. (1940). The effect of cradling practices upon the onset of walking in Hopi children. *Journal of Genetic Psychology*, **56**, 77-86.

Dennis, W. (1941). Infant development under conditions of restricted practice and of minimum social stimulation. *Genetic Psychology Monographs*, **23**, 143-189.

Dennis, W. (Ed.) (1951). *Readings in child psychology*. New York: Prentice-Hall.

Dennis, W. (1963). Environmental influences upon motor development. In W. Dennis (Ed.), *Readings in child psychology* (2nd ed., pp. 83-94). Englewood Cliffs, NJ: Prentice-Hall.

Dennis, W., & Dennis, M.G. (1951). Development under controlled environmental conditions. In W. Dennis (Ed.), *Readings in child psychology* (pp. 104-131). New York: Prentice-Hall.

DeOreo, K.L. (1971). *Dynamic and static balance in preschool children*. Unpublished doctoral dissertation, University of Illinois, Urbana.

DeOreo, K.L. (1974). The performance and development of fundamental motor skills in preschool children. In D.M. Landers (Ed.), *Psychology of motor behavior and sport*. Champaign, IL: Human Kinetics.

DeOreo, K., & Keogh, J. (1980). Performance of fundamental motor tasks. In C.B. Corbin (Ed.), *A textbook of motor development* (2nd ed., pp. 76-91). Dubuque, IA: W.C. Brown.

DeOreo, K., & Wade, M.G. (1971). Dynamic and static balancing ability of preschool children. *Journal of Motor Behavior*, **3**, 326-335.

DeOreo, K.L., & Williams, H.G. (1980). Characteristics of kinesthetic perception. In C.B. Corbin (Ed.), *A textbook of motor development* (2nd ed., pp. 174-196). Dubuque, IA: W.C. Brown.

DeVries, H.A. (1970). Physiological effects of an exercise training regimen upon men aged 52 to 88. *Journal of Gerontology*, **25**, 325-336.

Dickinson, J. (1974). *Proprioceptive control of human movement*. Princeton, NJ: Princeton Book.

DiNucci, J.M. (1976). Gross motor performance: A comprehensive analysis of age and sex differences between boys and girls ages six to nine years. In J. Broekhoff (Ed.), *Physical education, sports, and the sciences*. Eugene, OR: Microform.

DiNucci, J.M., & Shows, D.A. (1977). A comparison of the motor performance of black and caucasian girls age 6-8. *Research Quarterly*, **48**, 680-684.

DiPietro, J.A. (1981). Rough and tumble play: A function of gender. *Developmental Psychology*, **17**, 50-58.

DiSimoni, F.G. (1975). Perceptual and perceptual-motor characteristics of phonemic development. *Child Development*, **46**, 243-246.

Dittmer, J. (1962). *A kinematic analysis of the development of the running pattern of grade school girls and certain factors which distinguish good from poor performance at the observed ages*. Unpublished master's thesis, University of Wisconsin, Madison.

Dodwell, P.C., Muir, D.W., & DiFranco, D. (1976). Responses of infants visually presented objects. *Science*, **194**, 209-211.

Dorfman, P.W. (1977). Timing and anticipation: A developmental perspective. *Journal of Motor Behavior*, **9**, 67-80.

Doty, D. (1974). Infant speech perception. *Human Development*, **17**, 74-80.

Drillis, R. (1961). The influence of aging on the kinematics of gait. In *The Geriatric Amputee*, Publication 919. National Academy of Science, National Research Council.

Drinkwater, B.L., Horvath, S.M., & Wells, C.L. (1975). Aerobic power of females, age 10-68. *Journal of Gerontology*, **30**, 385-394.

Drowatzky, J.N., & Zuccato, F.C. (1967). Interrelationship between static and dynamic balance. *Research Quarterly*, **38**, 509-510.

Duda, J.L., & Tappe, M.K. (1988). Predictors of personal investment in physical activity among middle-aged and older adults. *Perception and Motor Skills*, **66**, 543-549.

Duda, J.L., & Tappe, M.K. (1989a). Personal investment in exercise among middle-aged and older adults. In A.C. Ostrow (Ed.), *Aging and motor behavior* (pp. 219-238). Indianapolis: Benchmark.

Duda, J.L., & Tappe, M.K. (1989b). Personal invest-ment in exercise among adults: The examination of age and gender-related differences in motiva-tional orientation. In A.C. Ostrow (Ed.), *Aging and motor behavior* (pp. 239-256). Indianapo-lis: Benchmark.

Dunham, P. (1977). Age, sex, speed and practice in coincidence-anticipation performance of children. *Perceptual and Motor Skills*, **45**, 187-193.

DuRandt, R. (1985). Ball catching proficiency among 4-, 6-, and 8-year-olds. In J.E. Clark & J.H. Humphrey (Eds.), *Motor development: Current selected research* (pp. 35-44). Princeton, NJ: Princeton Book.

Dustman, R.E., Ruhling, R.O., Russell, E.M., Shearer, D.E., Bonekat, H.W., Shigeoka, J.W., Wood, J.S., & Bradford, D.C. (1989). Aerobic exercise training and improved neuropsychologi-cal function of older individuals. In A.C. Ostrow (Ed.), *Aging and motor behavior* (pp. 67-83). Indianapolis: Benchmark.

Dwyer, J., & Mayer, J. (1973). The dismal condition: Problems faced by obese adolescent girls in Ameri-can society. In G.A. Bray (Ed.), *Obesity in per-spective* (pp. 103-110) (Fogarty Report No. 017-053-00046-9). Washington, DC: U.S. Govern-ment Printing Office.

Eaton, W.O., & Enns, L.R. (1986). Sex differences in human motor activity level. *Psychological Bul-letin*, **100**, 19-28.

Eaton, W.O., & Keats, J.G. (1982). Peer presence, stress, and sex differences in the motor activity levels of preschoolers. *Developmental Psychol-ogy*, **18**, 534-540.

Ebihara, O., Ikeda, M., & Myiashita, M. (1983). Birth order and children's socialization into sport. *International Review of Sport Sociology*, **18**, 69-89.

Edwards, R.G. (1981). *The beginnings of human life*. Burlington, NC: Carolina Biological Supply.

Ehsani, A.A. (1987). Cardiovascular adaptions to exercise training in the elderly. *Federation Pro-ceedings*, **46**, 1840-1843.

Einkauf, D.K., Gohdes, M.L., Jensen, G.M., & Jewell, M.J. (1987). Changes in spinal mobility with increasing age in women. *Physical Therapy*, **67**, 370-375.

Eisenberg, N., Wolchick, S.A., Hernandez, R., & Pasternack, J.F. (1985). Parental socialization of young children's play: A short-term longitudinal study. *Child Development*, **56**, 1506-1513.

Ekblom, B. (1969). Effect of physical training on oxygen transport system in man. *Acta Physiolog-ica Scandinavica Supplementum*, **328**, 1-76.

Elkind, D. (1975). Perceptual development in chil-dren. *American Scientist*, **63**, 533-541.

Elkind, D., Koegler, R., & Go, E. (1964). Studies in perceptual development: Whole-part perception. *Child Development*, **35**, 81-90.

Elliott, R. (1972). Simple reaction time in children: Effects of incentive, incentive shift, and other training variables. *Journal of Experimental Child Psychology*, **13**, 540-557.

Endler, N.S., Boulter, L.R., & Osser, H. (1976). *Contemporary issues in developmental psy-chology* (2nd ed.). New York: Holt, Rinehart, and Winston.

Eriksson, B.O. (1972). Physical training, oxygen supply and muscle metabolism in 11 to 15 year old boys. *Acta Physiologica Scandinavica Sup-plementum*, **384**, 1-48.

Eriksson, B.O. (1978). Physical activity from child-hood to maturity: Medical and pediatric considera-tions. In F. Landry & W.A.R. Orban (Eds.), *Physi-cal activity and human well-being*. Miami, FL: Symposia Specialists.

Eriksson, B., & Koch, G. (1973). Effect of physical training on hemodynamic response during sub-maximal exercise in 11-13 year old boys. *Acta Physiologica Scandinavica*, **87**, 27-39.

Espenschade, A.S. (1940). Motor performance in adolescence including the study of relationships with measures of physical growth and maturity. *Monograph of the Society for Research in Child Development*, **5**, 1-126.

Espenschade, A.S. (1947). Development of motor coordination in boys and girls. *Research Quar-terly*, **18**, 30-44.

Espenschade, A.S. (1960). Motor development. In W.R. Johnson (Ed.), *Science and medicine of exercise and sports* (pp. 419-439). New York: Harper & Row.

Espenschade, A., Dable, R.R., & Schoendube, R. (1953). Dynamic balance in adolescent boys. *Re-search Quarterly*, **24**, 270-274.

Espenschade, A., & Eckert, H. (1974). Motor devel-opment. In W.R. Johnson & E.R. Buskirk (Eds.), *Science and medicine of exercise and sport* (2nd ed., pp. 322-333). New York: Harper & Row.

Espenschade, A.S., & Eckert, H.D. (1980). *Motor development* (2nd ed.). Columbus, OH: Merrill.

Eston, R.G., Brodie, D.A., Burnie, J., Stokes, M., Griffiths, R.D., & Edwards, R.H.T. (1989). Meta-bolic cost of walking in boys with muscular dystro-phy. In S. Oseid & K. Carlsen (Eds.), *Children and exercise XIII* (pp. 405-414). Champaign, IL: Human Kinetics.

Ewart, C.K., Stewart, K.J., Gillilan, R.E., & Kelemen, M.H. (1986). Self-efficacy mediates strength gains during circuit weight training in men with coronary artery disease. *Medicine and Science in Sports and Exercise*, **18**, 531-540.

Exton-Smith, A.N. (1985). Mineral metabolism. In C.E. Finch & E.L. Schneider (Eds.), *Handbook of the biology of aging* (2nd ed., pp. 511-539). New York: Van Nostrand.

Fagard, J. (1990). The development of bimanual coordination. In C. Bard, M. Fleury, & L. Hay (Eds.), *Development of eye-hand coordination across the life span* (pp. 262-282). Columbia, SC: University of South Carolina Press.

Fagot, B.I. (1978). The influence of sex of child on parental reactions to toddler children. *Child Development*, **49**, 459-465.

Fagot, B.I. (1984). Teacher and peer reactions to boys' and girls' play styles. *Sex Roles*, **11**, 691-702.

Fagot, B.I., & Leinbach, M.D. (1983). Playstyles in early childhood: Social consequences for boys and girls. In M.B. Liss (Ed.), *Social and cognitive skills: Sex roles and children's play* (pp. 93-116). New York: Academic Press.

Falkner, F., & Tanner, J.M. (Eds.) (1978). *Human growth* (Vols. 1-3). New York: Plenum.

Feltz, D.L., & Petlichkoff, L. (1983). Perceived competence among interscholastic sport participants and dropouts. *Canadian Journal of Applied Sport Sciences*, **8**, 231-235.

Fieandt, K. von, Huhtala, A., Kullberg, P., & Saari, K. (1956). *Personal tempo and phenomenal time at different age levels* (Report No. 2). Helsinki: Psychological Institute, University of Helsinki.

Forssberg, H. (1982). Spinal locomotor functions and descending control. In B. Sjoland & A. Bjorklund (Eds.), *Brain stem control of spinal mechanisms*. New York: Fernstrom Foundation.

Forssberg, H., & Nashner, L. (1982). Ontogenetic development of postural control in man: Adaptation to altered support and visual conditions during stance. *Journal of Neuroscience*, **2**, 545-552.

Fox, K.R., & Corbin, C.B. (1989). The physical self-perception profile: Development and preliminary validation. *Journal of Sport & Exercise Psychology*, **11**, 408-430.

Frankenburg, W.K., & Dodds, J.B. (1967). The Denver developmental screening test. *Journal of Pediatrics*, **71**, 181-191.

Franks, B.D. (1989). *YMCA Youth Fitness Test manual*. Champaign, IL: Human Kinetics.

French, K.E., & Thomas, J.R. (1987). The relation of knowledge development to children's basketball performance. *Journal of Sport Psychology*, **9**, 15-32.

Frisch, R.E. (1972). Weight at menarche: Similarity for well-nourished and undernourished girls at differing ages, and evidence for historical constancy. *Pediatrics*, **50**, 445-450.

Frostig, M., Lefever, W., & Whittlesey, J. (1966). *Administration and scoring manual: Marianne Frostig developmental test of visual perception*. Palo Alto, CA: Consulting Psychologists Press.

Gabel, R.H., Johnston, R.C., & Crowinshield, R.D. (1979). A gait analyzer/trainer instrumentation system. *Journal of Biomedical Engineering*, **12**, 543-549.

Gabell, A., & Nayak, U.S.L. (1984). The effect of age on variability of gait. *Journal of Gerontology*, **39**, 662-666.

Gallagher, J.D., & Thomas, J.R. (1980a, April). *Adult-child differences in movement reproduction: Effects of kinesthetic sensory store and organization of memory*. Paper presented at the annual convention of the American Alliance for Health, Physical Education, Recreation and Dance, Detroit.

Gallagher, J.D., & Thomas, J.R. (1980b). Effects of varying post-KR intervals upon children's motor performance. *Journal of Motor Behavior*, **12**, 41-46.

Gallahue, D.L. (1982). *Understanding motor development in children*. New York: Wiley.

Gallahue, D.L. (1983, April). *Perceptual aspects of motor performance*. Paper presented at the annual convention of the American Alliance for Health, Physical Education, Recreation and Dance, Houston, TX.

Gatev, G. (1972). Role of inhibition in the development of motor coordination in early childhood. *Developmental Medicine and Child Psychology*, **14**, 336-341.

Germain, N.W., & Blair, S.N. (1983). Variability of shoulder flexion with age, activity, and sex. *American Corrective Therapy Journal*, **37**, 156-160.

Gesell, A. (1928). *Infancy and human growth*. New York: Macmillan.

Gesell, A. (1939). Reciprocal interweaving in neuromotor development. *Journal of Comparative Neurology*, **70**, 161-180.

Gesell, A. (1946). The ontogenesis of infant behavior. In L. Carmichael (Ed.), *Manual of child psychology* (pp. 295-331). New York: Wiley.

Gesell, A. (1954). The ontogenesis of infant behavior. In L. Carmichael (Ed.), *Manual of child psychology* (2nd ed.). New York: Wiley.

Gesell, A., & Amatruda, C.S. (1949). *Gesell developmental schedules*. New York: Psychological Company.

Gesell, A., & Ames, L.B. (1940). The ontogenetic organization of prone behavior in human infancy. *Journal of Genetic Psychology*, **56**, 247-263.

Gesell, A., & Thompson, H. (1929). Learning and growth in identical infant twins: An experimental study by the method of co-twin control. *Genetic Psychology Monographs*, **6**, 1-124.

Gesell, A., & Thompson, H. (1934). *Infant behavior: Its genesis and growth*. New York: McGraw-Hill.

Gesell, A., & Thompson, H. (1941). Twins T and C from infancy to adolescence: A biogenetic study of individual differences by the method of co-twin control. *Genetic Psychology Monographs*, **24**, 3-121.

Gesell, A., & Thompson, H. (1943). Learning and maturation in identical infant twins: An experimental analysis by the method of co-twin control. In R.G. Barker, J.S. Kounin, & H.F. Wright (Eds.), *Child behavior and development* (pp. 209-227). New York: McGraw-Hill.

Getchell, N., & Roberton, M.A. (1989). Whole body stiffness as a function of developmental level in children's hopping. *Developmental Psychology*, **25**, 920-928.

Getman, G.N. (1952). *How to develop your child's intelligence, a research publication*. Lucerne, MN: Author.

Getman, G.N. (1963). *The physiology of readiness experiment*. Minneapolis: P.A.S.S.

Gibson, J.J. (1966). *The senses considered as perceptual systems*. Boston: Houghton Mifflin.

Gibson, J.J. (1979). *An ecological approach to visual perception*. Boston: Houghton Mifflin.

Gibson, E.J., & Walk, R.D. (1960). The "visual cliff." *Scientific American*, **202**(4), 64-71.

Gilliam, T.B., & Freedson, P.S. (1980). Effects of a 12-week school physical fitness program on peak $VO_2$ body composition and blood lipids in 7 to 9 year old children. *International Journal of Sports Medicine*, **1**, 73-75.

Gilliam, T.B., Katch, V.L., Thorland, W., & Weltman, A. (1977). Prevalence of coronary heart disease risk factors in active children, 7 to 12 years of age. *Medicine and Science in Sports*, **9**, 21-25.

Glassow, R.B., & Kruse, P. (1960). Motor performance of girls age 6 to 14 years. *Research Quarterly*, **31**, 426-433.

Goldfield, E.C. (1989). Transition from rocking to crawling: Postural constraints on infant movement. *Developmental Psychology*, **25**, 913-919.

Goldfield, E.C., & Michel, G.F. (1986a). Spatiotemporal linkage in infant interlimb coordination. *Developmental Psychology*, **19**, 259-264.

Goldfield, E.C., & Michel, G.F. (1986b). The ontogeny of infant bimanual reaching during the first year. *Infant Behavior and Development*, **9**, 81-89.

Goodman, L., & Hamill, D. (1973). The effectiveness of the Kephart Getman activities in developing perceptual-motor and cognitive skills. *Focus on Exceptional Children*, **4**, 1-9.

Goodnow, J.J. (1971a). Eye and hand: Differential memory and its effect on matching. *Neuropsychologica*, **9**, 89-95.

Goodnow, J.J. (1971b). Matching auditory and visual series: Modality problem or translation problem? *Child Development*, **42**, 1187-1201.

Gordon, C.C., Chumlea, W.C., & Roche, A.F. (1988). Stature, recumbent, length, and weight. In T.G. Lohman, A.F. Roche, & R. Martorell (Eds.), *Anthropometric standardization reference manual* (pp. 3-8). Champaign, IL: Human Kinetics.

Gould, D., Feltz, D., Horn, T., & Weiss, M. (1982). Reasons for attrition in competitive youth swimming. *Journal of Sport Behavior*, **5**, 155-165.

Gould, D., Feltz, D., & Weiss, M. (1985). Motives for participating in competitive youth swimming. *International Journal of Sport Psychology*, **6**, 126-140.

Greendorfer, S.L. (1976, September). *A social learning approach to female sport involvement*. Paper presented at the annual convention of the American Psychological Association, Washington, DC.

Greendorfer, S.L. (1977). Role of socializing agents in female sport involvement. *Research Quarterly*, **48**, 304-310.

Greendorfer, S.L. (1979). Childhood sport socialization influences of male and female track athletes. *Arena Review*, **3**, 39-53.

Greendorfer, S.L. (1983). Shaping the female athlete: The impact of the family. In M.A. Boutilier & L. Sangiovanni (Eds.), *The sporting woman* (pp. 135-155). Champaign, IL: Human Kinetics.

Greendorfer, S.L., & Brundage, C.L. (1984, July). *Sex differences in children's motor skills: Toward a cross-disciplinary perspective*. Paper presented at the 1984 Olympic Scientific Congress, Eugene, OR.

Greendorfer, S.L., & Ewing, M.E. (1981). Race and gender differences in children's socialization into sport. *Research Quarterly for Exercise and Sport*, **52**, 301-310.

Greendorfer, S.L., & Lewko, J.H. (1978a). *Children's socialization into sport: A conceptual and empirical analysis*. Paper presented at the meeting of the 9th World Congress of Sociology, Uppsala, Sweden.

Greendorfer, S.L., & Lewko, J.H. (1978b). Role of family members in sport socialization of children. *Research Quarterly*, **49**, 146-152.

Greenough, W.T., Black, J.E., & Wallace, C.S. (1987). Experience and brain development. *Child Development*, **58**, 539-559.

Greulich, W.W., & Pyle, S.I. (1959). *Radiographic atlas of skeletal development of the hand and wrist* (2nd ed.). Stanford, CA: Stanford University Press.

Grillner, S. (1975). Locomotion in vertebrates: Central mechanisms and reflex interaction. *Physiological Review*, **55**, 247-304.

Grodjinovsky, A., Inbar, O., Dotan, R., & Bar-Or, O. (1980). Training effect on the anaerobic performance of children as measured by the Wingate anaerobic test. In K. Berg & B.O. Eriksson (Eds.), *Children and exercise IX* (pp. 139-145). Baltimore: University Park Press.

Gutteridge, M. (1939). A study of motor achievements of young children. *Archives of Psychology*, **244**, 1-178.

Hagburg, J.M., Allen, W.K., Seals, D.R., Hurley, B.F., Ehsani, A.A., & Holloszy, J.O. (1985). A hemodynamic comparison of young and older endurance athletes during exercise. *Journal of Applied Physiology*, **58**, 2041-2046.

Haith, M.M. (1966). The response of the human newborn to visual movement. *Journal of Experimental Child Psychology*, **3**, 235-243.

Halverson, H.M. (1931). An experimental study of prehension in infants by means of systematic cinema records. *Genetic Psychology Monographs*, **10**, 107-286.

Halverson, L. (1983). *Observing children's motor development in action*. Paper presented at the annual conference of the American Alliance for Health, Physical Education, Recreation and Dance. Eugene, OR: Microform Publications.

Halverson, L.E., Roberton, M.A., & Langendorfer, S. (1982). Development of the overarm throw: Movement and ball velocity changes by seventh grade. *Research Quarterly for Exercise and Sport*, **53**, 198-205.

Halverson, L.E., & Williams, K. (1985). Developmental sequences for hopping over distance: A prelongitudinal screening. *Research Quarterly for Exercise and Sport*, **56**, 37-44.

Hansman, C.F. (1962). Appearance and fusion of ossification centers in the human skeleton. *American Journal of Roentgenology*, **88**, 476-482.

Harris, G.J., & Burke, D. (1972). The effects of grouping on short-term serial recall of digits by children: Developmental trends. *Child Development*, **43**, 710-716.

Harrison, T.R., Dixon, K., Russell, R.O., Bidwai, P.S., & Coleman, H.N. (1964). The relation of age to the duration of contraction, ejection, and relaxation of the normal human heart. *American Heart Journal*, **67**, 189-199.

Harter, S. (1978). Effectance motivation reconsidered: Towards a developmental model. *Human Development*, **21**, 34-64.

Harter, S. (1981a). A model of intrinsic mastery motivation in children: Individual differences and developmental change. In W.A. Collins (Ed.), *Minnesota symposium on child psychology* (Vol. 14, pp. 215-255). Hillsdale, NJ: Erlbaum.

Harter, S. (1981b). The development of competence motivation in the mastery of cognitive and physical skills: Is there still a place for joy? In G.C. Roberts & D.M. Landers (Eds.), *Psychology of motor behavior and sport—1980* (pp. 3-29). Champaign, IL: Human Kinetics.

Harter, S. (1985). *Manual for the Self-Perception Profile for Children*. Denver: University of Denver.

Harter, S., & Pike, R. (1984). The pictorial scale of perceived competence and social acceptance for young children. *Child Development*, **55**, 1969-1982.

Hasselkus, B.R., & Shambes, G.M. (1975). Aging and postural sway in women. *Journal of Gerontology*, **30**, 661-667.

Haubenstricker, J.L., Branta, C.F., & Seefeldt, V.D. (1983). Standards of performance for throwing and catching. *Proceedings of the Annual Conference of the North American Society for Psychology in Sport and Physical Activity*, Asilomar, CA.

Haubenstricker, J., & Seefeldt, V. (1986). Acquisition of motor skills during childhood. In V. Seefeldt (Ed.), *Physical activity and well-being* (pp. 41-102). Reston, VA: American Alliance for Health, Physical Education, Recreation and Dance.

Haubenstricker, J.L., Seefeldt, V.D., & Branta, C.F. (1983, April). *Preliminary validation of a developmental sequence for the standing long jump*. Paper presented at the meeting of the American

Alliance for Health, Physical Education, Recreation and Dance, Houston, TX.

Haubenstricker, J., Seefeldt, V., Fountain, C., & Sapp, M. (1981, April). *The efficiency of the Bruininks-Oseretsky Test of Motor Proficiency in discriminating between normal children and those with gross motor dysfunction.* Paper presented at the annual conference of the American Alliance of Health, Physical Education, Recreation and Dance, Boston.

Hawn, P.R., & Harris, L.J. (1983). Hand differences in grasp duration and reaching in two- and five-month old infants. In G. Young, S. Segalowitz, C.M. Carter, & S.E. Trehub (Eds.), *Manual specialization and the developing brain* (pp. 331-348). New York: Academic Press.

Hay, J.G., & Reid, J.G. (1982). *The anatomical and mechanical bases of human motion.* Englewood Cliffs, NJ: Prentice-Hall.

Hay, L. (1978). Accuracy of children on an open-loop pointing task. *Perceptual and Motor Skills*, **47**, 1079-1082.

Hay, L. (1979). Spatial-temporal analysis of movements in children: Motor programs. *Journal of Motor Behavior*, **11**, 189-200.

Haywood, K.M. (1977). Eye movements during coincidence-anticipation performance. *Journal of Motor Behavior*, **9**, 313-318.

Haywood, K.M. (1980). Coincidence-anticipation accuracy across the life span. *Experimental Aging Research*, **6**, 451-462.

Haywood, K.M., Greenwald, G., & Lewis, C. (1981). Contextual factors and age group differences in coincidence-anticipation performance. *Research Quarterly for Exercise and Sport*, **52**, 458-464.

Haywood, K.M., & Patryla, V. (1978, May). *Relationship between growth and balance performance among normal and learning disabled children.* Paper presented at the meeting of the North American Society for Psychology of Sport and Physical Activity, Tallahassee, FL.

Haywood, K.M., & Trick, L.R. (1983). *Age-related visual changes and their implications for the motor skill performance of older adults.* Paper presented at the annual convention of the American Alliance for Health, Physical Education, Recreation and Dance (ERIC Document Reproduction Service No. ED 230 538).

Haywood, K. & Trick, L. (1990). Changes in visual functioning and perception with advancing age. *Missouri Journal of Health, Physical Education, Recreation and Dance*, pp. 51-73.

Haywood, K.M., Williams, K., & VanSant, A.

(1991). Qualitative assessment of the backswing in older adult throwing. *Research Quarterly for Exercise and Sport*, **62**, 340-343.

Hazen, N.L. (1982). Spatial exploration and spatial knowledge: Individual and developmental differences in young children. *Child Development*, **53**, 826-833.

Heath, G.W., Hagberg, J.M., Ehsani, A.A., & Holloszy, J.O. (1981). A physiological comparison of young and older endurance athletes. *Journal of Applied Physiology*, **51**, 634-640.

Hecaen, H. (1976). Acquired aphasia in children and the ontogenesis of hemispheric functional specialization. *Brain and Language*, **3**, 114-134.

Hecaen, H., & de Ajuriaguerra, J. (1964). *Left-handedness: Manual superiority and cerebral dominance.* New York: Grune & Stratton.

Hecox, K. (1975). Electro-physiological correlates of human auditory development. In L.B. Cohen & P. Salapatek (Eds.), *Infant perception: From sensation to cognition* (Vol. 2, pp. 151-191). New York: Academic Press.

Held, R., & Hein, A. (1963). Movement-produced stimulation in the development of visually guided behavior. *Journal of Comparative and Physiological Psychology*, **56**, 872-876.

Hellebrandt, F.A., & Braun, G.L. (1939). The influence of sex and age on the postural sway of man. *American Journal of Physical Anthropology*, **24**, Series 1, 347-360.

Heriza, C.B. (1986). *A kinematic analysis of leg movements in premature and fullterm infants.* Unpublished doctoral dissertation, Southern Illinois University at Edwardsville.

Herkowitz, J. (1978a). Assessing the motor development of children: Presentation and critique of tests. In M.V. Ridenour (Ed.), *Motor development* (pp. 165-187). Princeton, NJ: Princeton Book.

Herkowitz, J. (1978b). Developmental task analysis: The design of movement experiences and evaluation of motor development status. In M.V. Ridenour (Ed.), *Motor development* (pp. 139-164). Princeton, NJ: Princeton Book.

Herkowitz, J. (1978c). Instruments which assess the efficiency/maturity of children's fundamental motor pattern performance. In D.M. Landers & R.W. Christina (Eds.), *Psychology of motor behavior and sport—1977* (pp. 529-535). Champaign, IL: Human Kinetics.

Heyward, V.H. (1984). *Designs for fitness.* Minneapolis: Burgess.

Heyward, V.H. (1991). *Advanced fitness assessment and exercise prescription* (2nd ed.). Champaign, IL: Human Kinetics.

Higginson, D.C. (1985). The influence of socializing agents in the female sport-participation process. *Adolescence*, **20**, 73-82.

Hirsch, J., & Knittle, J.L. (1970). Cellularity of obese and nonobese human adipose tissue. *Federation Proceedings*, **29**, 1516-1521.

Hoeger, W.W.K., Hopkins, D.R., Button, S., & Palmer, T.A. (1990). Comparing the sit and reach with the modified sit and reach in measuring flexibility in adolescents. *Pediatric Exercise Science*, **2**, 156-162.

Hofsten, C. von (1979). Development of visually directed reaching: The approach phase. *Journal of Human Movement Studies*, **5**, 160-178.

Hofsten, C. von (1982). Eye-hand coordination in the newborn. *Developmental Psychology*, **18**, 450-461.

Hofsten, C. von (1984). Developmental changes in the organization of pre-reaching movements. *Developmental Psychology*, **3**, 378-388.

Hogan, P.I., & Santomeir, J.P. (1984). Effect of masters swim skills on older adults' self-efficacy. *Research Quarterly for Exercise and Sport*, **55**, 294-296.

Hohmann, A., & Creutzfeldt, O. (1975). Squint and the development of binocularity in humans. *Nature*, **254**, 613-614.

Horine, L.E. (1968). An investigation of the relationship of laterality to performance on selected motor ability tests. *Research Quarterly*, **39**, 90-95.

Horn, T.S. (1985). Coaches' feedback and changes in children's perceptions of their physical competence. *Journal of Educational Psychology*, **77**, 174-186.

Horn, T.S. (1986). The self-fulfilling prophecy theory: When coaches' expectations become reality. In J.M. Williams (Ed.), *Applied sport psychology: Personal growth to peak performance* (pp. 59-73). Palo Alto, CA: Mayfield.

Horn, T.S. (1987). The influence of teacher-coach behavior on the psychological development of children. In D. Gould & M.R. Weiss (Eds.), *Advances in pediatric sport science, Vol 2: Behavioral issues* (pp. 121-142). Champaign, IL: Human Kinetics.

Horn, T.S., & Hasbrook, C.A. (1986). Information components influencing children's perceptions of their physical competence. In M.R. Weiss & D. Gould (Eds.), *Sport for children and youths* (pp. 81-88). Champaign, IL: Human Kinetics.

Horn, T.S., & Hasbrook, C.A. (1987). Psychological characteristics and the criteria children use for self-evaluation. *Journal of Sport Psychology*, **9**, 208-221.

Horn, T.S., & Weiss, M.R. (1991). A developmental analysis of children's self-ability judgments in the physical domain. *Pediatric Exercise Science*, **3**, 310-326.

Howell, M.L., Loiselle, D.S., & Lucas, W.G. (1966). *Strength of Edmonton schoolchildren*. Unpublished manuscript, University of Alberta Fitness Research Unit, Edmonton.

Howell, M.L., & MacNab, R. (1966). *The physical work capacity of Canadian children*. Ottawa: Canadian Association for Physical Health Education and Recreation.

Howze, E.H., DiGilio, D.A., Bennett, J.P., & Smith, M.L. (1986). Health education and physical fitness for older adults. In B. McPherson (Ed.), *Sport and aging* (pp. 153-156). Champaign, IL: Human Kinetics.

Hupprich, F.L., & Sigerseth, P.O. (1950). The specificity of flexibility in girls. *Research Quarterly*, **21**, 25-33.

Huston, A. (1984). Sex typing. In P.H. Mussen (Ed.), *Carmichael's handbook of child psychology* (Vol. 4, pp. 387-469). New York: Wiley.

Hutinger, P.A. (1959). Differences in speed between American Negro and white children in performance of the 35-yard dash. *Research Quarterly*, **30**, 366-367.

Ikai, M. (1967). *Trainability of muscular endurance as related to age*. Proceedings of International Council of Health, Physical Education and Recreation 10th International Congress, Vancouver.

Inbar, O. (1978). *Acclimatization to dry and hot environment in young adults and children 8- to 10-years-old*. Ed. D. dissertation, Columbia University, New York.

Inbar, O., & Bar-Or, O. (1986). Anaerobic characteristics in male children and adolescents. *Medicine and Science in Sports and Exercise*, **18**, 264-269.

Inkeles, A. (1969). Social structure and socialization. In D.A. Goslin (Ed.), *Handbook of socialization theory and research* (pp. 615-632). Skokie, IL: Rand McNally.

Institute for Aerobics Research (1988). *The fitnessgram*. Dallas: Author.

Isaacs, L.D. (1980). Effects of ball size, ball color, and preferred color on catching by young children. *Perceptual and Motor Skills*, **51**, 583-586.

Isaacs, L.D. (1983). Coincidence-anticipation in simple catching. *Journal of Human Movement Studies*, **9**, 195-201.

Jenkins, L.M. (1930). *A comparative study of motor achievements of children five, six, and seven years of age.* New York: Teacher's College, Columbia University.

Jesse, J.P. (1977). Olympic lifting movements endanger adolescents. *The Physician and Sportsmedicine*, **5**, 60-67.

Johnson, M.L., Burke, B.S., & Mayer, J. (1956). Relative importance of inactivity and overeating in the energy balance of obese high school girls. *American Journal of Clinical Nutrition*, **4**, 37-44.

Johnsson, L.G., & Hawkins, J.E., Jr. (1972). Sensory and neural degeneration with aging, as seen in micro-dissections of the inner ear. *Annals of Otology, Rhinology, and Laryngology*, **81**, 179-193.

Jones, H.E. (1947). Sex differences in physical abilities. *Human Biology*, **19**, 12-25.

Jones, M.A., Buis, J.M., & Harris, I.D. (1986). Relationships of race and sex to physical and motor measures. *Perceptual and Motor Skills*, **63**, 169-170.

Julius, S., Amery, A., Whitlock, L.S., & Conway, J. (1967). Influence of age on the hemodynamic response to exercise. *Circulation*, **36**, 222-230.

Kaiser, S.B., & Phinney, J.S. (1983). Sex typing of play activities by girls' clothing style: Pants versus skirts. *Child Study Journal*, **13**, 115-132.

Kalil, R.E. (1989, December). Synapse formation in the developing brain. *Scientific American*, pp. 76-79, 82-85.

Karpovich, P.V. (1937). Textbook fallacies regarding the development of the child's heart. *Research Quarterly*, **8**, 33-37. (Reprinted in 1991 in *Pediatric Exercise Science*, **3**, 278-282)

Kasch, F.W., & Wallace, J.P. (1976). Physiological variables during 10 years of endurance exercise. *Medicine and Science in Sports*, **8**, 5-8.

Kausler, D.H. (1982). *Experimental psychology and human aging.* New York: Wiley.

Kavanagh, T., & Shephard, R.J. (1977). The effects of continued training on the aging process. *Annals of the New York Academy of Sciences*, **301**, 656-670.

Kelly, J.R. (1974). Socialization toward leisure: A developmental approach. *Journal of Leisure Research*, **6**, 181-193.

Kelso, J.A.S. (1982). Epilogue: Two strategies for investigating action. In J.A.S. Kelso (Ed.), *Human motor behavior: An introduction* (pp. 283-287). Hillsdale, NJ: Erlbaum.

Kelso, J.A.S., Holt, K.G., Kugler, P.N., & Turvey, M.T. (1980). On the concept of coordinative structures in dissipative structures: II. Empirical lines of convergence. In G.E. Stelmach & J.

Requin (Eds.), *Tutorials in motor behavior* (pp. 49-70). New York: North-Holland.

Kenshalo, D.R. (1977). Age changes in touch, vibration, temperature, kinesthesis, and pain sensitivity. In J.E. Birren & K.W. Schaie (Eds.), *Handbook of the psychology of aging* (pp. 562-579). New York: Van Nostrand Reinhold.

Kenyon, G.S., & McPherson, B.D. (1973). Becoming involved in physical activity and sport: A process of socialization. In G.L. Rarick (Ed.), *Physical activity: Human growth and development* (pp. 301-332). New York: Academic Press.

Kephart, N.C. (1964). Perceptual-motor aspects of learning disabilities. *Exceptional Children*, **31**, 201-206.

Kephart, N.C. (1971). *The slow learner in the classroom* (2nd ed.). Columbus, OH: Merrill.

Kermoian, R., & Campos, J.J. (1988). Locomotor experience: A facilitator of spatial cognitive development. *Child Development*, **59**, 908-917.

Kerr, R., & Booth, B. (1977). Skill acquisition in elementary school children and schema theory. In R.W. Christina & D.M. Landers (Eds.), *Psychology of motor behavior and sport—1976* (pp. 243-247). Champaign, IL: Human Kinetics.

Kidd, A.H., & Kidd, R.M. (1966). The development of auditory perception in children. In A.H. Kidd & J.L. Rivoire (Eds.), *Perceptual development in children*. New York: International Universities Press.

Klinger, A., Masataka, T., Adrian, M., & Smith, E. (1980, April). *Temporal and spatial characteristics of movement patterns of women over 60.* (Cited in Adrian, 1982.) AAHPERD Research Symposium, Detroit.

Klint, K.A., & Weiss, M.R. (1986). Dropping in and dropping out: Participation motives of current and former youth gymnasts. *Canadian Journal of Applied Sport Sciences*, **11**, 106-114.

Knittle, J.L. (1978). Adipose tissue development in man. In F. Falkner & J.M. Tanner (Eds.), *Human growth: Vol. 2. Postnatal growth.* New York: Plenum.

Knittle, J.L., & Hirsch, J. (1968). Effect of early nutrition on the development of rat epididymal fat pads: Cellularity and metabolism. *Journal of Clinical Investigation*, **47**, 2091-2098.

Knobloch, H., & Pasamanick, B. (1958). The relationship of race and socioeconomic status to the development of motor behavior patterns in infancy. *Psychiatric Research Reports of the American Psychiatric Association*, **10**, 123-133.

Kobayashi, K., Kitamura, K., Miura, M., Sodeyama,

H., Murase, Y., Miyashita, M., & Matsui, H. (1978). Aerobic power as related to body growth and training in Japanese boys: A longitudinal study. *Journal of Applied Physiology*, **44**, 666-672.

Koch, G., & Rocker, L. (1977). Plasma volume and intravascular protein masses in trained boys and fit young men. *Journal of Applied Physiology*, **43**, 1085-1088.

Koestler, A., & Smythies, J.R. (1969). *Beyond reductionism*. Boston: Beacon.

Komi, P.V. (1984). Physiological and biomechanical correlates of muscle function: Effects of muscle structure and stretch-shortening cycle on force and speed. In R.L. Terjung (Ed.), *Exercise and sport science reviews* (Vol. 12, pp. 81-121). Lexington, MA: Collamore.

Konczak, J. (1990). Toward an ecological theory of motor development: The relevance of the Gibsonian approach to vision for motor development research. In J.E. Clark & J.H. Humphrey (Eds.), *Advances in motor development research* (Vol 3, pp. 201-224). New York: AMS Press.

Korenman, S.G. (Ed.) (1982). *Endocrine aspects of aging*. New York: Elsevier Biomedical.

Kotulan, J., Reznickova, M., & Placheta, Z. (1980). Exercise and growth. In Z. Placheta (Ed.), *Youth and physical activity* (pp. 61-117). Brno, Czechoslovakia: J.E. Purkyne University.

Krahenbuhl, G.S., & Martin, S.L. (1977). Adolescent body size and flexibility. *Research Quarterly*, **48**, 797-799.

Krahenbuhl, G.S., Pangrazi, R.P., Petersen, G.W., Burkett, L.N., & Schneider, M.J. (1978). Field testing of cardiorespiratory fitness in primary school children. *Medicine and Science in Sports*, **10**, 208-213.

Kreighbaum, E., & Barthels, K.M. (1990). *Biomechanics* (3rd ed.). New York: Macmillan.

Krolner, B., Tondevold, E., Toft, B., Berthelsen, B., & Nielsen, S.P. (1982). Bone mass of the axial and the appendicular skeleton in women with Colles' fracture: Its relation to physical activity. *Clinical Physiology*, **2**, 147-157.

Kuczaj, S.A., II, & Maratsos, M.P. (1975). On the acquisition of front, back, and side. *Child Development*, **46**, 202-210.

Kuffler, S.W., Nicholls, J.G., & Martin, A.R. (1984). *From neuron to brain* (2nd ed.). Sunderland, MA: Sinauer.

Kugler, P.N., Kelso, J.A.S., & Turvey, M.T. (1980). On the concept of coordinative structures in dissipative structures. I. Theoretical lines of convergence. In G.E. Stelmach & J. Requin (Eds.), *Tutorials in motor behavior* (pp. 3-47). New York: North-Holland.

Kugler, P.N., Kelso, J.A.S., & Turvey, M.T. (1982). On the control and coordination of naturally developing systems. In J.A.S. Kelso & J.E. Clark (Eds.), *The development of movement control and coordination* (pp. 5-78). New York: Wiley.

Kukla, A. (1978). An attributional theory of choice. In L. Berkowitz (Ed.), *Advances in experimental social psychology* (Vol. 2). New York: Academic Press.

Laidlaw, R.W., & Hamilton, M.A. (1937). A study of thresholds in appreciation of passive movement among normal control subjects. *Bulletin of the Neurological Institute*, **6**, 268-273.

Landahl, H.D., & Birren, J.E. (1959). Effects of age on the discrimination of lifted weights. *Journal of Gerontology*, **14**, 48-55.

Langendorfer, S. (1980). *Longitudinal evidence for developmental changes in the preparatory phase of the overarm throw for force*. Paper presented at the annual convention of the American Alliance for Health, Physical Education, Recreation and Dance, Detroit.

Langendorfer, S. (1982). *Developmental relationships between throwing and striking: A prelongitudinal test of motor stage theory*. Unpublished doctoral dissertation, University of Wisconsin, Madison.

Langendorfer, S. (1987). Prelongitudinal screening of overarm striking development performed under two environmental conditions. In J.E. Clark & J.H. Humphrey (Eds.), *Advances in motor development research* (Vol. 1, pp. 17-47). New York: AMS Press.

Langlois, J.H., & Downs, A.C. (1980). Mothers, fathers, and peers as socialization agents of sex-typed play behaviors in young children. *Child Development*, **51**, 1237-1247.

Larsson, L. (1982). Physical training effects on muscle morphology in sedentary males at different ages. *Medicine and Science in Sports and Exercise*, **14**, 203-206.

Lasky, R.E. (1977). The effect of visual feedback of the hand on the reaching and retrieval behavior of young infants. *Child Development*, **48**, 112-117.

Lawrence, D.G., & Hopkins, D.A. (1972). Developmental aspects of pyramidal motor control in the rhesus monkey. *Brain Research*, **40**, 117-118.

Lawrence, D.G., & Kuypers, H.G.J.M. (1968). The functional organization of the motor system in the monkey. I. The effects of bilateral pyramidal lesions. *Brain*, **91**, 1-14.

Leavitt, J. (1979). Cognitive demands of skating and stickhandling in ice hockey. *Canadian Journal of Applied Sport Science, 4,* 46-55.

Lee, D.N., & Aronson, E. (1974). Visual proprioceptive control of standing in human infants. *Perception & Psychophysics, 15,* 529-532.

Lehman, H.C. (1953). *Age and achievement.* Princeton, NJ: Princeton University Press.

Lemanski, R.F., & Henke, K.G. (1989). Exercise-induced asthma. In C.V. Gisolfi & D.R. Lamb (Eds.), *Perspectives in exercise science and sports medicine Vol 2: Youth, exercise, and sport* (pp. 465-512). Indianapolis: Benchmark.

Leme, S., & Shambes, G. (1978). Immature throwing patterns in normal adult women. *Journal of Human Movement Studies, 4,* 85-93.

Lemon, P.W.R. (1989). Nutrition for muscular development of young athletes. In C.V. Gisolfi & D.R. Lamb (Eds.), *Perspectives in exercise science and sports medicine Vol. 2: Youth, exercise, and sport* (pp. 369-400). Indianapolis: Benchmark.

Lengyel, M., & Gyarfas, I. (1979). The importance of echocardiography in the assessment of left ventricular hypertrophy in trained and untrained school children. *Acta Cardiologica, 34,* 63-69.

Lenneberg, E. (1967). *The biological foundations of language.* New York: Wiley.

Leuhring, S.K. (1989). *Component movement patterns of two groups of older adults in the task of rising to standing from the floor.* Master's thesis, Virginia Commonwealth University, Richmond.

Lewis, M. (1972). Culture and gender roles: There is no unisex in the nursery. *Psychology Today, 5,* 54-57.

Lewko, J.H., & Ewing, M.E. (1980). Sex differences and parental influences in sport involvement of children. *Journal of Sport Psychology, 2,* 62-68.

Lewko, J.H., & Greendorfer, S.L. (1988). Family influences in sport socialization of children and adolescents. In F.L. Smoll, R.A. Magill, & M.J. Ash (Eds.), *Children in sport* (3rd ed., pp. 287-300). Champaign, IL: Human Kinetics.

Liberty, C., & Ornstein, P.A. (1973). Age differences in organization and recall: The effects of training in categorization. *Journal of Experimental Child Psychology, 15,* 169-186.

Liss, M.B. (1983). Learning gender-related skills through play. In M.B. Liss (Ed.), *Social and cognitive skills: Sex roles and children's play* (pp. 147-166). New York: Academic Press.

Little, M.A., & Hochner, D.H. (1973). *Human thermoregulation, growth, and mortality* (Module in

Anthropology No. 36). Reading, MA: Addison-Wesley.

Lloyd, B., & Smith, C. (1985). The social representation of gender and young children's play. *British Journal of Developmental Psychology, 3,* 65-73.

Lockman, J.J. (1984). The development of detour ability during infancy. *Child Development, 55,* 482-491.

Lohman, T.G. (1989). Assessment of body composition in children. *Pediatric Exercise Science, 1,* 19-30.

Lohman, T.G., Roche, A.F., & Martorell, R. (Eds.) (1988). *Anthropometric standardization reference manual.* Champaign, IL: Human Kinetics.

Long, A.B., & Looft, W.R. (1972). Development of directionality in children: Ages six through twelve. *Developmental Psychology, 6,* 375-380.

Loovis, E.M. (1976). Model for individualizing physical education experiences for the preschool moderately retarded child (Doctoral dissertation, The Ohio State University, 1975). *Dissertation Abstracts International, 36,* 5126A. (University Microfilms No. 76-3485)

Lowrey, G.H. (1973). *Growth and development of children.* Chicago: Year Book Medical.

Loy, J.W., McPherson, B.D., & Kenyon, G. (1978). *Sport and social systems.* Reading, MA: Addison-Wesley.

Lussier, L., & Buskirk, E.R. (1977). Effects of endurance training regimen on assessment of work capacity in prepubertal children. *New York Academy of Science, 301,* 734-744.

Maehr, M.L. (1984). Meaning and motivation. In R. Ames & C. Ames (Eds.), *Research on motivation in education* (Vol. 1, pp. 115-144). New York: Academic Press.

Makrides, S.C. (1983). Protein synthesis and degradation during ageing and senescence. *Biological Review of the Cambridge Philosophical Society, 58,* 343-422.

Malina, R.M. (1969). Growth, maturation, and performance of Philadelphia Negro and White elementary school children (Doctoral dissertation, University of Pennsylvania, 1968). *Dissertation Abstracts International, 30,* 951B. (University Microfilms No. 69-15091)

Malina, R.M. (1973). Ethnic and cultural factors in the development of motor abilities and strength in American children. In G.L. Rarick (Ed.), *Physical activity: Human growth and development* (pp. 333-363). New York: Academic Press.

Malina, R.M. (1975). *Growth and development: The first twenty years in man.* Minneapolis: Burgess.

Malina, R.M. (1978). Growth of muscle tissue and muscle mass. In F. Falkner & J.M. Tanner (Eds.), *Human growth: Vol. 2. Postnatal growth* (pp. 273-294). New York: Plenum.

Malina, R.M. (1980). Adolescent growth, maturity, and development. In C.B. Corbin (Ed.), *A textbook of motor development* (2nd ed., pp. 268-273). Dubuque, IA: Brown.

Malina, R.M., & Bouchard, C. (1991). *Growth, maturation, and physical activity*. Champaign, IL: Human Kinetics.

Malina, R.M., Bouchard, C., Shoup, R.F., & Lariviere, G. (1982). Age, family size and birth order in Montreal Olympic athletes. In J.E.L. Carter (Ed.), *Physical structure of Olympic athletes, Part I* (pp. 13-24). Basel, Switzerland: S. Karger.

Malina, R.M., & Roche, A.F. (1983). *Manual of physical status and performance in childhood: Vol. 2. Physical performance*. New York: Plenum.

Maloney, S.K., Fallon, B., & Wittenberg, C.K. (1984). *Aging and health promotion: Market research for public education, executive summary* (Contract No. 282-83-0105). Washington, DC: Public Health Service, Office of Disease Prevention and Health Promotion.

Martin, A.D., Carter, J.E.L., Hendy, K.C., & Malina, R.M. (1988). Segment lengths. In T.G. Lohman, A.F. Roche, & R. Martorell (Eds.), *Anthropometric standardization reference manual* (pp. 9-26). Champaign, IL: Human Kinetics.

Martin, R.W. (1966). *Selected anthropometric, strength, and power characteristics of White and Negro boys*. Unpublished master's thesis, University of Toledo.

Martino, A. (1966). *Anthropometric measurements in the lower leg of White and Negro high school boys in relation to vertical jumping ability*. Unpublished master's thesis, University of Oklahoma, Norman.

Martorell, R., Malina, R.M., Castillo, R.O., Mendoza, F.S., & Pawson, I.G. (1988). Body proportions in three ethnic groups: Children and youths 2–17 years in NHANES II and HHANES. *Human Biology*, **60**, 205-222.

Mathews, D.K. (1963). *Measurement in physical education*. Philadelphia: W.B. Saunders.

Mayer, J. (1968). *Overweight: Causes, cost, and control*. Englewood Cliffs, NJ: Prentice Hall.

McCarver, R.B. (1972). A developmental study of the effect of organization cues on short-term memory. *Child Development*, **43**, 1317-1325.

McCaskill, C.L., & Wellman, B.L. (1938). A study of common motor achievements at the preschool ages. *Child Development*, **9**, 141-150.

McClenaghan, B.A., & Gallahue, D.L. (1978). *Fundamental movement: A developmental and remedial approach*. Philadelphia: W.B. Saunders.

McConnell, A. & Wade, G. (1990). Effects of lateral ball location, grade, and sex on catching. *Perceptual and Motor Skills*, **70**, 59-66.

McDonnell, P.M. (1975). The development of visually guided reaching. *Perception and Psychophysics*, **18**, 181-185.

McDonnell, P.M. (1979). Patterns of eye-hand coordination in the first year of life. *Canadian Journal of Psychology*, **33**, 253-267.

McGraw, M.B. (1935). *Growth: A study of Johnny and Jimmy*. New York: Appleton-Century. (Reprinted in 1975 by Arno Press)

McGraw, M.B. (1939). Later development of children specially trained during infancy. *Child Development*, **10**, 1-19.

McGraw, M.B. (1940). Neuromuscular development of the human infant as exemplified in the achievement of erect locomotion. *Journal of Pediatrics*, **17**, 747-771.

McGraw, M.B. (1943). *The neuromuscular maturation of the human infant*. New York: Columbia University Press. (Reprinted in 1963 by Hafner)

McKenzie, B.E., & Bigelow, E. (1986). Detour behavior in young human infants. *British Journal of Developmental Psychology*, **4**, 139-148.

McPherson, B.D. (1978). The child in competitive sport: Influence of the social milieu. In R.A. Magill, M.J. Ash, & F.L. Smoll (Eds.), *Children in sport: A contemporary anthology* (pp. 219-249). Champaign, IL: Human Kinetics.

McPherson, B.D. (1983). *Aging as a social process. An introduction to individual and population aging*. Toronto: Butterworths.

McPherson, B.D. (1986). Sport, health, well-being and aging: Some conceptual and methodological issues and questions for sport scientists. In B. McPherson (Ed.), *Sport and aging* (pp. 3-23). Champaign, IL: Human Kinetics.

McPherson, B., Marteniuk, R., Tihanyi, J., & Clark, W. (1980). The social system of age group swimmers: The perception of swimmers, parents, and coaches. *Canadian Journal of Applied Sciences*, **5**, 142-145.

Messick, J.A. (1991). Prelongitudinal screening of hypothesized developmental sequences for the overhead tennis serve in experienced tennis players 9-19 years of age. *Research Quarterly for Exercise and Sport*, **62**, 249-256.

Michel, G.F. (1983). Development of hand-use preference during infancy. In G. Young, S. Segalowitz,

C.M. Carter, & S.E. Trehub (Eds.), *Manual specialization and the developing brain* (pp. 33-70). New York: Academic Press.

Michel, G.F. (1988). A neuropsychological perspective on infant sensorimotor development. In C. Rovee-Collier & L.P. Lipsitt (Eds.), *Advances in infancy research* (Vol. 5, pp. 1-37). Norwood, NJ: Ablex.

Michel, G.F., & Goodwin, R.A. (1979). Intrauterine birth position predicts new born supine head position preferences. *Infant Behavior and Development*, **2**, 29-38.

Michel, G.F., & Harkins, D.A. (1986). Postural and lateral asymmetries in the ontogeny of handedness during infancy. *Developmental Psychobiology*, **19**, 247-258.

Micheli, L.J. (1984). Sport injuries in the young athlete: Questions and controversies. In L.J. Micheli (Ed.), *Pediatric and adolescent sports medicine* (pp. 1-9). Boston: Little, Brown.

Micheli, L.J. (1989). The exercising child: Injuries. *Pediatric Exercise Science*, **1**, 329-335.

Milani-Comparetti, A. (1981). The neurophysiologic and clinical implications of studies on fetal motor behavior. *Seminars in Perinatology*, **5**, 183-189.

Milani-Comparetti, A., & Gidoni, E.A. (1967). Routine developmental examination in normal and retarded children. *Developmental Medicine and Child Neurology*, **9**, 631-638.

Miller, F.S. (1968). *A comparative analysis of physical performance between male Caucasian and non-Caucasian (Mexican) students at the seventh and eighth grade level*. Unpublished master's thesis, California State College at Long Beach.

Miller, P.H. (1983). *Theories of developmental psychology*. San Francisco: W.H. Freeman.

Milne C., Seefeldt, V., & Reuschlein, P. (1976). Relationship between grade, sex, race, and motor performance in young children. *Research Quarterly*, **47**, 726-730.

Mirwald, R.L., & Bailey, D.A. (1986). *Maximal aerobic power: A longitudinal analysis*. London, Ontario: Sports Dynamics.

Mirwald, R.L., Bailey, D.A., Cameron, N., & Rasmussen, R.L. (1981). Longitudinal comparison of aerobic power in active and inactive boys aged 7.0 to 17.0 years. *Annals of Human Biology*, **8**, 405-414.

Molen, H.H. (1973). *Problems on the evaluation of gait*. Unpublished doctoral dissertation, The Institute of Biomechanics and Experimental Rehabilitation, Free University, Amsterdam.

Molnar, G. (1978). Analysis of motor disorder in retarded infants and young children. *American Journal of Mental Deficiency*, **83**, 213-222.

Moritani, T., & DeVries, H.A. (1980). Potential for gross muscle hypertrophy in older men. *Journal of Gerontology*, **35**, 672-682.

Morris, G.S.D. (1976). Effects ball and background color have upon the catching performance of elementary school children. *Research Quarterly*, **47**, 409-416.

Morrongiello, B.A. (1984). Auditory temporal pattern perception in 6- and 12-month-old infants. *Developmental Psychology*, **20**, 441-448.

Morrongiello, B.A. (1986). Infants' perception of multiple-group auditory patterns. *Infant Behavior and Development*, **9**, 307-320.

Morrongiello, B.A. (1988). The development of auditory pattern perception skills. In C. Rovee-Collier & L.P. Lipsitt (Eds.), *Advances in infancy research* (Vol. 6, pp. 135-172). Norwood, NJ: Ablex.

Morrongiello, B.A., & Clifton, R.K. (1984). Effects of sound frequency on behavioral and cardiac orienting in newborn and five-month-old infants. *Journal of Experimental Child Psychology*, **38**, 429-446.

Morrongiello, B.A., Trehub, S.E., Thorpe, L.A., & Capodilupo, S. (1985). Children's perceptions of melodies: The role of contour, frequency, and rate of presentation. *Journal of Experimental Child Psychology*, **40**, 279-292.

Munns, K. (1981). Effects of exercise on the range of joint motion in elderly subjects. In E.L. Smith & R.C. Serfass (Eds.), *Exercise and aging: The scientific basis* (pp. 149-166). Hillside, NJ: Enslow.

Murphy, G.L., & Wright, J.C. (1984). Changes in conceptual structure with expertise: Differences between real-world experts and novices. *Journal of Experimental Psychology: Learning, Memory, and Cognition*, **10**, 144-155.

Murray, M.P. (1985). Shoulder motion and muscle strength of normal men and women in two age groups. *Clinical Orthopedics and Related Research*, **192**, 268-273.

Murray, M.P., Drought, A.B., & Kory, R.C. (1964). Walking patterns of normal men. *Journal of Bone and Joint Surgery*, **46-A**, 335-360.

Murray, M.P., Gardner, G.M., Mollinger, L.A., & Sepic, S.B. (1980). Strength of isometric and isokinetic contractions. *Physical Therapy*, **60**, 412-419.

Murray, M.P., Kory, R.C., Clarkson, B.H., & Sepic, S.B. (1966). Comparison of free and fast speed walking patterns of normal men. *American Journal of Physical Medicine*, **45**, 8-24.

Murray, M.P., Kory, R.C., & Sepic, S.B. (1970).

Walking patterns of normal women. *Archives of Physical Medicine and Rehabilitation*, **51**, 637-650.

Napier, J. (1956). The prehensile movements of the human hand. *Journal of Bone and Joint Surgery*, **38B**, 902-913.

Naus, M., & Shillman, R. (1976). Why a Y is not a V: A new look at the distinctive features of letters. *Journal of Experimental Psychology: Human Perception and Performance*, **2**, 394-400.

Needleman, H.L., Gunnoe, C., Leviton, A., Reed, R., Peresie, H., Maher, C., & Barrett, P. (1979). Deficits in psychologic and classroom performance of children with elevated dentine lead levels. *The New England Journal of Medicine*, **300**, 689-695.

Needleman, H.L., Schell, A., Bellinger, D., Leviton, A., & Allred, E.N. (1990). The long-term effects of exposure to low doses of lead in childhood: An 11-year follow-up report. *The New England Journal of Medicine*, **322**, 83-88.

Nelson, C.J. (1981). *Locomotor patterns of women over 57*. Unpublished master's thesis, Washington State University, Pullman.

Newell, K.M., Scully, D.M., McDonald, P.V., & Baillargeon, R. (1989). Task constraints and infant grip configurations. *Developmental Psychobiology*, **22**, 817-832.

Nicklas, T.A., Webber, L.S., Koschak, M., & Berenson, G.S. (1992). Nutrient adequacy of low fat intakes for children: The Bogalusa Heart Study. *Pediatrics*, **89**, 221-228.

Nielsen, B., Nielsen, K., Hansen, M.B., & Asmussen, E. (1980). Training of "functional muscle strength" in girls 7-19 years old. In K. Berg & B.O. Eriksson (Eds.), *Children and exercise IX* (pp. 69-78). Baltimore: University Park Press.

Nilsson, B.E., & Westlin, N.E. (1971). Bone density in athletes. *Clinical Orthopedics*, **77**, 179-182.

Norris, A.H., Shock, N.W., Landowne, M., & Falzone, J.A. (1956). Pulmonary function studies: Age differences in lung volume and bellows function. *Journal of Gerontology*, **11**, 379-387.

Northman, J.E., & Black, K.N. (1976). An examination of errors in children's visual and haptic-tactual memory for random forms. *Journal of Genetic Psychology*, **129**, 161-165.

Novotny, V. (1981). Veranderungen des Knochenalters im Verlauf einer mehrjahrigen sportlichen Belastung [Variation in bone age caused by the stress of sport over the course of several years]. *Medizin und Sport*, **21**, 44-47.

Nyhan, N.L. (1990). Structural abnormalities. *Clinical Symposia*, **42**(2), 1-32.

Oettingen, G. (1985). The influence of the kindergarten teacher on sex differences in behavior. *International Journal of Behavioral Development*, **8**, 3-13.

Orlick, T.D. (1973, January/February). Children's sport—A revolution is coming. *Canadian Association for Health, Physical Education and Recreation Journal*, pp. 12-14.

Orlick, T.D. (1974, November/December). The athletic dropout: A high price for inefficiency. *Canadian Association for Health, Physical Education and Recreation Journal*, pp. 21-27.

Ornstein, P.A., & Naus, M.J. (1978). Rehearsal processes in children's memory. In P.A. Ornstein (Ed.), *Memory development in children* (pp. 69-99). Hillsdale, NJ: Erlbaum.

Ornstein, P.A., & Naus, M.J. (1984). *Effects of the knowledge base on children's processing*. Unpublished manuscript, University of North Carolina, Chapel Hill.

Oscai, L.B. (1989). Exercise and obesity: Emphasis on animal models. In C.V. Gisolfi & D.R. Lamb (Eds.), *Perspectives in exercise science and sports medicine Vol. 2: Youth, exercise, and sport* (pp. 273-292). Indianapolis: Benchmark.

Oscai, L.B., Babirak, S.P., Dubach, F.B., McGarr, J.A., & Spirakis, C.N. (1974). Exercise or food restriction: Effect on adipose tissue cellularity. *American Journal of Physiology*, **227**, 901-904.

Oyster, N., Morton, M., & Linnell, S. (1984). Physical activity and osteoporosis in post-menopausal women. *Medicine and Science in Sports and Exercise*, **16**, 44-50.

Parizkova, J. (1963). Impact of age, diet, and exercise on man's body composition. *Annals of the New York Academy of Sciences*, **110**, 661-674.

Parizkova, J. (1968). Longitudinal study of the development of body composition and body build in boys of various physical activity. *Human Biology*, **40**, 212-225.

Parizkova, J. (1972). Somatic development and body composition changes in adolescent boys differing in physical activity and fitness: A longitudinal study. *Anthropologie*, **10**, 3-36.

Parizkova, J. (1973). Body composition and exercise during growth and development. In G.L. Rarick (Ed.), *Physical activity: Human growth and development* (pp. 97-124). New York: Academic Press.

Parizkova, J. (1977). *Body fat and physical fitness*. The Hague, The Netherlands: Martinus Nijhoff B.V.

Parizkova, J., & Carter, J.E.L. (1976). Influence of physical activity on stability of somatotypes in boys. *American Journal of Physical Anthropology*, **44**, 327-340.

Parizkova, J., & Eiselt, E. (1968). Longitudinal study of changes in anthropometric indicators and body composition in old men of various physical activity. *Human Biology*, **40**, 331-344.

Pascual-Leone, J. (1970). A mathematical model for the transition rule in Piaget's developmental stages. *Acta Psychologica*, **32**, 301-345.

Pate, R.R. (1989). The case for large-scale physical fitness testing in American youth. *Pediatric Exercise Science*, **1**, 290-294.

Patterson, C.J., & Mischel, W. (1975). Plans to resist distraction. *Developmental Psychology*, **11**, 369-378.

Patriksson, G. (1981). Socialization to sports involvement. *Scandinavian Journal of Sports Sciences*, **3**, 27-32.

Payne, V.G. (1982). Simultaneous investigation of effects of distance of projection and object size on object reception by children in grade 1. *Perceptual and Motor Skills*, **54**, 1183-1187.

Payne, V.G., & Koslow, R. (1981). Effects of varying ball diameters on catching ability of young children. *Perceptual and Motor Skills*, **53**, 739-744.

Peiper, A. (1963). *Cerebral function in infancy and childhood*. New York: Consultants Bureau.

Perelle, I.B. (1975). Difference in attention to stimulus presentation mode with regard to age. *Developmental Psychology*, **11**, 403-404.

Pew, R.W., & Rupp, G. (1971). Two quantitative measures of skill development. *Journal of Experimental Psychology*, **90**, 1-7.

Pfeiffer, R., & Francis, R.S. (1986). Effects of strength training on muscle development in prepubescent, pubescent, and postpubescent males. *The Physician and Sportsmedicine*, **14**, 134-143.

Phillips, M., Bookwalter, C., Denman, C., McAuley, J., Sherwin, H., Summers, D., & Yeakel, H. (1955). Analysis of results from the Kraus-Weber test of minimum muscular fitness in children. *Research Quarterly*, **26**, 314-323.

Piaget, J. (1952). *The origins of intelligence in children*. New York: International Universities Press.

Pick, A.D. (Ed.) (1979). *Perception and its development: A tribute to Eleanor J. Gibson*. Hillsdale, NJ: Erlbaum.

Pick, H.L. (1989). Motor development: The control of action. *Developmental Psychology*, **25**, 867-870.

Pikler, E. (1968). Some contributions to the study of gross motor development in children. *Journal of Genetic Psychology*, **113**, 27-39.

Plowman, S.A. (1992). Criterion referenced standards for neuromuscular physical fitness tests: An analysis. *Pediatric Exercise Science*, **4**, 10-19.

Pollock, M.L. (1974). Physiological characteristics of older champion track athletes. *Research Quarterly*, **45**, 363-373.

Pomerance, A. (1965). Pathology of the heart with and without failure in the aged. *British Heart Journal*, **27**, 697-710.

Pope, M.J. (1984). *Visual proprioception in infant postural development*. Unpublished doctoral dissertation, University of Southampton, Highfield, Southampton, United Kingdom.

Powell, R.R. (1974). Psychological effects of exercise therapy upon institutionalized geriatric mental patients. *Journal of Gerontology*, **29**, 157-161.

Power, T.G. (1985). Mother- and father-infant play: A developmental analysis. *Child Development*, **56**, 1514-1524.

Power, T.G., & Parke, R.D. (1983). Pattens of mother and father play with their 8-month-old infant: A multiple analyses approach. *Infant Behavior and Development*, **6**, 453-459.

Power, T.G., & Parke, R.D. (1986). Patterns of early socialization: Mother- and father-infant interactions in the home. *International Journal of Behavioral Development*, **9**, 331-341.

Prader, A., Tanner, J.M., & von Harnack, G.A. (1963). Catch-up growth following illness or starvation: An example of developmental canalization in man. *Journal of Pediatrics*, **62**, 646-659.

President's Council on Physical Fitness and Sports. (1987). *The Presidential Physical Fitness Award program*. Washington, DC: Author.

Prohaska, T.R., Leventhal, E.A., Leventhal, H., & Keller, M.L. (1985). Health practices and illness cognition in young, middle aged, and elderly adults. *Journal of Gerontology*, **40**, 569-578.

Raab, D.M., Agre, J.C., McAdam, M., & Smith, E.L. (1988). Light resistance and stretching exercise in elderly women: Effect upon flexibility. *Archives of Physical Medicine and Rehabilitation*, **69**, 268-272.

Rabbitt, P. (1965). An age decrement in the ability to ignore irrelevant information. *Journal of Gerontology*, **20**, 233-238.

Ramsay, D. (1980). Onset of unimanual handedness in infants. *Infant Behavior and Development*, **3**, 377-386.

Ramsay, D.S. (1985). Infants' block banging at midline: Evidence for Gesell's principle of "reciprocal interweaving" in development. *British Journal of Developmental Psychology*, **3**, 335-343.

Ramsay, D., Campos, J.J., & Fenson, L. (1979). Onset of bimanual handedness in infants. *Infant Behavior and Development*, **2**, 69-76.

Ramsay, D.S., & Willis, M.P. (1984). Organization and lateralization of reaching in infants: An extension of Bresson et al. *Neuropsychologia*, **22**, 639-641.

Rarick, G.L. (Ed.) (1973). *Physical activity: Human growth and development*. New York: Academic Press.

Rarick, G.L., & Smoll, F.L. (1967). Stability of growth in strength and motor performance from childhood to adolescence. *Human Biology*, **39**, 295-306.

Razel, M. (1985). A reanalysis of the evidence for the genetic nature of early motor development. *Advances in Applied Developmental Psychology*, **1**, 171-211.

Razel, M. (1988). Call for a follow-up study of experiments on long-term deprivation of human infants. *Perceptual and Motor Skills*, **67**, 147-158.

Reid, L. (1967). *The pathology of emphysema*. London: Lloyd-Luke.

Rhodes, A. (1937). A comparative study of motor abilities of Negroes and whites. *Child Development*, **8**, 369-371.

Rhodes, P. (1981). *Childbirth*. Burlington, NC: Carolina Biological Supply.

Rians, C.B., Weltman, A., Cahill, B.R., Janney, C.A., Tippett, S.R., & Katch, F.I. (1987). Strength training for prepubescent males: Is it safe? *The American Journal of Sports Medicine*, **15**, 483-489.

Ridenour, M.V. (1978). Programs to optimize infant motor development. In M.V. Ridenour (Ed.), *Motor development: Issues and applications* (pp. 39-61). Princeton, NJ: Princeton Book.

Rikli, R., & Busch, S. (1986). Motor performance of women as a function of age and physical activity level. *Journal of Gerontology*, **41**, 645-649.

Risser, W.L., & Preston, D. (1989). Incidence and causes of musculoskeletal injuries in adolescents training with weights. *Pediatric Exercise Science*, **1**, 84. (abstract)

Roach, E.G., & Kephart, N.C. (1966). *The Purdue perceptual-motor survey*. Columbus, OH: Merrill.

Roberton, M.A. (1977). Stability of stage categorizations across trials: Implications for the "stage theory" of overarm throw development. *Journal of Human Movement Studies*, **3**, 49-59.

Roberton, M.A. (1978a). Longitudinal evidence for developmental stages in the forceful overarm throw. *Journal of Human Movement Studies*, **4**, 167-175.

Roberton, M.A. (1978b). Stability of stage categorizations in motor development. In D.M. Landers & R.W. Christina (Eds.), *Psychology of motor behavior and sport—1977* (pp. 494-506). Champaign, IL: Human Kinetics.

Roberton, M.A. (1978c). Stages in motor development. In M.V. Ridenour (Ed.), *Motor development: Issues and applications* (pp. 63-81). Princeton, NJ: Princeton Book.

Roberton, M.A. (1984). Changing motor patterns during childhood. In J.R. Thomas (Ed.), *Motor development during childhood and adolescence* (pp. 48-90). Minneapolis: Burgess.

Roberton, M.A. (1988). The weaver's loom: A developmental metaphor. In J.E. Clark & J.H. Humphrey (Eds.), *Advances in motor development research* (Vol. 2, pp. 129-141). New York: AMS Press.

Roberton, M.A., & DiRocco, P. (1981). Validating a motor skill sequence for mentally retarded children. *American Corrective Therapy Journal*, **35**, 148-154.

Roberton, M.A., & Halverson, L.E. (1977). The developing child—his changing movement. In B. Logsdon (Ed.), *Physical education for children: A focus on the teaching process*. Philadelphia: Lea & Febiger.

Roberton, M.A., & Halverson, L.E. (1984). *Developing children—their changing movement*. Philadelphia: Lea & Febiger.

Roberton, M.A., & Halverson, L.E. (1988). The development of locomotor coordination: Longitudinal change and invariance. *Journal of Motor Behavior*, **20**, 197-241.

Roberton, M.A., Halverson, L., Langendorfer, S., & Williams, K. (1979). Longitudinal changes in children's overarm throw ball velocities. *Research Quarterly*, **50**, 256-264.

Roberton, M.A., & Langendorfer, S. (1980). Testing motor development sequences across 9-14 years. In D. Nadeau, W. Halliwell, K. Newell, & G. Roberts (Eds.), *Psychology of motor behavior and sport—1979* (pp. 269-279). Champaign, IL: Human Kinetics.

Roberts, S.B., Savage, J., Coward, W.A., Chew, B., & Lucas, A. (1988). Energy expenditure and intake in infants born to lean and overweight mothers. *New England Journal of Medicine*, **318**, 461-466.

Rogers, D. (1982). *Life-span human development*. Monterey, CA: Brooks/Cole.

Rolland-Cachera, M.F., & Bellisle, F. (1986). No correlation between adiposity and food intake: Why are working class children fatter? *American Journal of Clinical Nutrition, 44*, 779-787.

Rose, H.E., & Mayer, J. (1968). Activity, caloric intake, fat storage, and the energy balance of infants. *Pediatrics, 41*, 18-29, s.

Rose, S.A., Gottfried, A.W., & Bridger, W.H. (1981). Cross-modal transfer in 6-month-old infants. *Developmental Psychology, 17*, 661-669.

Rosenhall, V., & Rubin, W. (1975). Degenerative changes in the human sensory epithelia. *Acta Otolaryngologica, 79*, 67-81.

Rosinski, R.R. (1977). *The development of visual perception.* Santa Monica, CA: Goodyear.

Ross, A.O. (1976). *Psychological aspects of learning disabilities and reading disorders.* New York: McGraw-Hill.

Ross, J.G., Pate, R.R., Delpy, L.A., Gold, R.S., & Svilar, M. (1987). New health-related fitness norms. *Journal of Physical Education, Recreation and Dance, 58*, 66-70.

Rothstein, A.L. (1977). Information processing in children's skill acquisition. In R.W. Christina & D.M. Landers (Eds.), *Psychology of motor behavior and sport—1976* (pp. 218-227). Champaign, IL: Human Kinetics.

Rotstein, A., Dotan, R., Bar-Or, O., & Tenenbaum, G. (1986). Effect of training on anaerobic threshold, maximal power, and anaerobic performance of preadolescent boys. *International Journal of Sports Medicine, 7*, 281-286.

Rowland, T.W. (1989a). Oxygen uptake and endurance fitness in children: A developmental perspective. *Pediatric Exercise Science, 1*, 313-328.

Rowland, T.W. (1989b). On trainability and heart rates. *Pediatric Exercise Science, 1*, 187-188.

Rudel, R., & Teuber, H. (1971). Pattern recognition within and across sensory modalities in normal and brain injured children. *Neuropsychologia, 9*, 389-400.

Rudman, W. (1986). Life course socioeconomic transitions and sport involvement: A theory of restricted opportunity. In B. McPherson (Ed.), *Sport and aging* (pp. 25-35). Champaign, IL: Human Kinetics.

Ruff, H.A. (1984). Infants' manipulative exploration of objects: Effects of age and objects' characteristics. *Developmental Psychology, 29*, 9-20.

Ruff, H.A., & Halton, A. (1978). Is there directed reaching in the human neonate? *Developmental Psychology, 4*, 425-426.

Rutenfranz, J. (1986). Longitudinal approach to assessing maximal aerobic power during growth: The European experience. *Medicine and Science in Sports and Exercise, 15*, 486-490.

Sabatino, D.A., & Becker, J.T. (1971). Relationship between lateral preference and selected behavioral variables for children failing academically. *Child Development, 42*, 2055-2060.

Sady, S.P. (1986). Cardiorespiratory exercise in children. In F. Katch & P.F. Freedson (Eds.), *Clinics in sports medicine* (pp. 493-513). Philadelphia: Saunders.

Safrit, M.J. (1990). The validity and reliability of fitness tests for children: A review. *Pediatric Exercise Science, 2*, 9-28.

Sale, D.G. (1989). Strength training in children. In G.V. Gisolfi & D.R. Lamb (Eds.), *Perspectives in exercise science and sports medicine. Vol 2: Youth, exercise and sport* (pp. 165-222). Indianapolis: Benchmark.

Salkind, N.J. (1981). *Theories of human development.* New York: D. Van Nostrand.

Salthouse, T.A. (1980). Age and memory: Strategies for localizing the loss. In L.W. Poon, J.L. Fozard, L.S. Cermak, D. Arenberg, & L.W. Thompson (Eds.), *New directions in memory and aging* (pp. 47-65). Hillsdale, NJ: Erlbaum.

Saltin, B., & Grimby, G. (1968). Physiological analysis of middle-aged and old former athletes: Comparison with still active athletes of the same ages. *Circulation, 38*, 1104-1115.

Sandler, L., Van Campen, J., Ratner, G., Stafford, C., & Weismar, R. (1970). Responses of urban preschool children to a developmental screening test. *Journal of Pediatrics, 77*, 775-781.

Sapp, M., & Haubenstricker, J. (1978). *Motivation for joining and reasons for not continuing in youth sport programs in Michigan.* Paper presented at the American Alliance for Health, Physical Education, Recreation and Dance national conference, Kansas City, MO.

Scanlan, T.K. (1988). Social evaluation and the competition process: A developmental perspective. In F.L. Smoll, R.A. Magill, & M.J. Ash (Eds.), *Children in sport* (3rd ed., pp. 135-148). Champaign, IL: Human Kinetics.

Scanlan, T.K., & Lewthwaite, R. (1986). Social psychological aspects of competition for male youth sport participants: IV. Predictors of enjoyment. *Journal of Sport Psychology, 8*, 25-35.

Scanlan, T.K., Stein, G.L., & Ravizza, K. (1988). An in-depth study of former elite figure skaters: II. Sources of enjoyment. *Journal of Sport & Exercise Psychology, 11*, 65-83.

Schaie, K.W. (1965). A general model for the study of developmental problems. *Psychological Bulletin, 64*, 92-107.

Schellenberger, B. (1981). The significance of social relations in sport activity. *International Review of Sport Sociology*, **16**, 69-77.

Schmidt, R.A. (1977). Schema theory: Implications for movement education. *Motor Skills: Theory Into Practice*, **2**, 36-48.

Schwanda, N.A. (1978). *A biomechanical study of the walking gait of active and inactive middle-age and elderly men*. Unpublished doctoral dissertation, Springfield College, Springfield, MA.

Schwartz, L.A., & Markham, W.T. (1985). Sex stereotyping in children's toy advertisements. *Sex Roles*, **12**, 157-170.

Seefeldt, V. (1973). *Developmental sequences in fundamental motor skills*. Unpublished paper, Michigan State University, East Lansing.

Seefeldt, V., & Haubenstricker, J. (1982). Patterns, phases, or stages: An analytical model for the study of developmental movement. In J.A.S. Kelso & J.E. Clark (Eds.), *The development of movement control and coordination* (pp. 309-318). New York: Wiley.

Seefeldt, V., Reuschlein, S., & Vogel, P. (1972, April). *Sequencing motor skills within the physical education curriculum*. Paper presented at the annual convention of the American Association for Health, Physical Education, and Recreation, Houston, TX.

Seils, L.G. (1951). The relationship between measures of physical growth and gross motor performance of primary-grade school children. *Research Quarterly*, **22**, 244-260.

Sepic, S.B., Murray, M.P., Mollinger, L.A., Spurr, G.B., & Gardner, G.M. (1986). Strength and range of motion in the ankle in two age groups of men and women. *American Journal of Physical Medicine*, **65**, 75-84.

Servedio, F.J., Barels, R.L., Hamlin, R.L., Teske, D., Shaffer, T., & Servedio, A. (1985). The effects of weight training using Olympic style lifts, on various physiological variables in prepubescent boys. *Medicine and Science in Sports and Exercise*, **17**, 288. (abstract)

Sessoms, J.E. (1942). *Common motor abilities of Negro preschool children*. Unpublished master's thesis, Iowa State University, Ames.

Sewall, L., & Micheli, L.J. (1986). Strength training for children. *Journal of Pediatric Orthopedics*, **6**, 143-146.

Shambes, G.M. (1976). Static postural control in children. *American Journal of Physical Medicine*, **55**, 221-252.

Sharkey, B.J. (1990). *Physiology of fitness* (3rd ed.). Champaign, IL: Human Kinetics.

Shea, E.J. (1986a). Older Americans in sport. *Illinois Journal of Health, Physical Education, Recreation and Dance*, **26**, 20-22.

Shea, E.J. (1986b). *Swimming for seniors*. Champaign, IL: Human Kinetics.

Sheffield, L.T., & Roitman, D. (1973). Systolic blood pressure, heart rate, and treadmill work at anginal threshold. *Chest*, **63**, 327-335.

Sheldon, J.H. (1963). The effect of age on the control of sway. *Gerontologia Clinica*, **5**, 129-138.

Shephard, R.J. (1978a). Human physiological work capacity. In *IBP Human Adaptability Project, Synthesis: Vol. 4*. New York: Cambridge University Press.

Shephard, R.J. (1978b). *Physical activity and aging*. Chicago: Year Book Medical.

Shephard, R.J. (1979). Recurrence of myocardial infarction. *British Heart Journal*, **42**, 133-138.

Shephard, R.J. (1981). Cardiovascular limitations in the aged. In E.L. Smith & R.C. Serfass (Eds.), *Exercise and aging: The scientific basis* (pp. 19-29). Hillside, NJ: Enslow.

Shephard, R.J. (1982). *Physical activity and growth*. Chicago: Year Book Medical.

Shephard, R.J., & Kavanagh, T. (1978). The effects of training on the aging process. *The Physician and Sportsmedicine*, **6**, 33-40.

Shirley, M.M. (1931). *The first two years: A study of twenty-five babies. Postural and locomotor development* (Vol. 1). Minneapolis: University of Minnesota Press.

Shirley, M.M. (1933). *The first two years: A study of twenty-five babies. Intellectual development* (Vol. 2). Minneapolis: University of Minnesota Press.

Shirley, M.M. (1963). The motor sequence. In D. Wayne (Ed.), *Readings in child psychology*. Englewood Cliffs, NJ: Prentice-Hall.

Shock, N.W., & Norris, A.H. (1970). Neuromuscular coordination as a factor in age changes in muscular exercise. In D. Brunner & E. Jokl (Eds.), *Physical activity and aging*. Baltimore: University Park Press.

Shuleva, K.M., Hunter, G.R., Hester, D.J., & Dunaway, D.L. (1990). Exercise oxygen uptake in 3- through 6-year-old children. *Pediatric Exercise Science*, **2**, 130-139.

Shumway-Cook, A., & Woollacott, M. (1985). The growth of stability: Postural control from a developmental perspective. *Journal of Motor Behavior*, **17**, 131-147.

Sidney, K.H., Shephard, R.J., & Harrison, J.E. (1977). Endurance training and body composition of the elderly. *American Journal of Clinical Nutrition*, **30**, 326-333.

Siegel, J.A., Camaione, D.N., & Manfredi, T.G.

(1989). The effects of upper body resistance training on pre-pubescent children. *Pediatric Exercise Science, 1*, 145-154.

Siegler, R.S., & Jenkins, E.A. (1989). *How children discover new strategies.* Hillsdale, NJ: Erlbaum.

Simard, T. (1969). Fine sensorimotor control in healthy children. *Pediatrics, 43*, 1035-1041.

Simons, J., Beunen, G.P., Renson, R., Claessens, A.L.M., Vanreusel, B., & Lefevre, J.A.V. (1990). *Growth and fitness of Flemish girls: The Leuven growth study.* Champaign, IL: Human Kinetics.

Simons-Morton, B.G., Baranowski, T., O'Hara, N.M., Parcel, G.S., Huang, I.W., & Wilson, B. (1990). Children's frequency of participation in moderate to vigorous physical activities. *Research Quarterly for Exercise and Sport, 61*, 307-314.

Sinclair, C. (1971). Dominance pattern of young children, a follow-up study. *Perceptual and Motor Skills, 32*, 142.

Sinclair, C.B. (1973). *Movement of the young child: Ages two to six.* Columbus, OH: Merrill.

Singleton, W.T. (1955). Age and performance timing on simple skills. In *Old age and the modern world* (Report of the Third Congress of the International Association of Gerontology). London: E. & S. Livingstone.

Skrobak-Kaczynski, J., & Andersen, K.L. (1975). The effect of a high level of habitual physical activity in the regulation of fatness during aging. *International Archives of Occupational and Environmental Health, 36*, 41-46.

Slaughter, M.H., Lohman, T.G., Boileau, R.A., Horswill, C.A., Stillman, R.J., VanLoan, M.D., & Bemben, D.A. (1988). Skinfold equations for estimation of body fatness in children and youth. *Human Biology, 60*, 709-723.

Sloan, W. (1955). The Lincoln-Oseretsky motor development scale. *Genetic Psychology Monographs, 51*, 183-252.

Smith, A.B. (1985). Teacher modeling and sex-types play preferences. *New Zealand Journal of Educational Studies, 20*, 39-47.

Smith, A.D. (1980). Age differences in encoding, storage, and retrieval. In L.W. Poon, J.L. Fozard, L.S. Cermak, D. Arenberg, & L.W. Thompson (Eds.), *New directions in memory and aging* (pp. 23-45). Hillsdale, NJ: Erlbaum.

Smith, E.L., Reddan, W., & Smith, P.E. (1981). Physical activity and calcium modalities for bone mineral increase in aged women. *Medicine and Science in Sports and Exercise, 13*, 60-64.

Smith, E.L., Sempos, C.T., & Purvis, R.W. (1981). Bone mass and strength decline with age. In E.L. Smith & R.C. Serfass (Eds.), *Exercise and aging: The scientific basis* (pp. 59-87). Hillside, NJ: Enslow.

Smith, E.L., & Serfass, R.C. (Eds.) (1981). *Exercise and aging: The scientific basis.* Hillside, NJ: Enslow.

Smith, J., & Walker, J.M. (1983). Knee and elbow range of motion in healthy older individuals. *Physical and Occupational Therapy in Geriatrics, 2*, 31-38.

Smith, L.B., Kemler, D.G., & Aronfried, J. (1975). Developmental trends in voluntary selective attention: Differential aspects of source distinctiveness. *Journal of Experimental Child Psychology, 20*, 353-362.

Smith, M.D. (1979). Getting involved in sport: Sex differences. *International Review of Sport Sociology, 14*, 93-99.

Smith, R.E., Smoll, F.L., & Curtis, B. (1979). Coach effectiveness training: A cognitive-behavioral approach to enhancing relationship skills in youth sport coaches. *Journal of Sport Psychology, 1*, 59-75.

Smoll, F.L., & Schutz, R.W. (1990). Quantifying gender differences in physical performance: A developmental perspective. *Developmental Psychology, 26*, 360-369.

Smoll, F.L., & Smith, R.E. (1989). Leadership behaviors in sport: A theoretical model and research paradigm. *Journal of Applied Social Psychology, 19*, 1522-1551.

Snyder, E.E., & Spreitzer, E.A. (1973). Family influence and involvement in sports. *Research Quarterly, 44*, 249-255.

Snyder, E., & Spreitzer, E. (1976). Correlates of sport participation among adolescent girls. *Research Quarterly, 47*, 804-809.

Snyder, E.E., & Spreitzer, E. (1978). Socialization comparisons of adolescent female athletes and musicians. *Research Quarterly, 49*, 342-350.

Snyder, E.E., & Spreitzer, E.A. (1983). *Social aspects of sport* (2nd ed.). Englewood Cliffs, NJ: Prentice-Hall.

Spelke, E.S. (1979). Exploring audible and visible events in infancy. In A.D. Pick (Ed.), *Perception and its development: A tribute to Eleanor J. Gibson.* Hillsdale, NJ: Erlbaum.

Spetner, N.B., & Olsho, L.W. (1990). Auditory frequency resolution in human infancy. *Child Development, 61*, 632-652.

Spilich, G.J., Vesonder, G.T., Chiesi, H.L., & Voss, J.F. (1979). Text processing of individuals with high and low domain knowledge. *Journal of Verbal Learning and Verbal Behavior, 18*, 275-290.

Spirduso, W.W. (1975). Reaction and movement time as a function of age and physical activity level. *Journal of Gerontology*, **30**, 435-440.

Spirduso, W.W. (1980). Physical fitness and psychomotor speed: A review. *Journal of Gerontology*, **35**, 850-865.

Spirduso, W.W., Gilliam, P., & Wilcox, R.E. (1984). Speed of movement initiation performance predicts differences in [3H] spiroperiodol receptor bings in normal rats. *Psychopharmacology*, **83**, 205-209.

Spreitzer, E., & Snyder, E. (1983). Correlates of participation in adult recreational sports. *Journal of Leisure Research*, **15**, 28-38.

Sprynarova, S., & Reisenauer, R. (1978). Body dimensions and physiological indications of physical fitness during adolescence. In R.J. Shepard & H. Lavallee (Eds.), *Physical fitness assessment* (pp. 32-37). Springfield, IL: Charles C Thomas.

Stadulis, R.I. (1971). *Coincidence-anticipation behavior of children*. Unpublished doctoral dissertation, Teachers College, Columbia University, New York.

Stafanik, P.A., Heald, F.P., & Mayer, J. (1959). Caloric intake in relation to energy output of obese and non-obese adolescent boys. *American Journal of Clinical Nutrition*, **7**, 55-62.

Stamford, B.A. (1973). Effects of chronic institutionalization on the physical working capacity and trainability of geriatric men. *Journal of Gerontology*, **28**, 441-446.

Stamford, B.A. (1988). Exercise and the elderly. In K.B. Pandolf (Ed.), *Exercise and sport sciences reviews* (Vol. 16, pp. 341-379). New York: Macmillan.

Stanish, W.D. (1984). Overuse injuries in athletes: A perspective. *Medicine and Science in Sport and Exercise*, **16**, 1-7.

Steben, R.E., & Steben, A.H. (1981). The validity of the strength shortening cycle in selected jumping events. *Journal of Sports Medicine and Physical Fitness*, **21**, 28-37.

Sterritt, G., Martin, V., & Rudnick, M. (1971). Auditory-visual and temporal-spatial integration as determinants of test difficulty. *Psychonomic Science*, **23**, 289-291.

Stewart, K.J., & Gutin, B. (1976). Effects of physical training on cardiorespiratory fitness in children. *Research Quarterly*, **47**, 110-120.

Stolz, H.R., & Stolz, L.M. (1951). *Somatic development of adolescent boys*. New York: Macmillan.

Stratton, R.K. (1978a). Information processing deficits in children's motor performance: Implications for instruction. *Motor Skills: Theory into Practice*, **3**, 49-55.

Stratton, R.K. (1978b, May). *Selective attention deficits in children's motor performance: Can we help?* Paper presented at the annual conference of the North American Society for Psychology of Sport and Physical Activity, Tallahassee, FL.

Strohmeyer, H.S., Williams, K., & Schaub-George, D. (1991). Developmental sequences for catching a small ball: A prelongitudinal screening. *Research Quarterly for Exercise and Sport*, **62**, 257-266.

Stunkard, A., & Mendelson, M. (1967). Obesity and the body image. I. Characteristics of disturbances in the body image of some obese persons. *American Journal of Psychiatry*, **123**, 1296-1300.

Super, C.M. (1976). Environmental effects on motor development: The case of 'African infant precocity.' *Developmental Medicine and Child Neurology*, **18**, 561-567.

Sutherland, D.H., Olshen, R., Cooper, L., & Woo, S. (1980). The development of mature gait. *Journal of Bone and Joint Surgery*, **62-A**, 336-353.

Swanson, R., & Benton, A.L. (1955). Some aspects of the genetic development of right-left discrimination. *Child Development*, **26**, 123-133.

Szafran, J. (1951). Changes with age and with exclusion of vision in performance at an aiming task. *Quarterly Journal of Experimental Psychology*, **3**, 111-118.

Tanner, J. (1961). *Education and physical growth*. London: University of London Press.

Tanner, J.M. (1962). *Growth at adolescence* (2nd ed.). Oxford: Blackwell Scientific.

Teeple, J.B. (1978). Physical growth and maturation. In M.V. Ridenour (Ed.), *Motor development: Issues and applications* (pp. 3-27). Princeton, NJ: Princeton Book.

Temple, A.L. (1952). *Motor abilities of White and Negro children seven, eight, and nine years of age*. Unpublished master's thesis, University of California–Berkeley.

Temple, I.G., Williams, H.G., & Bateman, N.J. (1979). A test battery to assess intrasensory and intersensory development of young children. *Perceptual and Motor Skills*, **48**, 643-659.

Thelen, E. (1981). Kicking, rocking, and waving: Contextual analysis of rhythmical stereotypes in normal human infants. *Animal Behaviour*, **29**, 3-11.

Thelen, E. (1983). Learning to walk is still an "old" problem: A reply to Zelazo. *Journal of Motor Behavior*, **15**, 139-161.

Thelen, E. (1985). Developmental origins of motor coordination: Leg movements in human infants. *Developmental Psychobiology, 18*, 1-22.

Thelen, E. (1986). Treadmill-elicited stepping in seven-month-old infants. *Child Development, 57*, 1498-1506.

Thelen, E. (1989). Self-organization in developmental processes: Can systems approaches work? In M.R. Gunnar & E. Thelen (Eds.), *System and development. The Minnesota symposia on child psychology* (Vol. 22, pp. 77-117). Hillsdale, NJ: Erlbaum.

Thelen, E., Bradshaw, G., & Ward, J.A. (1981). Spontaneous kicking in month-old infants: Manifestations of a human central locomotor program. *Behavioral and Neural Biology, 32*, 45-53.

Thelen, E., & Fisher, D.M. (1982). Newborn stepping: An explanation for a "disappearing reflex." *Developmental Psychology, 18*, 760-775.

Thelen, E., & Fisher, D.M. (1983). The organization of spontaneous leg movements in newborn infants. *Journal of Motor Behavior, 15*, 353-377.

Thelen, E., Kelso, J.A.S., & Fogel, A. (1987). Self-organizing systems and infant motor development. *Developmental Review, 7*, 37-65.

Thelen, E., Ridley-Johnson, R., & Fisher, D.M. (1983). Shifting patterns of bilateral coordination and lateral dominance in the leg movements of young infants. *Developmental Psychobiology, 16*, 29-46.

Thelen, E., & Ulrich, B.D. (1991). Hidden skills. *Monographs of the Society for Research in Child Development, 56* (1, Serial No. 223).

Thelen, E., Ulrich, B.D., & Jensen, J.L. (1989). The developmental origins of locomotion. In M.H. Woollacott & A. Shumway-Cook (Eds.), *Development of posture and gait across the life span* (pp. 25-47). Columbia, SC: University of South Carolina Press.

Thomas, J.R. (1980). Acquisition of motor skills: Information processing differences between children and adults. *Research Quarterly for Exercise and Sport, 51*, 158-173.

Thomas, J.R., & French, K.E. (1985). Gender differences across age in motor performance: A meta-analysis. *Psychological Bulletin, 98*, 260-282.

Thomas, J.R., French, K.E., Thomas, K.T., & Gallagher, J.D. (1988). Children's knowledge development and sport performance. In F.L. Smoll, R.A. Magill, & M.J. Ash (Eds.), *Children in sport* (3rd ed., pp. 179-202). Champaign, IL: Human Kinetics.

Thomas, J.R., Gallagher, J.D., & Purvis, G.J. (1981). Reaction time and anticipation time: Effects of development. *Research Quarterly, 52*, 359-367.

Thomas, J.R., Mitchell, B., & Solomon, M.A. (1979). Precision knowledge of results and motor performance: Relationship to age. *Research Quarterly, 50*, 687-698.

Thomas, J.R., Thomas, K.T., & Gallagher, J.D. (1981). Children's processing of information in physical activity and sport. *Motor Skills: Theory into Practice Monographs,* (No. 3, 1-8).

Thompson, M.E. (1944). An experimental study of racial differences in general motor ability. *Journal of Educational Psychology, 35*, 49-54.

Thompson, M.E., & Dove, C.C. (1942). A comparison of physical achievement of Anglo and Spanish American boys in junior high school. *Research Quarterly, 13*, 341-346.

Timiras, P.S. (1972). *Developmental physiology and aging.* New York: Macmillan.

Trehub, S.E. (1973). *Auditory linguistic sensitivity in infants.* Unpublished doctoral dissertation, McGill University, Montreal.

Trehub, S.E., Bull, D., & Thorpe, L.A. (1984). Infants' perception of melodies: The role of melodic contour. *Child Development, 55*, 821-830.

Tremblay, A., Despres, J.-P., & Bouchard, C. (1988). Alternation in body fat and fat distribution with exercise. In C. Bouchard & F.E. Johnston (Eds.), *Fat distribution during growth and later health outcomes.* New York: Liss.

Trevarthan, C. (1984). How control of movement develops. In H.T.A. Whiting (Ed.). *Human motor actions: Bernstein reassessed* (pp. 223-261). Amsterdam: North-Holland.

Turner, J.M., Mead, J., & Wohl, M.E. (1968). Elasticity of human lungs in relation to age. *Journal of Applied Physiology, 35*, 664-671.

Ulrich, B.D., Thelen, E., & Niles, D. (1990). Perceptual determinants of action: Stair-climbing choices of infants and toddlers. In J.E. Clark & J.H. Humphrey (Eds.), *Advances in motor development research* (Vol. 3, pp. 1-15). New York: AMS Press.

Ulrich, D.A. (1985). *Test of Gross Motor Development.* Austin, TX: Pro-Ed.

Vaccaro, P., & Clarke, D.H. (1978). Cardiorespiratory alterations in 9- to 11-year-old children following a season of competitive swimming. *Medicine and Science in Sports, 10*, 204-207.

Van Duyne, H.J. (1973). Foundations of tactical perception in three to seven year olds. *Journal of the Association for the Study of Perception, 8*, 1-9.

Van Praagh, E., Fellmann, N., Bedu, M., Falgairette,

G., & Coudert, J. (1990). Gender difference in the relationship of anaerobic power output to body composition in children. *Pediatric Exercise Science*, **2**, 336-348.

VanSant, A.F. (1989). A life span concept of motor development. *Quest*, **41**, 224-234.

VanSant, A.F. (1990). Life-span development in functional tasks. *Physical Therapy*, **70**, 788-798.

VanSant, A. (in press). A life-span perspective of age differences in righting movements. In Roberton, M.A. (Ed.), *Advances in motor development research* (Vol. 4). New York: AMS Press.

Van Wieringen, J.C. (1978). Secular growth changes. In F. Falkner & J.M. Tanner (Eds.), *Human growth. Vol. 2: Postnatal growth* (pp. 445-473). New York: Plenum.

Victors, E. (1961). *A cinematrographical analysis of catching behavior of a selected group of seven and nine year old boys*. Unpublished doctoral dissertation, University of Wisconsin, Madison.

Vobecky, J.S., Vobecky, J., Shapcott, D., & Demers, P.P. (1983). Nutrient intake patterns and nutritional status with regard to relative weight in early infancy. *American Journal of Clinical Nutrition*, **38**, 730-738.

Vrijens, J. (1978). Muscle strength development in the pre- and post-pubescent age. *Medicine and Sport*, **11** 152-158.

Wadden, T.A., & Stunkard, A.J. (1985). Social and psychological consequences of obesity. *Annals of Internal Medicine*, **103**, 1062-1067.

Wade, M.G. (1980). Coincidence-anticipation of young normal and handicapped children. *Journal of Motor Behavior*, **12**, 103-112.

Wagner, J.A., Robinson, S., Tzankoff, S.P., & Marino, R.P. (1972). Heat tolerance and acclimatization to work in the heat in relation to age. *Journal of Applied Physiology*, **33**, 616-622.

Walk, R.D. (1969). Two types of depth discrimination by the human infant. *Psychonomic Science*, **14**, 253-254.

Walk, R.D., & Gibson, E.J. (1961). A comparative and analytical study of visual depth perception. *Psychological Monographs*, **75** (15, Whole No. 519).

Walker, J.M., Sue, D., Miles-Elkousy, N., Ford, G., & Trevelyan, H. (1984). Active mobility of the extremities in older subjects. *Physical Therapy*, **64**, 919-923.

Walker, L. (1938). *Comparison of selected athletic abilities of White and Negro boys*. Unpublished master's thesis, George Peabody College for Teachers, Nashville.

Walker, R. (1965). *The effect of a controlled program of physical activity on the physical efficiency, respiratory function, airway obstruction and dependency on drugs of the asthmatic child. Report I. Physical work capacity and respiratory function*. Toronto: Tuberculosis and Respiratory Disease Association.

Walker-Andrews, A.S., & Gibson, E.J. (1986). What develops in bimodal perception? In L.P. Lipsitt & C. Rovee-Collier (Eds.), *Advances in infancy research* (Vol. 4, pp. 171-181). Norwood, NJ: Ablex.

Warren, W.H. (1984). Perceiving affordances: Visual guidance of stair-climbing. *Journal of Experimental Psychology: Human Perception and Performance*, **10**, 683-703.

Washington, R.L. (1989). Anaerobic threshold in children. *Pediatric Exercise Science*, **1**, 244-256.

Weiner, J., & Lourie, J.A. (1981). *Practical human biology*. New York: Academic Press.

Weiss, M.R. (1983). Modeling and motor performance: A developmental perspective. *Research Quarterly for Exercise and Sport*, **54**, 190-197.

Weiss, M.R. (1993). Psychological effects of intensive sport participation on children and youth: Self-esteem and motivation. In B.R. Cahill & A.J. Pearl (Eds.), *Intensive participation in children's sports* (pp. 39-69). Champaign, IL: Human Kinetics.

Weiss, M.R., & Horn, T.S. (1990). The relation between children's accuracy estimates of their physical competence and achievement-related characteristics. *Research Quarterly for Exercise and Sport*, **61**, 250-258.

Weiss, M.R., & Knoppers, A. (1982). The influence of socializing agents on female collegiate volleyball players. *Journal of Sport Psychology*, **4**, 267-279.

Weiss, M.R., McAuley, E., Ebbeck, V., & Wiese, D.M. (1990). Self-esteem and causal attributions for children's physical and social competence in sport. *Journal of Sport & Exercise Psychology*, **12**, 21-36.

Welford, A.T. (1977a). Causes of slowing of performance with age. *Interdisciplinary Topics in Gerontology*, **11**, 23-51.

Welford, A.T. (1977b). Motor performance. In J.E. Birren & K.W. Schaie (Eds.), *Handbook of the psychology of aging* (pp. 450-496). New York: Van Nostrand Reinhold

Welford, A.T. (1977c). Serial reaction times, continuity of task, single-channel effects, and age. In

S. Dornic (Ed.), *Attention and performance VI*. Hillside, NJ: Erlbaum.

Welford, A.T. (1980a). Memory and age: A perspective view. In L.W. Poon, J.L. Fozard, L.S. Cermak, D. Arenberg, & L.W. Thompson (Eds.), *New directions in memory and aging* (pp. 1-17). Hillside, NJ: Erlbaum.

Welford, A.T. (1980b). Motor skill and aging. In C.H. Nadeau, W.R. Halliwell, K.M. Newell, & G.C. Roberts (Eds.), *Psychology of motor behavior and sport—1979* (pp. 253-268). Champaign, IL: Human Kinetics.

Welford, A.T., Norris, A.H., & Shock, N.W. (1969). Speed and accuracy of movement and their changes with age. *Acta Psychologica*, **30**, 3-15.

Weltman, A., Janney, C., Rians, C.B., Strand, K., Berg, B., Tippitt, S., Wise, J., Cahill, B.R., & Katch, F.I. (1986). The effects of hydraulic resistance strength training in prepubertal males. *Medicine and Science in Sports and Exercise*, **18**, 629-638.

Whitall, J. (1988a). The development of visual directed reaching: From description to explanation. In J.E. Clark & J.H. Humphrey (Eds.), *Advances in motor development research* (Vol. 2, pp. 143-163). New York: AMS Press.

Whitall, J. (1988b). *A developmental study of interlimb coordination in running and galloping*. Unpublished doctoral dissertation, University of Maryland, College Park.

White, B.L., Castle, P., & Held, R. (1964). Observations on the development of visually-directed reaching. *Child Development*, **35**, 349-364.

Wickens, C.D. (1974). Temporal limits of human information processing: A developmental study. *Psychological Bulletin*, **81**, 739-755.

Wickstrom, R.L. (1983). *Fundamental motor patterns* (3rd ed.). Philadelphia: Lea & Febiger.

Wickstrom, R.L. (1987). Observations on motor pattern development in skipping. In J.E. Clark & J.H. Humphrey (Eds.), *Advances in motor development research* (Vol. 1, pp. 49-60). New York: AMS Press.

Wild, M. (1937). *The behavior pattern of throwing and some observations concerning its course of development in children*. Unpublished doctoral dissertation, University of Wisconsin, Madison.

Wild, M. (1938). The behavior pattern of throwing and some observations concerning its course of development in children. *Research Quarterly*, **9**, 20-24.

Williams, H. (1968). *Effects of systematic variation of speed and direction of object flight and of age and skill classification on visuo-perceptual judgments of moving objects in three-dimensional space*. Unpublished doctoral dissertation, University of Wisconsin, Madison.

Williams, H. (1973). Perceptual-motor development in children. In C. Corbin (Ed.). *A textbook of motor development* (pp. 111-148). Dubuque, IA: W.C. Brown.

Williams, H.G. (1981). Neurophysiological correlates of motor development: A review for practitioners. *Motor Skills: Theory into Practice Monographs* (No. 3, 31-40)

Williams, H. (1983). *Perceptual and motor development*. Englewood Cliffs, NJ: Prentice-Hall.

Williams, H. (1986). The development of sensory-motor function in young children. In V. Seefeldt (Ed.), *Physical activity and well-being* (pp. 104-122). Reston, VA: American Alliance for Health, Physical Education, Recreation and Dance.

Williams, J.R., & Scott, R.B. (1953). Growth and development of Negro infants: IV. Motor development and its relationship to child rearing practices in two groups of Negro infants. *Child Development*, **24**, 103-121.

Williams, K. (1980). The developmental characteristics of a forward roll. *Research Quarterly for Exercise and Sport*, **51**, 703-713.

Williams, K., Goodman, M., & Green, R. (1985). Parent-child factors in gender role socialization in girls. *Journal of the American Academy of Child Psychiatry*, **24**, 720-731.

Williams, K., Haywood, K., & VanSant, A. (1990). Movement characteristics of older adult throwers. In J.E. Clark & J.H. Humphrey (Eds.), *Advances in motor development research* (Vol. 3, pp. 29-44). New York: AMS Press.

Williams, K., Haywood, K., & VanSant, A. (1991). Throwing patterns of older adults: A follow-up investigation. *International Journal of Aging and Human Development*, **33**, 279-294.

Wilmore, J.H., Frisancho, R.A., Gordon, C.C., Himes, J.H., Martin, A.D., Martorell, R., & Seefeldt, V.D. (1988). Body breadth equipment and measurement techniques. In T.G. Lohman, A.F. Roche, & R. Martorell (Eds.), *Anthropometric standardization reference manual* (pp. 27-38). Champaign, IL: Human Kinetics.

Winter, D.A. (1983). Biomechanical motor patterns in normal walking. *Journal of Motor Behavior*, **15**, 302-330.

Winterhalter, C. (1974). *Age and sex trends in the development of selected balancing skills*. Unpublished master's thesis, University of Toledo.

Wohlwill, J.F. (1973). *The study of behavioral development*. New York: Academic Press.

Woollacott, M.H. (1983). *Children's changing capacity to process information*. Paper presented at the annual convention of the American Alliance for Health, Physical Education, Recreation and Dance. (Available through Microform Publications, Eugene, OR)

Woollacott, M.H. (1986). Gait and postural control in the aging adult. In W. Bles & Th. Brandt (Eds.), *Disorders of posture and gait* (pp. 326-336). New York: Elsevier.

Woollacott, M., Debu, B., & Mowatt, M. (1987). Neuromuscular control of posture in the infant and child. *Journal of Motor Behavior*, **19**, 167-186.

Woollacott, M., Shumway-Cook, A.T., & Nashner, L.M. (1982). Postural reflexes and aging. In J.A. Mortimer (Ed.), *The aging motor system* (pp. 98-119). New York: Praeger.

Woollacott, M., Shumway-Cook, A., & Nashner, L.M. (1986). Aging and posture control: Changes in sensory organization and muscular coordination. *International Journal of Aging and Human Development*, **23**, 97-114.

Woollacott, M.H., Shumway-Cook, A., & Williams, H. (1989). The development of posture and balance control in children. In M.H. Woollacott & A. Shumway-Cook (Eds.), *Development of posture and gait across the life span* (pp. 77-96). Columbia, SC: University of South Carolina Press.

Yamaguchi, Y. (1984). A comparative study of adolescent socialization into sport: The case of Japan and Canada. *International Review for Sociology of Sport*, **19**(1), 63-82.

Yarmolenko, A. (1933). The motor sphere of school age children. *Journal of Genetic Psychology*, **42**, 298-318.

Yoshida, T., Ishiko, I., & Muraoka, I. (1980). Effect of endurance training on cardiorespiratory functions of 5-year-old children. *International Journal of Sports Medicine*, **1**, 91-94.

Young, A., Stokes, M., & Crowe, M. (1985). The size and strength of the quadriceps muscles of old and young men. *Clinical Physiology*, **5**, 145-154.

Zaichkowsky, L.D., Zaichkowsky, L.B., & Martinek, T.J. (1980). *Growth and development: The child and physical activity*. St. Louis: Mosby.

Zelazo, P.R. (1983). The development of walking: New findings and old assumptions. *Journal of Motor Behavior*, **15**, 99-137.

Zelazo, P.R., Konner, M., Kolb, S., & Zelazo, N.A. (1974). Newborn walking: A reply to Pontius. *Perceptual and Motor Skills*, **39**, 423-428.

Zelazo, P.R., Zelazo, N.A., & Kolb, S. (1972a). Newborn walking. *Science*, **177**, 1058-1059.

Zelazo, P.R., Zelazo, N.A., & Kolb, S. (1972b). "Walking" in the newborn. *Science*, **176**, 314-315.

Zimmerman, H.M. (1956). Characteristic likenesses and differences between skilled and non-skilled performance of the standing broad jump. *Research Quarterly*, **27**, 352.

Zwiren, L.D. (1989). Anaerobic and aerobic capacities of children. *Pediatric Exercise Science*, **1**, 31-44.

# Credits

Figure 1.4 is from "The Developmental Origins of Locomotion" by E. Thelen, B.D. Ulrich, and J.L. Jensen. In *Development of Posture and Gait Across the Life Span* (p. 28) by M.H. Woolacott and A. Shumway-Cook (Eds.), 1989, Columbia, SC: University of South Carolina Press. Adapted by permission.

Figures 2.2 and 2.3 are from *NCHS Growth Curves for Children* by P.V.V. Hamill, 1977, Washington, DC: National Center for Health Studies, DHEW Publication No. (PHS) 78-1650.

Figure 2.7 is from *Anthropometric Standardization Reference Manual* (p. 18) by T.G. Lohman, A.F. Roche, and R. Martorell (Eds.), 1988, Champaign, IL: Human Kinetics. Copyright 1988 by T.G. Lohman, A.F. Roche, and R. Martorell. Reprinted by permission.

Figures 2.8a and 2.8b are from *A Radiographic Standard of Reference for the Growing Hand and Wrist* (pp. 53, 73) by S.I. Pyle, 1971, Chicago, IL: Yearbook Medical Publishers. Copyright 1971 by Bolton-Brush Growth Center. Reprinted by permission.

Figure 2.9 is from *Advances in Reproductive Physiology* by A. Maclaren (Ed.), 1967, London: Elek Books. Copyright 1967 by Grafton Books division of Collins Publishing Group. Reprinted by permission.

Figures 2.10 and 2.11 are reproduced with permission from *The Beginnings of Human Life* (pp. 12, 14) by R.G. Edwards, 1981, Burlington, NC: Carolina Biology Reader Series. Copyright 1981 by Finestride Ltd. and Carolina Biological Supply Co.

Figure 2.12 is from *Reproductive Physiology for Medical Students* (p. 191) by P. Rhodes, 1969, London: J. & A. Churchill Ltd. Copyright 1969 by Churchill Livingston. Reprinted by permission.

Figure 2.13 is from "Standards From Birth to Maturity for Height, Weight, Velocity, and Weight Velocity: British Children, 1965—1" by J.M. Tanner, R.H. Whitehouse, and M. Taikishi, 1966, *Archives of Disease in Childhood*, **41**, pp. 454-471. Copyright 1966 by the British Medical Association. Reprinted by permission.

Figure 2.14 is from *Osteoporosis* by J.F. Aloia, 1989, Champaign, IL: Leisure Press. Copyright 1989 by J.F. Aloia. Reprinted by permission.

Figures 2.16 and 2.17 are from *Developmental Physiology and Aging* (pp. 283, 284) by P.S. Timiras, 1972, New York, NY: Macmillan. Copyright 1972 by Macmillan. Reprinted by permission.

Figure 2.18 is provided by Carolina Biological Supply Company of Burlington, North Carolina, from their Human Development slide series.

Figure 2.20 is reproduced with permission from *Bones* (2nd ed.) by J.J. Pritchard, 1979, Burlington, NC: Carolina Biology Reader Series. Copyright 1979 by Carolina Biological Supply Co.

Figure 2.21 is from *Physical Activity: Human Growth and Development* (p. 44) by G.L. Rarick (Ed.), 1973, New York, NY: Academic Press. Copyright 1973 by Academic Press. Reprinted by permission.

Figures 2.22, 2.23, 2.24, and 7.3 are from *Physiology of Fitness* (2nd ed.) (pp. 237, 238, 249, 275) by B.J. Sharkey, 1984, Champaign, IL: Human Kinetics. Copyright 1984 by B.J. Sharkey. Reprinted by permission.

Figure 2.25 is from "Subcutaneous Fat Distribution During Growth" by R.M. Malina & C. Bouchard. In *Fat Distribution During Growth and Later Health Outcomes* (p. 70), by C. Bouchard and F.E. Johnston (Eds.), 1988, New York, NY: Liss. Copyright © 1988 by Alan R. Liss. Reprinted by permission of Wiley-Liss, a division of John Wiley & Sons, Inc.

Figures 2.27, 2.35, 7.1, 7.7, 7.8, and 9.7 are from *Growth, Maturation, and Physical Activity* (pp. 222, 347, 375, 385, 386, 422) by R.M. Malina and C. Bouchard, 1991, Champaign, IL: Human Kinetics. Copyright 1991 by R.M. Malina and C. Bouchard. Reprinted by permission.

Figure 2.28 is from *Functional Human Anatomy* (4th ed.) (p. 274) by J.E. Crouch, 1985, Philadelphia: Lea & Febiger. Copyright 1985 by Lea & Febiger. Reprinted by permission.

Figures 2.29 and 2.33 are from *Dynamic Anatomy and Physiology* (5th ed.) (pp. 234, 294) by L.L. Langley, I.R. Telford, and J.B. Christensen, 1980, New York, NY: McGraw-Hill. Copyright 1980 by Mosby-Year Book, Inc., St. Louis. Reprinted by permission.

Figure 2.30 is from *The Human Organism* (5th ed.) (p. 260) by R.M. DeCoursey and J.L. Renfro,

1980, New York, NY: McGraw-Hill. Copyright 1980 by McGraw-Hill. Reprinted by permission.

**Figure 2.31** is from *Dynamic Anatomy and Physiology* (3rd ed.) (p. 256) by L.L. Langley, I.R. Telford, and J.B. Christensen, 1969, New York, NY: McGraw-Hill. Copyright 1969 by McGraw-Hill. Reprinted by permission.

**Figures 2.32 and 2.33** are from *Illustrated Physiology* (4th ed.) (pp. 256, 301) by A.B. McNaught and R. Callander, 1983, Edinburgh, Scotland: Churchill Livingstone. Copyright 1983 by Churchill Livingstone. Reprinted by permission.

**Figure 2.34** is from *The Birth Atlas*, New York, NY: The Maternity Center Assn. Copyright by the Maternity Center Association. Reprinted by permission.

**Figure 3.1** is drawn from "Spontaneous Kicking in Month-Old Infants: Manifestation of a Human Central Locomotor Program" by E. Thelen, G. Bradshaw, and J.A. Ward, 1981, *Behavioral and Neural Biology*, **32**, p. 47.

**Figure 3.6** is from "An Experimental Study of Prehension in Infants by Means of Systematic Cinema Records" by H.M. Halverson, 1931, *Genetic Psychology Monographs*, **10**, pp. 212-215. Copyright 1931 by Helen Dwight Reid Educational Foundation. Reprinted by permission.

**Figure 3.8** is from "Developmental Changes in Eye-Hand Coordination Behaviors: Preprogramming Versus Feedback Control" by L. Hay. In *Development of Eye-Hand Coordination Across the Life Span* (p. 235) by C. Bard, M. Fleury, and L. Hay (Eds.), 1990, Columbia, SC: University of South Carolina Press. Copyright 1990 by the University of South Carolina. Reprinted by permission 1992.

**Figures 4.1a, 4.1c, 4.3a, 4.6, 4.10-4.13, 4.18-4.31, 4.35, 4.39, and 4.40** are redrawn from film tracings provided by the Motor Development and Child Study Laboratory, Department of Physical Education and Dance, University of Wisconsin-Madison.

**Figures 4.1b, 4.5, and 4.8** are redrawn from *Fundamental Motor Patterns* (3rd ed.) (pp. 29, 74, 77) by R.L. Wickstrom, 1983, Philadelphia, PA: Lea & Febiger.

**Figure 4.14** is reprinted by permission from the *Research Quarterly for Exercise and Sport*, Vol. 56, March, 1985, "Developmental Sequences for Hopping Over Distance: A Prelongitudinal Screening" (p. 38) by L. Halverson & K. Williams. The *Research Quarterly for Exercise and Sport* is a publication of the American Alliance for Health, Physical Education, Recreation and Dance, 1900 Association Drive, Reston, VA 22091.

**Figure 4.15** is redrawn from "Changing Patterns of Locomotion: From Walking to Skipping" by J.E. Clark and J. Whitall. In *Development of Posture and Gait Across the Life Span* (p. 132) by M.H. Woollacott & A. Shumway-Cook (Eds.), 1989, Columbia, SC: University of South Carolina Press.

**Figure 4.41** is from *Developing Children—Their Changing Movement* (p. 54) by M.A. Roberton and L.E. Halverson, 1984, Philadelphia, PA: Lea & Febiger. Copyright 1984 by Lea & Febiger. Reprinted by permission.

**Figures 5.1-5.3** are from "Acquisition of Motor Skills During Childhood" by J. Haubenstricker and V. Seefeldt. In *Physical Activity and Well-Being* (p. 70) by V. Seefeldt (Ed.), 1986, Reston, VA: American Alliance for Health, Physical Education, and Dance. Copyright 1986 by AAHPERD. Reprinted by permission.

**Figures 5.4-5.6** are from "Gender Differences Across Age in Motor Performance: A Meta-Analysis" by J.R. Thomas and K.E. French, 1985, *Psychological Bulletin*, **98**, pp. 268, 269, 270, 272. Copyright 1985 by the American Psychological Association. Reprinted by permission.

**Figure 5.7** is from "Quantifying Gender Differences in Physical Performance: A Developmental Perspective" by F.L. Smoll and R.W. Schutz, 1990, *Developmental Psychology*, **26**, p. 366. Copyright 1990 by the American Psychological Association. Reprinted by permission.

**Figures 5.8 and 5.9** are from "Developmental Task Analysis: The Design of Movement Experiences and Evaluation of Motor Development Status" by J. Herkowitz. In *Motor Development* (pp. 141, 149) by M.V. Ridenour (Ed.), 1978, Princeton, NJ: Princeton Book Company. Copyright 1978 by Princeton Book Company. Reprinted by permission.

**Figure 5.10** is from *Swimming for Seniors* (pp. 5, 6) by E.J. Shea, 1986, Champaign, IL: Human Kinetics. Copyright 1986 by Edward J. Shea. Reprinted by permission.

**Figure 5.13** is from "Throwing Patterns of Older Adults: A Follow-Up Investigation" by K. Williams, K. Haywood, and A. VanSant, 1991, *The International Journal of Aging and Human Development*, **33**, p. 286. Copyright 1991 by Baywood Publishing Company, Inc. Reprinted by permission.

**Figure 6.2** is from *Eye and Brain* (2nd ed.) (p. 151) by R.L. Gregory, 1972, New York: World

University Library, McGraw-Hill. Reprinted by permission of George Weidenfeld & Nicolson Limited, London.

**Figure 6.3** Copyright 1972 by Western Psychological Services. Not to be reproduced without written permission of copyright owner. All rights reserved. Reprinted by permission of Western Psychological Services, 12031 Wilshire Blvd., Los Angeles, CA 90025.

**Figure 6.4** is from "Studies of Perceptual Development: II. Part-Whole Perception" by D. Elkind, R.R. Koegler, and E. Go, 1964, *Child Development*, **35**, pp. 81-90. Copyright 1964 by Society for Research in Child Development, Inc. Reprinted by permission.

**Figure 6.5** is from *Perception: The World Transformed* by Lloyd Kaufman. Copyright 1979 by Oxford University Press, Inc. Reprinted by permission.

**Figure 6.6** is redrawn from "Detour Behavior in Young Infants" by B.E. McKenzie and E. Bigelow, 1986, *British Journal of Developmental Psychology*, **4**, pp. 139-148.

**Figure 6.8** is from *A Primer of Infant Development* by T.G.R. Bower, 1977, San Francisco: W.H. Freeman. Copyright 1977 by W.H. Freeman. Reprinted by permission.

**Figure 6.9** is based on Morrongiello, 1988.

**Figure 6.10** is from "Children's Development of Posture and Balance Control: Changes in Motor Coordination and Sensory Integration" by M.H. Woollacott, B. Debu, and A. Shumway-Cook. In *Advances in Pediatric Sport Sciences* (Vol. 2) (p. 214) by D. Gould and M.R. Weiss (Eds.), 1987, Champaign, IL: Human Kinetics. Copyright 1987 by Human Kinetics. Reprinted by permission.

**Figure 6.11** is from "Development of Postural Control in Children: Effects of Gymnastics Training" by B. Debu, M. Woollacott, and M. Mowatt. In *Advances in Motor Development Research* (Vol. 2) (p. 46) by J.E. Clark and J.H. Humphrey (Eds.), 1988, New York, NY: AMS Press. Copyright 1988 by AMS Press. Reprinted by permission.

**Figure 6.12** is from "Movement-Produced Stimulation in the Development of Visually Guided Behavior" by R. Held and A. Hein, 1963, *Journal of Comparative and Physiological Psychology*, **56**, p. 873. Copyright 1963 by the American Psychological Association. Reprinted by permission.

**Figure 6.13** is from "Locomotor Experience: A Facilitator of Spatial Cognitive Development" by R. Kermoian and J.J. Campos, 1988, *Child Development*, **59**, p. 911. Copyright 1988 by the Society for Research in Child Development, Inc. Reprinted by permission.

**Figure 6.14** is provided by B.D. Ulrich of Indiana University.

**Figure 7.2** is from *Pediatric Sports Medicine for the Practitioner* (pp. 4, 5) by O. Bar-Or, 1983, New York, NY: Springer. Copyright 1983 by Springer-Verlag. Reprinted by permission.

**Figure 7.4** is from "Exercise and the Elderly" by B.A. Stamford. In *Exercise and Sport Sciences Reviews* (Vol. 16) (p. 344) by K.B. Pandolf (Ed.), 1988, New York, NY: Macmillan Publishing Company. Copyright 1988 by McGraw-Hill, Inc. Reprinted by permission. Redrawn from Dehn and Bruce (1972). Data plotted are from: (a) Dehn and Bruce (1972), (b) Dill et al. (1967), (c) Hollmann (1965), all cited in Dehn and Bruce, and (d) Dehn and Bruce.

**Figure 7.5** is from "Anaerobic and Aerobic Capacities of Children" by L.D. Zwiren, 1989, *Pediatric Exercise Science*, **1**, p. 40. Copyright 1989 by Human Kinetics Publishers. Reprinted by permission.

**Figure 7.6** is from "Muscle Morphology, Enzymatic Activity, and Muscle Strength in Elderly Men: A Follow-Up Study" by A. Aniansson, M. Hedberg, G.B. Henning, and G. Grimby, 1986, *Muscle & Nerve*, **9**, p. 588. Copyright © by John Wiley & Sons, Inc. Reprinted by permission.

**Figure 7.9** is from "Comparing the Sit and Reach With the Modified Sit and Reach in Measuring Flexibility in Adolescents" by W.W.K. Hoeger, D.R. Hopkins, S. Button, and T.A. Palmer, 1990, *Pediatric Exercise Science*, **2**, p. 158. Copyright 1990 by Human Kinetics Publishers. Reprinted by permission.

**Figure 7.10** is redrawn after Bovend'eerdt et al., 1980, and Branta et al., 1984. From *Growth and Fitness of Flemish Girls* (p. 118) by J. Simons, G.P. Beunen, R. Renson, A.L.M. Claessens, B. Vanreusel, and J.A.V. Lefevre, 1990, Champaign, IL: Human Kinetics. Copyright 1990 by Human Kinetics Publishers. Reprinted by permission.

**Figure 7.11** Data are from Parizkova (1963, 1965). From *Body Fat and Physical Fitness* (p. 154) by J. Parizkova, 1977, The Hague, The Netherlands: Martinus Nijhoff B.V. Publishers. Copyright 1977 by Martinus Nijhoff B.V. Publishers. Reprinted by permission.

**Figure 8.1** is adapted from "Information Processing in Children's Skill Acquisition" by A.L. Rothstein. In *Psychology of Motor Behavior and*

*Sport* (p. 219) by R.W. Christina and D.M. Landers (Eds.), 1977, Champaign, IL: Human Kinetics. Copyright 1977 by Human Kinetics Publishers. Reprinted by permission.

**Figure 8.2** is from "Aerobic Exercise Training and Improved Neuropsychological Function of Older Individuals" by R.E. Dustman et al. In *Aging and Motor Behavior* (p. 75), by A.C. Ostrow (Ed.), 1989, Indianapolis: Benchmark Press. Copyright 1989 by Pergamon Press. Reprinted by permission.

**Figure 8.4** is drawn from data reported in "The Relation of Knowledge Development to Children's Basketball Performance" by K.E. French and J.R. Thomas, 1987, *Journal of Sport Psychology*, **9**, p. 27. Copyright 1987 by Human Kinetics Publishers, Inc.

**Figure 8.5** is from "Precision Knowledge of Results and Motor Performance: Relationship to Age" by J.R. Thomas, B. Mitchell, and M.A. Solomon, 1979, *Research Quarterly*, **50**, p. 696. Copyright 1979 by the American Alliance for Health, Physical Education and Dance. Reprinted by permission.

**Figure 8.6** is from "Effects of Varying Post-KR Intervals Upon Children's Motor Performance" by J.D. Gallagher and J.R. Thomas, 1980, *Journal of Motor Behavior*, **12**, p. 44. Copyright 1980 by J.D. Gallagher and J.R. Thomas. Reprinted by permission.

**Figure 9.1** is based on Kenyon and McPherson (1973).

**Figure 9.4** is based on Horn (1987).

**Figure 9.5** is based on Duda and Tappe (1989a) and Maehr (1984).

**Figure 9.6** is from "Personal Investment in Exercise Among Adults: The Examination of Age and Gender-Related Differences in Motivational Orientation" by J.L. Duda and M.K. Tappe. In *Aging and Motor Behavior* (pp. 246, 248) by A.C. Ostrow (Ed.), 1989, Indianapolis, IN: Benchmark Press. Reprinted by permission of Wm. C. Brown Communications, Inc., Dubuque, Iowa. All rights reserved.

**Table 1.3** is based on Clark and Whitall (1989a).

**Tables 2.1 and 2.2** are from *Developmental Physiology and Aging* (pp. 63-64, 382) by P.S. Timiras, 1972, New York, NY: Macmillan. Copyright 1972 by Macmillan. Adapted by permission.

**Tables 4.1 and 4.2** are from *Fundamental Motor Patterns* (3rd ed.) (pp. 68, 69) by R.L. Wickstrom, 1983, Philadelphia PA: Lea & Febiger.

**Table 4.2** is also adapted from information in studies by Bayley (1935) (B) and McCaskill & Wellman (1938) (M&W).

**Table 4.3** is from "Sequencing Motor Skills Within the Physical Education Curriculum" by V. Seefeldt, S. Reuschlein, and P. Vogel, 1972. Paper presented to the annual conference of the American Association for Health, Physical Education and Recreation. Adapted by permission.

**Table 4.4** is from "A Developmental Sequence of the Standing Long Jump" (pp. 73-85) by J.E. Clark and S.J. Phillips. In *Motor Development: Current Selected Research (Volume 1)* by J.E. Clark and J.H. Humphrey (Eds.), 1985, Princeton, NJ: Princeton Book Company. Copyright 1985 by Princeton Book Company, Publishers. Adapted by permission.

**Tables 4.5, 4.6, 4.7, and 4.11** are from *Developing Children—Their Changing Movement* (pp. 56, 63, 88, 92-93, 103, 106, 107, 118, 122-123) by M.A. Roberton and L.E. Halverson, 1984, Philadelphia, PA: Lea & Febiger. Copyright 1984 by Lea & Febiger. Reprinted by permission.

**Table 4.8.** The preparatory trunk action and the parenthetical information in Step 3 of Racket Action are from "Prelongitudinal Screening of Hypothesized Developmental Sequences for the Overhead Tennis Serve in Experienced Tennis Players 9-19 Years of Age" by J.A. Messick, 1991, *Research Quarterly for Exercise and Sport*, **62**, September, 249-256. *Research Quarterly for Exercise and Sport* is a publication of the American Alliance for Health, Physical Education, Recreation, and Dance, Reston, VA 22091. The remaining components are from "Prelongitudinal Screening of Overarm Striking Development Performed Under Two Environmental Conditions" (p. 26) by S. Langendorfer. In *Advances in Motor Development Research* (Vol. 1) by J.E. Clark and J.H. Humphrey (Eds.), 1987, New York, NY: AMS Press. Copyright 1987 by AMS Press. Reprinted by permission.

**Table 4.9.** The arm action component is adapted from "Standards of Performance for Throwing and Catching" by J.L. Haubenstricker, C.F. Branta, and V.D. Seefeldt, 1983. Paper presented at the annual conference of the North American Society for Psychology of Sport and Physical Activity, Asilomar, California. Based on "Sequencing Motor Skills Within the Physical Education Curriculum" by V. Seefeldt, S. Reuschlein, and P. Vogel, 1972. Paper presented at the annual conference of the American Association for Health, Physical Education, and Recreation, Houston, Texas. The hand and body action components are from "Developmental Sequences for Catching a Small Ball: A Prelongitudinal Screening" by H.S. Strohmeyer, K. Williams, and D. Schaub-George. Reprinted with permission from *Research Quarterly for Exercise and Sport*, vol. 62, (September, 1991). *Research Quarterly for Exercise and Sport* is a publication of the American Alliance for Health, Physical Education, Recreation. and Dance, Reston, VA 22091.

Table 4.10 is from "Life Span Development of Righting" by A. VanSant, in press. In *Advances in Motor Development Research* (Vol. 4) by J.E. Clark and J.H. Humphrey (Eds.), New York, NY: AMS Press. Copyright by AMS Press. Reprinted by permission.

Tables 5.1 and 7.4 are from "Stability of Growth in Strength in Motor Performance From Childhood to Adolescence," 1967, by G.L. Rarick and F.L. Smoll, *Human Biology*, **39**, pp. 299, 301, 302. Copyright 1966 by Wayne State University Press. Reprinted by permission.

Table 5.2 is adapted from data in *Genetic and Anthropological Studies of Olympic Athletes* (pp. 82-145) by A.L. deGaray, L. Levine, and J.E.L. Carter, 1974, New York, NY: Academic Press, and from "Age, Family Size and Birth Order in Montreal Olympic Athletes" (p. 20) by R.M. Malina, C. Bouchard, R.F. Shoup, and G. Lariviere, 1982, in *Physical Structure of Olympic Athletes, Part I*, by J.E.L. Carter (Ed.), Basel, Switzerland: S. Karger.

Table 5.3 is from *Age and Achievement* (p. 256)

by H.C. Lehman, 1953, Princeton, NJ: Princeton University Press. Copyright 1953 by the American Philosophical Society. Reprinted by permission.

Tables 7.1, 7.2, and 7.3 are reproduced with permission from Shephard, R.J.: *Physical Activity and Growth* (pp. 70, 80, 104). Copyright 1982 by Yearbook Medical Publishers, Inc., Chicago.

Table 7.5 is adapted from "The Specificity of Flexibility in Girls" by F.L. Hupprich and P.O. Sigerseth, 1950, *Research Quarterly*. **39**, pp. 30-32.

Table 7.6 Data are from Parizkova (1968a, b). From *Body Fat and Physical Fitness* (p. 130) by J. Parizkova, 1977, The Hague, The Netherlands: Martinus Nijhoff B.V. Publishers. Copyright 1977 by Martinus Nijhoff B.V. Publishers. Reprinted by permission.

Table 9.1 is from "Sex Differences and Parental Influence in Sport Involvement of Children" by J.H. Lewko and M.E. Ewing, 1980, *Journal of Sport Psychology*, **2**, p. 66. Copyright 1980 by Human Kinetics. Adapted by permission.

Table 9.2 is from "Comparisons of Mental and Motor Test Scores for Ages 1-15 Months by Sex, Birth Order, Race, Geographic Location, and Education of Parents" by N. Bayley, 1965, *Child Development*, **36**, p. 405. Copyright 1965 by University of Chicago Press.

## Chapter Opening Photos

Chapter 1 opening photo (p. 3) is from *Parenting Your Superstar* (p. 92), by R.J. Rotella and L.K. Bunker, 1987, Champaign, IL: Leisure Press. Copyright 1987 by Robert J. Rotella and Linda K. Bunker. Reprinted by permission.

Chapter 2 opening photo (p. 29) courtesy of Lee, Michelle, and baby Reifsteck.

Chapter 3 opening photo (p. 87) is from *The Baby Swim Book* (p. 122), by C.L. Kochen and J. McCabe, 1986, Champaign, IL: Leisure Press. Copyright 1986 by Cinda L. Kochen and Janet McCabe. Photograph by Fred M. Bonnett. Reprinted by permission.

Chapter 4, chapter 6, chapter 8, and chapter 9 opening photos (pp. 119, 203, 281, and 303) are from *Physical Education for Children: Concepts Into Practice* (pp. 100,

48, 68, 60), by J.R. Thomas, A.M. Lee, and K.T. Thomas, 1988, Champaign, IL: Human Kinetics. Copyright 1988 by Jerry R. Thomas, Katherine T. Thomas, and Amelia M. Lee. Reprinted by permission.

Chapter 5 opening photo (p. 175) is from "Program Factors That Influence Adherence" by B.A. Franklin. In *Exercise Adherence* (p. 243), by R.K. Dishman (Ed.), 1988, Champaign, IL: Human Kinetics. Copyright 1988 by Rod K. Dishman. Reprinted by permission.

Chapter 7 opening photo (p. 239) is from *I'll Meet You at the Finish!* (p. 20), by C.P. Shipman, 1987, Champaign, IL: Life Enhancement Publications. Copyright 1987 by Chris Pepper Shipman. Reprinted by permission.

# Index